TECHNICAL
REPORT

# National Evaluation of Safe Start Promising Approaches

## Assessing Program Implementation

Dana Schultz, Lisa H. Jaycox, Laura J. Hickman,
Anita Chandra, Dionne Barnes-Proby,
Joie Acosta, Alice Beckman, Taria Francois,
Lauren Honess-Morreale

Sponsored by the U.S. Department of Justice's Office of Juvenile Justice and Delinquency Prevention

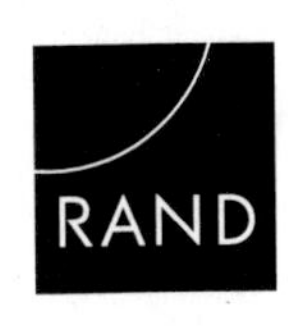


HEALTH and
INFRASTRUCTURE, SAFETY, AND ENVIRONMENT

This research was sponsored by the U.S. Department of Justice's Office of Juvenile Justice and Delinquency Prevention and was conducted under the auspices of the Safety and Justice Program within RAND Infrastructure, Safety, and Environment and under RAND Health's Health Promotion and Disease Prevention Program.

**Library of Congress Cataloging-in-Publication Data**

National evaluation of Safe Start Promising Approaches : assessing program implementation / Dana Schultz ... [et al.].
p. cm.
Includes bibliographical references.
ISBN 978-0-8330-4968-1 (pbk. : alk. paper)
1. Safe Start Promising Approaches (Program)--Evaluation. 2. Children and violence--United States--Prevention. 3. Children--Services for--United States--Evaluation. 4. Child welfare--United States. I. Schultz, Dana (Dana J.)

HQ784.V55N35 2010
362.76--dc22

2010011742



Published 2010 by the RAND Corporation
1776 Main Street, P.O. Box 2138, Santa Monica, CA 90407-2138
1200 South Hayes Street, Arlington, VA 22202-5050
4570 Fifth Avenue, Suite 600, Pittsburgh, PA 15213-2665
RAND URL: http://www.rand.org/
To order RAND documents or to obtain additional information, contact
Distribution Services: Telephone: (310) 451-7002;
Fax: (310) 451-6915; Email: order@rand.org

## Preface

Safe Start Promising Approaches (SSPA) was the second phase of a planned four-phase initiative focusing on preventing and reducing the impact of children's exposure to violence and sponsored by the U.S. Department of Justice's Office of Juvenile Justice and Delinquency Prevention (OJJDP). The RAND Corporation conducted the national evaluation of the SSPA phase of the initiative, in collaboration with the national evaluation team: OJJDP, the Safe Start Center, the Association for the Study and Development of Communities, and the 15 program sites. The evaluation design involved three components: a process evaluation, including a cost analysis; an evaluation of training; and an outcomes evaluation.

This document provides the results for the process and training evaluations. It documents the activities of the 15 SSPA programs for the first two years of implementation. In the main body of this report, we synthesize information across all 15 sites to describe the program and community settings, interventions, and implementations. In the appendixes, we provide a detailed description of each SSPA program and the results of the training evaluation.

These results will be of interest to clinicians, practitioners, policymakers, community leaders, and others interested in implementing programs for children exposed to violence.

This research was conducted under the auspices of the Safety and Justice Program within RAND Infrastructure, Safety, and Environment (ISE) and under RAND Health's Health Promotion and Disease Prevention Program.

The mission of RAND Infrastructure, Safety, and Environment is to improve the development, operation, use, and protection of society's essential physical assets and natural resources and to enhance the related social assets of safety and security of individuals in transit and in their workplaces and communities. Safety and Justice Program research addresses occupational safety, transportation safety, food safety, and public safety—including violence, policing, corrections, substance abuse, and public integrity. Information about the Safety and Justice Program is available online (http://www.rand.org/ise/safety).

RAND Health, a division of the RAND Corporation, is one of the largest private health research groups in the world. The projects within RAND Health address a wide range of health care policy issues, with an emphasis on policy research that can improve the health of people around the world. This project was conducted within the Health Promotion and Disease Prevention Program (HPDP) of RAND Health. RAND HPDP addresses issues related to measuring healthy and unhealthy behaviors, examining the distribution of health behaviors across population subgroups, identifying what causes or influences such behaviors, and designing and evaluating interventions to improve health behaviors. A profile of RAND Health, abstracts of its publications, and ordering information can be found at www.rand.org/health.

Questions or comments about this report should be sent to the project leader, Lisa Jaycox (Lisa_Jaycox@rand.org). Inquiries about research projects should be sent to the following address:

Greg Ridgeway, Director
Safety and Justice Program, ISE
RAND Corporation
1776 Main Street
Santa Monica, CA 90407-2138
310-393-0411, x7734
gregr@rand.org

## Contents

# Summary

Nationally, approximately 61 percent of children have been exposed to violence during the past year, and there is reason to believe that the problem has grown worse in recent decades (Finkelhor et al., 2009). Children's exposure to violence (CEV) can have serious consequences, including a variety of psychiatric disorders and behavioral problems, such as posttraumatic stress disorder (PTSD), depression, and anxiety. School performance has also been shown to suffer as a result of CEV. Moreover, research suggests that the effects of exposure to violence may persist well into adulthood. Fortunately, research has also shown that early childhood interventions can substantially improve children's chances of future social and psychological well-being.

## Background: The Safe Start Program

Safe Start is a community-based initiative focused on developing and fielding interventions to prevent and reduce the impact of CEV. Sponsored by the U.S. Department of Justice's Office of Juvenile Justice and Delinquency Prevention (OJJDP), the initiative consists of four phases:

- **Phase One:** Expanding the system of care for children exposed to violence by conducting demonstration projects. Now complete, this phase involved demonstrations of various innovative promising practices in the system of care for children who have been exposed to violence.
- **Phase Two:** Building on Phase One, this phase was intended to implement and evaluate promising and evidence-based programs in community settings to identify how well programs worked in reducing and preventing the harmful effects of CEV.
- **Phases Three:** Still in the planning stages, the aim of this phase is to build a knowledge base of effective interventions in the field of CEV.
- **Phase Four:** The goal of this phase is to "seed" on a national scale the effective strategies identified in the earlier phases.

Each phase also includes an evaluation component, intended to assess the implementation of the various interventions and their impact on children's outcomes.

This report focuses on Phase Two of the Safe Start program. For this phase, known as Safe Start Promising Approaches (SSPA), OJJDP selected 15 program sites across the country to implement a range of interventions for helping children and families cope with the effects of CEV. Sites were located in the following communities:

Bronx, New York
Broward County, Florida
Chelsea, Massachusetts
Dallas, Texas
Dayton, Ohio
Erie, Pennsylvania
Kalamazoo, Michigan
Miami, Florida
Multnomah County, Oregon
Oakland, California
Providence, Rhode Island
San Diego County, California
San Mateo County, California
Toledo, Ohio
Washington Heights/Inwood, New York

The program sites varied in numerous ways. First, they focused on multiple types of violence exposure and interventions for such exposure, including variations in ages and age-appropriate practices. The 15 sites also varied in size, location, and population characteristics. Each of the communities had identified barriers to services for children exposed to violence and viewed SSPA as an opportunity to increase capacity, coordinate services, and address gaps in the array of services in the community. The SSPA programs were situated locally within a variety of different kinds of lead agencies or organizations, including health clinics or hospitals, human services agencies, organizational units within universities, domestic violence or child maltreatment services agencies, and county-level government offices. In developing their programs, the lead agencies partnered with the specific agencies in the community that work with children exposed to violence: law enforcement agencies, child protective services agencies, human services agencies, behavioral health organizations, and other community nonprofit agencies. The programs received their referrals from a variety of sources, including the clinic or hospital system, child welfare system, domestic violence shelters, human services agencies, Head Start, or a combination of the above.

The 15 Safe Start programs comprised a range of intervention components. All included a therapeutic component; about two-thirds focused on dyadic or family therapy, while the rest used individual or group therapy approaches. In some cases, the modality varied by age, with dyadic or family therapy for younger children and group therapy for older children. Many of the sites also used case management or coordination. Some of the sites had other intervention components, such as advocacy, parent groups, or other services (e.g., multidisciplinary evaluation of family needs, an in-home safety assessment, etc.). The intervention setting also varied, with interventions offered in families' homes, clinics, shelters, child centers, or Head Start classrooms. The interventions varied in length from three months to more than one year. At all of the sites, the interventions were conducted in the context of a rigorous evaluation, as required by OJJDP.

## Evaluation Approach

RAND Corporation researchers evaluated the SSPA phase of the initiative in collaboration with the national evaluation team: OJJDP, the Safe Start Center, the Association for the Study and Development of Communities (ASDC), and the 15 program sites. The evaluation design involved three components: a process evaluation, including a cost analysis; an evaluation of training; and an outcomes evaluation. This report presents the results of our implementation process evaluation as well as the cost and training evaluation results.

Our evaluation of the SSPA programs drew on a framework that focused on three domains: the program context, the intervention, and the process of implementation followed by the programs.

The **program context** domain includes community setting, program setting, and evaluation design. This domain encompasses factors such as community support and readiness for a program and the fit between the program and the community that influence the implementation of community-based violence prevention programs. The **intervention** domain includes the intervention setting and approach, therapeutic content, case management or coordination, and other intervention components. Finally, the **implementation process** includes referral and recruitment into the program and service delivery in addition to the family/child characteristics and provider characteristics. Provider-level factors include staff selection, facilitative administration, and financial, organizational, and human resources systems.

To collect information about the sites and the interventions, we examined the inputs into SSPA projects, such as the planning and start-up processes, organizational and program characteristics, staff, costs, and collaboration with community partners. We also examined each site's activities, including the specific services provided, the implementation process, adjustments made during implementation, the barriers and facilitators to program implementation, and any unexpected developments.

Data collection for this process evaluation included site visits; quarterly activity reports on services, training, policies, and advocacy; document review; regular email and telephone communication; and evaluation of staff training activities. During the site visits, we collected data from a variety of sources, including key informant interviews with program staff and community partners, case reviews of randomly selected cases, tours of facilities, a quality assurance checklist completed by the clinical supervisor, and observations of relevant meetings. We used the information from these data collection efforts to develop the program descriptions for each site that appear in Appendix B of this report. In addition, a separate analysis of staff trainings conducted by the sites is provided in Appendix C. For the cross-site analyses in the main body of this report, we synthesized the information from the program descriptions to describe the program context, interventions, and implementation processes at the SSPA sites.

## Findings: Factors Affecting SSPA Implementation

Our assessment of the program context, interventions, and implementation processes identified factors that were related to implementation of the SSPA programs. The programs' focus on children exposed to violence led to the identification of some unique factors that are most relevant to other such programs, but we also identified factors that are generic to rolling out any mental health program in community settings. Some factors helped implementation, and some hindered it. We summarize these factors below, highlighting those that were evident across more than one site or that offered particularly clear implications for future work with children exposed to violence.

## Program Context

The following contextual factors were found to affect program implementation at some sites:

- **Widespread recognition of need.** When there was widespread recognition among community agencies and service providers of the need to increase capacity and coordinate services, the lead agencies/organizations were better able to develop an intervention that addressed the gaps in the array of services for children exposed to violence.
- **Strong individual leadership at the lead agency.** Strong individual leaders at some SSPA programs served as program advocates in the community and within the lead agency/organization. These leaders were able to increase the program's visibility both externally and internally and provide support and direction for program implementation.
- **Clear division of responsibility for program implementation.** The structure of some of the lead agencies or organizations meant that they could take responsibility for providing the staff and resources for program implementation. In turn, partner agencies were not burdened with responsibilities related to implementing the programs.
- **Close working relationships among partner agencies and referral sources.** Some SSPA programs took advantage of existing relationships and trust developed through prior experiences with partner agencies or organizations to smooth the way for implementing a new program in the community. These types of relationships were evidenced by strong buy-in from partner organizations, demonstrated by up-front support and understanding of the potential program benefits.
- **Burden of research requirements.** SSPA's research component posed challenges for program implementation. The reluctance of referral sources and families to participate when the program involved a control or comparison group negatively influenced the referral and recruitment processes, even though the services being offered were not otherwise available in the community.

Based on these factors, we drew implications for program context that other communities seeking to implement similar interventions can use to facilitate implementation. Table S.1 recaps the factors discussed above and pairs them with relevant implications.

**Table S.1**
**Program Context: Factors and Implications**

| Factor | Implication |
|---|---|
| **Importance of widespread recognition of need** | **Provide opportunities to bring community agencies and service providers together to identify and address gaps and barriers to services for children exposed to violence.** A promising avenue is collaboration to develop a program that addresses gaps in the existing network of services and supports and fits the needs of children exposed to violence. |
| **Importance of strong individual leadership at the lead agency** | **Dedicate a staff leader with power to make program-level decisions and adjustments.** A program leader with adequate time to lead can effectively develop collaborative relationships with community partners and implement the program. Ideally, the program lead person would have decisionmaking authority for program activities and modifications. |
| **Importance of a clear division of responsibility for program implementation** | **Design a program that places primary responsibility for implementation with a lead agency or organization.** It is important for the program to be structured with a clearly delineated lead agency/organization to take primary responsibility for program implementation. |

**Table S.1—Continued**

| Factor | Implication |
|---|---|
| **Importance of close working relationships among partner agencies and referral sources** | **Capitalize on existing strong relationships with partner agencies and referral sources.** It is important for those involved in the program's design and planning phases to take advantage of existing collaborative efforts and relationships and prior experiences together. Trust between agencies appears to be particularly important for interventions for children exposed to violence. This can increase initial buy-in and ensure that the partner agencies understand why the supports and services are needed and how the planned program is expected to affect outcomes for participating families and children. **Select known or internal referral sources.** To the extent possible, take advantage of existing relationships with community agencies/organizations or internal referral sources. Structuring the program with referral sources that are known or internal to the lead agency/organization can also help ease program implementation. |
| **Burden of research requirements** | **Assess the impact of the evaluation design on program staff, families, and referral sources.** If an evaluation component is included, a first step is to recognize and understand how the specific research plan affects different parties, including the program staff providing services and supports, the participating families, and the staff at the referral sources. **Develop tools to increase buy-in for the evaluation component and minimize the negative impact.** A next step is to educate all parties about the benefits of the research project, including its role in augmenting services available in the community and ensuring effective treatment. Education tools might include program brochures or fact sheets geared toward the intended audience that use nontechnical language to explain the research design and the importance of the research component to the overall program. |

### Intervention

The following factors related to the interventions themselves were found to affect implementation across more than one site:

- **Differences between the intervention approaches and the families' needs and priorities.** While the intervention approaches were developed to fill a gap in mental health services in the community as perceived by community partners, the focus on mental health services did not necessarily fit with families' own priorities, which were often directed toward addressing safety and basic needs before turning to mental health. This issue with sequencing of services created challenges with service delivery, as families had other priorities at the time of their referral into the programs.
- **Convenience of intervention setting.** Many of the SSPA programs delivered the services in families' homes that enabled them to address some of the logistical challenges related to successful engagement of families in treatment and provide a safe environment for families to receive services.
- **Use of needs assessment or developmental screenings.** SSPA programs that included a needs assessment or development screening as one of their intervention components found that this approach helped them engage families.
- **Ability to provide for families' immediate and basic needs.** The case management or coordination component enabled the SSPA programs to connect with families and address their basic needs. Doing so helped providers engage with families who were unfamiliar with mental health and begin to establish trust and increase comfort with the intervention.
- **Wide array of therapy options.** By offering a wide range of therapy options, some SSPA programs were able to tailor the therapeutic component to the families' needs and circumstances. This sort of flexible approach helped these programs be responsive to the unique needs of families.

- **Adaptable components of the therapy models.** Some therapy models provided guidelines rather than manuals. This enabled the clinicians to tailor the therapeutic strategies and techniques to the families' circumstances.
- **Inability to monitor adherence to the therapy models.** Because of resource constraints, most SSPA programs were unable to systematically ascertain whether individual project staff were following the therapeutic guidelines or standards when delivering the intervention services. This made it difficult to assess whether the therapy was delivered as intended by the model developers.

The factors and their implications for developing and implementing community-based programs for children exposed to violence are summarized in the Table S.2.

**Table S.2**
**Intervention: Factors and Implications**

| Factor | Implication |
|---|---|
| **Problem with differences between the intervention approaches and the families' needs and priorities** | **Understand the priorities and needs of families in the program's target population.** When selecting the intervention components, it is important to align the overall intervention approach and the mix of services and supports offered with the needs and issues of the families with a child exposed to violence. Despite the identified violence exposure, families may have more pressing basic needs that the program needs to tackle before addressing the violence exposure. |
| **Importance of a convenient intervention setting** | **Consider the intervention setting.** The location of service delivery has implications for implementation. In an effort to help engage families and address some of the safety, transportation, and child care issues related to participating in a mental health program, it may be beneficial to offer the program in the home or in a school or day care setting. Particularly for families with small children, the location of service delivery can help ease the burden of participating in mental health treatment and increase the families' engagement. |
| **Importance of needs assessments or developmental screenings** | **Conduct needs assessments or developmental screening to engage families.** An intervention approach that includes a thorough assessment of the families' needs can help ensure that the overall intervention approach aligns with families' circumstances, including their safety issues related to violence. |
| **Importance of provision for families' immediate and basic needs** | **Ensure that families are provided or connected to sources of assistance to meet their basic needs.** Many of the families with children exposed to violence have multiple stressors in their lives. The complexity of their situations may make it difficult to focus on and engage in mental health treatment. At the outset of the program, assess families' basic needs for services and supports and either provide them with case management or coordination as part of the program or refer them to an agency or organizations that can help address some of their immediate needs. |
| **Importance of an array of therapy options** | **Offer more than one therapeutic approach to facilitate the matching of the services to individual families' needs and circumstances.** There is no one therapeutic approach that is appropriate for all families with children exposed to violence. By assessing the therapeutic needs of families and offering differing therapeutic options that can meet those needs, the program can better address the unique needs of different families. |
| **Importance of adaptable components of the therapy models** | **Modify the selected therapeutic model to offer activities or curriculum most suitable for the target population.** Certain therapeutic models offer flexibility in the guidelines for their use. If the therapeutic model allows, tailoring certain activities, examples, or techniques can help the program better meet the needs of families with children exposed to violence. It is important to consult with experts before making any modifications to make sure that the core components of the model are retained. |
| **Problem with monitoring adherence to the therapy models** | **Develop a process for monitoring adherence to the therapy model over time.** To maximize the effectiveness of the therapeutic models, it is important to integrate methods for monitoring how program staff who are providing the treatment are following the intervention guidelines or standards. By designating someone to take responsibility for adherence, the program can assess whether the program staff delivering the intervention are adequately trained, demonstrate acceptable skills level in delivering the intervention services, and adhere to the intervention standards described in the site's model. |

#### Implementation Process

The following factors related to the process of implementing the interventions were commonly found to affect implementation at the sites:

- **Close physical proximity of referral sources and program staff.** Some SSPA programs were structured so that referral sources were located at the program office or program staff regularly went on-site to the referral agency to identify referrals. Referrals from internal or co-located staff at the referral source made it easier for program staff and referral sources to communicate and resulted in a steadier flow of referrals.
- **Provision of incentives (e.g., training) to the referral sources.** Some referral sources had been trained by program staff about the issues of CEV and the program's benefits and understood the potential positive impact of the program on families. These referral sources were better positioned to maintain a steady flow of referrals.
- **Stable referral sources.** Some SSPA referral agencies experienced frequent staff turnover, making it difficult to maintain a steady flow of referrals and necessitating efforts to re-educate new staff.
- **Cumbersome referral processes.** The referral processes for some SSPA programs were complicated and/or new. This meant that the referring agencies were sometimes slow to start making referrals or were reluctant to refer into the program.
- **Highly mobile families.** After initial referral, some families were difficult to enroll because of their residential mobility. Some of this mobility was undoubtedly related to their violence exposure. This prevented the programs from completing the intake process and/or determining eligibility for referred families. The mobility of some families also made completing therapy sessions difficult.
- **Families' negative views or experiences with mental health services referrals.** Some referral sources faced problems with families' negative experiences or perceptions about mental health services, and sometimes around issues of mandatory reporting of child abuse and a desire to keep violence exposure private. These factors affected families' willingness to accept a referral for mental health services.
- **Complexity of families' treatment needs.** Many SSPA programs found that the families had multiple and complex situations and difficulties meeting day-to-day needs, including safety issues. These immediate needs often took precedence for families and made it difficult for service providers to deliver the therapy component of the program.
- **Close relationships with families.** The referral sources and program staff at some SSPA programs invested time and resources into building close relationships with families. These close relationships helped the referral sources engage families in discussions about violence exposure and the SSPA program. The program staff felt that the closer relationships helped engage families in the intervention.
- **Culturally inconsistent services.** Some of the SSPA programs struggled with a lack of cultural consistency related to race/ethnicity, socioeconomic status, and other demographic characteristics between those providing services and the families being served. These differences posed challenges in service delivery if families could not be served by providers proficient in their culture or primary language.
- **Clearly defined program parameters.** Some SSPA programs had problems clarifying the roles and responsibilities of different program staff and determining when to end

services for individual families. This confusion within the program sometimes made if difficult for the program to engage and retain families in the program.

- **Flexible service delivery model.** Some SSPA programs had flexibility within the service delivery model that allowed them to adjust caseloads, the intervention setting, or program staff roles. This flexibility helped the programs be responsive to families' circumstances.
- **Staffing issues among service providers.** Some of the service providers experienced issues with staff turnover, ongoing training needs, and staff burnout. These types of staffing issues made it challenging to maintain consistent, quality services.
- **Close communication and coordination between program staff and other service providers.** Some SSPA programs worked to establish and maintain clear lines of communication between program staff and other service providers working with the families. Coordination strategies, such as multidisciplinary or case coordination meetings, provided opportunities for sharing information, coordinating services and supports, and planning next steps.
- **Strained relationships between child welfare and domestic violence agencies.** Historically, collaboration between child welfare and domestic violence agencies has been difficult because of different priorities. Traditionally, child welfare agencies focus on the needs and safety of the child, whereas domestic violence agencies focus on the battered woman and her needs. Some of the SSPA programs found it challenging to navigate these divergent perspectives and integrate the different approached to families.

Table S.3 summarizes these factors and describes the implications for designing programs and providing services to families.

**Table S.3**
**Implementation Process: Factors and Implications**

| Factor | Implication |
|---|---|
| **Importance of close physical proximity of referral sources and program staff** | **Develop internal agency referral sources or co-locate program staff with the referral source.** Close physical proximity of the referring party to the program staff can help ensure a steady stream of referrals. For programs that receive some or all referrals internally, the staff can be educated about the program and the mechanics of the referral process. For programs that receive external referrals, consider placing program staff on-site with the referral agency or organization to facilitate referrals. |
| **Importance of incentivizing the referral sources** | **Provide training and outreach to referral sources.** The agencies and organizations that are providing referrals or conducting recruitment for the program need to understand how the planned program is expected to affect outcomes related to violence exposure for participating families and children and how it benefits their agency or organization. Education and outreach efforts can include program materials, training sessions, or one-on-one meetings with staff making referrals. |
| **Importance of stable referral sources** | **Prepare for staff turnover at referral agencies.** To plan for turnover, develop program materials and referral processes that can be transferred as referral agency staff turn over. The program materials, referral forms, contact information, and communication pathways need be clear, concise, and readily accessible and transferable for existing and new staff at the referral agency or organization. |
| **Importance of ongoing training of staff members** | **Plan for training over time rather than simply at the beginning.** Our training evaluation revealed that early gains in knowledge in serving children exposed to violence do not sustain over time; therefore booster sessions to maintain skills and comfort levels may be needed, particularly in the areas of family engagement. |
| **Problem of cumbersome referral processes** | **Streamline referral processes.** It is important to make the referral process as simple and straightforward as possible for the referring agencies, so as to bring interested families into the intervention as quickly as possible after referral for or detection of violence exposure. |

**Table S.3—Continued**

| Factor | Implication |
|---|---|
| **Problem of highly mobile families** | **Recruit families from multiple systems of care and use multiple approaches to track and locate families.** High rates of family transience, partially related to violence exposure, can reduce program recruitment and retention. Recruitment from more than one system of care may broaden outreach to eligible families and increase the number of families served. Also, collect abundant information on families at intake so as to be able to "track and locate" them over time. |
| **Problem of families' negative views or experiences with mental health services referrals** | **Work with referral agencies to address issues around the stigma of mental health services.** To reduce the stigma associated with mental health services and increase families' interest in accepting mental health services referrals, those who are making referrals or recruiting families to participate need to frame the program as something that will help their children. |
| **Problem of families' complex treatment needs** | **Develop a complete treatment plan to address all of a family' needs.** To address families' complex treatment needs, program staff and service providers should develop a comprehensive plan for services and supports with clearly defined responsibilities and lines of communication to coordinate among the different social service organizations involved with these families. It is also important to provide up-front case management and support to families to address the immediate and basic needs of families related to exposure to violence and other disadvantages. |
| **Importance of close relationships with families** | **Work with the referral sources and service providers on strategies to build relationships, establish trust, and help families understand the potential benefits of mental health services.** Those making referrals need to be educated on recognizing CEV and the symptoms of trauma so they feel comfortable discussing these issues with families. It is also important for the referral process to allow enough time for those making referrals to establish a trusting relationship with families. To help develop strong connections between families and the program's service providers, it is important to consider including an assessment and relationship-building component that enables families to become familiar with and accepting of the providers. |
| **Problem of culturally inconsistent services** | **Educate program staff about cultural differences and develop service delivery approaches that respect cultural issues.** To address the cultural aspects of service delivery for the target population, the lead agency or organization should employ staff and partner with agencies with different cultural and language competencies. |
| **Problem of unclear program parameters** | **Define the roles of different service providers for families.** The program can be structured such that those providing services to families have clearly defined roles and the criteria for ending services are clear. It is important that the families understand who is responsible for the different intervention components and the conditions under which the intervention will end. |
| **Importance of a flexible service delivery model** | **Adjust the service delivery processes to help program staff manage time and caseloads.** A flexible service delivery model can enable the program's service providers to change the setting, staff hours, staff roles, or caseloads to allow them to serve more families and better manage their time and caseloads. |
| **Problem of staffing issues among service providers** | **Maintain regular contact with program staff and provide routine refresher training and supervision.** Program management can improve service delivery by maintaining regular contact with those providing services and providing opportunities for refresher or supplemental training. The program's clinical supervisors should also monitor caseloads, staff morale and burnout, and the quality of the services being offered. |
| **Importance of close communication and coordination between program staff and service providers** | **Plan multidisciplinary or case coordination meetings.** To facilitate understanding and communication and provide a forum for troubleshooting, the program's staff and service providers can plan regular case management or coordination meetings that allow those involved with the family to share information, discuss the family's situation, ask questions of one another, and plan next steps. |
| **Problem of strained relationship among partner agencies** | **Recognize the different perspectives of partner agencies/organizations.** In planning the program, it is important to recognize that some partner agencies have differing perspectives and orientations about children exposed to violence. |

## Conclusions

Looking across the SSPA programs, it is clear that the only feature shared by the interventions was their goal: providing interventions for children exposed to violence. Otherwise, the programs varied across every dimension, complicating the challenge of evaluating the process of implementing them. Therefore, it is necessary to be cautious about the conclusions drawn from this assessment of the implementation processes.

Given these limitations, however, it is possible to detect broad patterns across the sites' implementation experiences. Despite successes in launching programs and delivering needed services to children exposed to violence, most programs faced difficulties getting referrals, engaging families in treatment, and providing a program that aligned with the families' individual priorities. We briefly discuss each of these points in more detail below.

For many reasons, most sites struggled with lower-than-expected referrals throughout implementation. Some programs experienced difficulties establishing or enhancing collaborative relationships with the partner agencies/organizations that were providing referrals into the program. In some cases, the agency's own services to the family took precedence over identifying and referring for violence exposure. In other situations, the research component of the intervention made referral sources reluctant to refer, knowing that some families would not receive the program. The structure of the referral process itself also provided challenges, with proximity and the burden on referral sources playing a role in the flow of referrals into the program. These challenges suggest that, when designing programs for children exposed to violence, it is important to develop strategies for educating, collaborating, and maintaining strong relationships with referral sources.

The SSPA programs also struggled with engaging the families in the interventions being offered. The challenges arose for a variety of reasons, including the multitude of stressors faced by families, perceived stigma of mental health treatment, cultural differences, and families' reluctance to participate in a research project. The experiences of the SSPA programs highlight the critical role that engagement and retention strategies play in providing community-based programs for children exposed to violence.

Finally, with multiple and complex treatment needs in addition to pressing basic needs, families of children exposed to violence may need interventions with flexibility in the array of services and in the sequencing of components, focusing first on addressing basic needs. Among the diversity of program setting, population, and intervention types, this may be the most consistent experience of the 15 SSPA interventions and therefore potentially the most central lesson for future undertakings focused on addressing the needs of children exposed to violence.

While we do not yet know the impact of the interventions on child and family outcomes, the findings from this process evaluation provide guidance for future community-based programs for children exposed the violence. The upcoming report on the outcome evaluation component of the national evaluation will address the questions related to the effect of the programs on child and family outcomes.

# Acknowledgments

This report would not have been possible without the many contributions of the Safe Start program staff and leadership at each of the 15 sites. We are extremely grateful for their generosity with their time and support during the data collection for this report and reviews of earlier drafts. Within RAND, we are indebted to David Adamson for his thorough and careful review of the report and his draft of the executive summary. Priya Sharma provided invaluable research assistance in the early phases of the project. Molly Scott and Al Crego provided programming assistance with the training evaluation data and quarterly reports. Scot Hickey set up the database and reporting functions for this project. We also thank Kristen Kracke and Jeffrey Gersh of OJJDP for their assistance and support with this effort. We also appreciate the important contributions of the RAND quality assurance peer reviewers, Bradley Stein and Abigail Gerwitz. Their thoughtful comments helped improve the quality of this report.

## Abbreviations

| | |
|---|---|
| ACS | Administration for Children's Services |
| ARC | attachment, regulation, competency (or attachment, self-regulation, and competency) |
| BDVP | Bronx Domestic Violence Program |
| CAC | Child Advocacy Center |
| CBCL | Child Behavior Checklist |
| CEV | children's exposure to violence |
| CFDA | Catalog of Federal Domestic Assistance |
| CM/MH | case management/mental health |
| CPP | Child-Parent Psychotherapy |
| CTAC | Children's Trauma Assessment Center |
| CVC | Crime Victim Center |
| DCYF | Rhode Island Department of Children, Youth, and Families |
| DOVE | Domestic and Other Violence Emergencies |
| DVERT | Domestic Violence Enhanced Response Team |
| FAHIS | Florida Abuse Hotline Information System |
| FCT | Family-Centered Treatment® |
| FSRI | Family Service of Rhode Island |
| HAC | Homeless Assistance Center |
| HPDP | Health Promotion and Disease Prevention Program |
| HSSIP | Head Start School Intervention Project |
| IFCS | Institute for Family Centered Services, Inc. |
| IRB | Institutional Review Board |
| ISE | RAND Infrastructure, Safety, and Environment |
| MDE | multidisciplinary evaluation |
| MGH | Massachusetts General Hospital |
| NMIC | Northern Manhattan Improvement Corporation |
| OCY | Office of Children and Youth |
| OJJDP | Office of Juvenile Justice and Delinquency Prevention |
| PCIT | Parent Child Interaction Therapy |
| PEACE | Promoting, Educating, Advocacy, Collaboration, and Empowerment |
| PREVENT | Prevention and Evaluation of Early Neglect and Trauma Project |
| PTSD | posttraumatic stress disorder |
| QAR | quarterly activity report |

| | |
|---|---|
| REVOC | Kalamazoo Collaborative Initiative for Reducing the Effects of Violence on Children |
| SMU | Southern Methodist University |
| SSPA | Safe Start Promising Approaches |
| TERM | Treatment and Evaluation Resource Management |
| TF-CBT | Trauma-Focused Cognitive-Behavioral Therapy |
| VIP | Violence Intervention Program, Inc. |
| YCATS | Young Children's Assessment and Treatment Services |

CHAPTER ONE

# Introduction

## Background: Children Exposed to Violence

In recent years, the risk to children exposed to violence at home and in communities has gained wider recognition (Kracke and Hahn, 2008). Evidence suggests that only a minority, 29 percent, of children ages 2 through 17 experienced no direct or indirect victimization in the given study year (Finkelhor et al., 2005). A recent national study of the prevalence of children's exposure to violence (CEV) found that 61 percent of children had experienced or witnessed violence in the last year (Finkelhor et al., 2009). Research has shown, however, that early childhood interventions can substantially improve children's chances of future social and psychological well-being (Mercy and Saul, 2009).

### Incidence and Prevalence of Children's Exposure to Violence

Common sources of CEV are direct child maltreatment (i.e., abuse and neglect), witnessing domestic violence, and witnessing community and school violence. The most recent national estimates of child maltreatment show that state and local child protective services agencies accepted 3.2 million referrals for neglect and abuse in 2007. From these referrals, 794,000 children were found to be victims of abuse or neglect, representing a national rate of 10.6 per 1,000 children. Children from birth to age 3 represented the largest portion of the total, with 32 percent of all victims in this age group. An estimated 1,760 children died as a result of their maltreatment, with more than three-quarters of them younger than age 4 (Department of Health and Human Services, 2009).

Witnessing violence in their home may also adversely impact children. While estimates vary considerably, a growing body of literature attests that a high proportion of children are exposed to domestic violence situations, referring to violence between adult intimate partners (Zinzow et al., 2009). Studies of police data have found that nearly half of domestic violence incidents include child witnesses (Fantuzzo, 2007; Fusco and Fantuzzo, 2009). The most widely known self-report survey of family violence found that one-third of children had witnessed parental violence (Straus and Gelles, 1990).

Children are also victimized and exposed to violence outside the home. A study of preschool age children living in a low-income neighborhood found that more than three-quarters had been exposed to violence at home or in the community (Graham-Bermann and Seng, 2005). Our own work in Los Angeles middle schools showed that 40 percent of children had been victimized in the community and 63 percent had witnessed community violence in the prior year (Jaycox et al., 2002). Among adolescents, 55 percent report exposure to community violence (McCart, 2007). Youth are also the victims of violent crime such as rape, sexual assault, robbery, and assault in their communities at a rate of 26.5 per 1,000 (Baum, 2005). Data on school-age children indicate that 32 percent reported being bullied at school and 4 percent reported being a victim of crime at school (Dinkes, Kemp, and Baum, 2009). About 6 percent of high school students in the United States report not going to school on one or more days in the past month because they fear for their safety at school or on their way to and from school (Centers for Disease Control and Prevention, 2008).

### Effects on Children of Exposure to Violence

A variety of psychiatric disorders and behavioral problems may result from direct or indirect exposure to violence, of which posttraumatic stress disorder (PTSD) is perhaps the most well known (Morris, 2009). Other consequences include depression, anxiety, behavioral problems, and other disorders (Jaycox et al., 2002; Lansford et al., 2002; Gilbert et al., 2009). School performance has also been shown to suffer as a result of violence exposure (Schwartz and Gorman, 2003; Morris, 2009).

The consequences of exposure to violence are likely to be felt well into adulthood (Morris, 2009). Research suggests that exposed individuals are at greater risk for persistent mental health problems (Kracke and Hahn, 2008), such as substance abuse and major depressive disorder (Widom and Hiller-Sturmhofel, 2001; Lynch, 2003). There is also risk of revictimization (Finkelhor et al., 2005). Early abuse is also linked to later delinquency and violent behavior (Kernic et al., 2002; Gilbert et al., 2009). For example, a recent study found that teenagers who had witnessed gun violence were twice as likely to engage in violent acts (Bingenheimer, Brennan, and Earls, 2005).

## Safe Start Initiative Overview

Given the prevalence of exposure to violence among children, and the impact violence exposure has on children, the need for intervention is clear. Safe Start Promising Approaches (SSPA) was the second phase of a planned four-phase initiative focusing on preventing and reducing the impact of CEV and sponsored by the U.S. Department of Justice's Office of Juvenile Justice and Delinquency Prevention (OJJDP). The ultimate goals of the Safe Start Initiative, by phase, are:

- **Phase One:** Expanding the system of care for children exposed to violence by conducting demonstration projects. Now complete, this phase involved demonstrations of various innovative promising practices in the system of care for children who have been exposed to violence.
- **Phase Two:** Building on Phase One, this phase was intended to implement and evaluate promising and evidence-based programs in community settings to identify how well programs worked in reducing and preventing the harmful effects of CEV.
- **Phases Three:** Still in the planning stages, the aim of this phase is to build a knowledge base of effective interventions in the field of CEV.
- **Phase Four:** The goal of this phase is to "seed" on a national scale the effective strategies identified in the earlier phases.

The initiative's first phase involved demonstrations of various innovative promising practices for intervention with children who have been exposed to violence. It targeted system-level outcomes, including local agency and community engagement and collaboration, service integration, and new/expanded/enhanced programming in 11 different sites across the country and also encouraged innovative practices for children identified as exposed to violence. This demonstration was designed to create a "continuum of care" across the full spectrum of prevention, intervention, treatment, and response for children exposed to violence and to generate an understanding of how communities can successfully develop and implement innovative policy and practice interventions to reduce CEV (Hyde et al., 2007). The first phase of the Safe Start Initiative culminated in a report detailing which processes had been effective and generating additional questions that still needed to be answered in subsequent phases of the initiative (ASDC, 2007).

The second phase, SSPA, focused on reducing and preventing the impact of CEV by implementing evidence-based and theory-based interventions, referred to as "promising approaches." OJJDP selected 15 program sites across the country that proposed a range of approaches, focused on multiple types of violence, included variations in ages and age-appropriate practices, and would be implemented in different settings. Each site participated in a national evaluation in which the intervention practices were evaluated using experimental or quasi-experimental studies, with the goal of building knowledge about the effectiveness of specific intervention strategies intended to reduce the harmful effects of CEV (Safe Start Center, 2008). In addition, detailed documentation of the planning and start-up process, implementation of services, and costs attributed to running the interventions was conducted to describe the context in which the sites planned and implemented the practices.

Phases three and four, which focus on applying the lessons learned from the previous phases, have yet to be launched.

## Evaluation Overview

The RAND Corporation conducted the national evaluation of the SSPA phase of the initiative in collaboration with the national evaluation team: OJJDP, the Safe Start Center, the Association for the Study and Development of Communities, and the 15 program sites. The national evaluation was designed to:

- assess the effectiveness of the SSPA interventions for children,
- examine variability in the intervention effects, and
- identify plausible reasons for that variability.

The evaluation design involved three components: an outcome evaluation; a process evaluation, including a cost analysis; and an evaluation of training.

### Outcome Evaluation

The outcome evaluation was designed to examine whether interventions are associated with individual-level changes in specific outcome domains at a particular site or cluster of sites. For this component, a rigorous controlled evaluation design was developed at each site, either with a randomized control group (wait-list or alternative intervention) or a comparison group selected on similar characteristics. Longitudinal data on families were collected for within-site and cross-site analysis of the impact of these programs on child outcomes. The data included demographic, violence exposure, outcome, and resilience data at the child level. As of spring 2010, the outcome evaluation is under way. Findings from the outcome evaluation will be reported in a separate report.

### Process Evaluation

The process evaluation, designed to describe the sites and their activities, is the focus of this report. The purpose of the process evaluation was to describe the context in which the 15 sites planned and implemented their specific SSPA programs. Data were collected for the process evaluation from a variety of sources, including site visits, quarterly activity reports (QARs), document review, and regular email and telephone communication.

**Site visits**. During the first two years of implementation, members of the RAND research team visited each site twice. The site visits allowed the team to gather detailed qualitative information about the program's implementation from a variety of perspectives. The site visits involved:

- **Key informant interviews.** For the key informant interviews, we used a semistructured interview protocol that focused on the planning process, implementation, training, quality assurance monitoring, policies and protocols, costs, collaboration in the community, program administration, and next steps.
- **Structured case reviews.** We conducted structured case reviews with therapists, case managers, advocates, or other program staff on a random sample of treatment and control or comparison cases to obtain more details on the process that the program staff used with families to deliver services and treat families.
- **Quality assurance reviews.** The quality assurance checklist was completed with the person responsible for clinical supervision of the therapists providing the Safe Start services. The checklist was designed to document the quality assurance processes and procedures the sites used to assure quality implementation of the therapy component of their interventions.
- **Observations.** We also toured facilities and observed staff meetings, clinical processes, training sessions, multidisciplinary team meetings, and group therapy sessions to gather information on how the programs were implemented.

**Quarterly activity reports.** The QARs were designed to collect information on study enrollment, service delivery, training, policies and protocols, and advocacy. The forms were standard but customized for each site so that at each site and across sites we would be able to report on the amount and types of services delivered, trainings conducted or attended, and policies created or changed.

**Document review.** We gathered a library of materials from the sites about their inputs and activities, including the original proposal, agency and program brochures and descriptions, training presentations, budgets, agency annual reports, and policy manuals.

**Regular email and telephone communication.** We also gathered descriptive and contextual information about implementation via regular email and telephone communications with program staff.

We used information from these sources to develop the cross-site analyses in the main body of this report and the detailed program descriptions that appear in Appendix B. The program descriptions were developed to describe the development and implementation of the

Safe Start program at each site. These descriptions synthesize the information gathered on the different aspects of the intervention from each source, including the key informant interviews with key program staff and community partners, structured case reviews, quality assurance reviews, observations, document review, and regular email and telephone communication.

After completing all 15 program descriptions, we used them to synthesize information and identify the factors related to the program context, interventions, and implementation processes. In Chapters Three, Four, and Five of this report, we describe the program and community settings, interventions, and implementations across all sites. Information from the QARs provides the basis for Chapter Six. The process evaluation components and methods are described further in Appendix A.

### Training Evaluation

The training evaluation was designed to assess the impact of training on staff knowledge and attitudes and to help us understand how training may have changed practice in working with children and families. We collected data on a sample of training sessions across sites using pre- and post-trainee surveys, follow-up trainee surveys, and key informant interviews when possible. For these analyses, we describe the content of site-specific trainings, provide site-specific data on participant characteristics, and detail changes in knowledge and perspectives where appropriate. We also briefly summarize pooled data across sites with attention to changes in attitudes and practices in working with children exposed to violence. Findings from the training evaluation are found in Appendix C of this report.

## Framework for Understanding Implementation in Community-Based Settings

Our understanding of the implementation of the SSPA programs was guided by a general conceptual framework about how programs are implemented in community settings. As shown in Figure 1.1, we utilized a framework adapted from Greenberg and colleagues (Greenberg et al., 2005; Chen, 1990) about the implementation of community-based mental health programs. In this model, a "planned program" includes components such as the program design and target population. "Planned implementation support" includes pre-planning activities, quality of program materials, technical support, and implementer readiness. Both the planned program and the planned implementation support then feed into the program as it is actually implemented. For instance, implementation support factors include pre-service and in-service training, ongoing coaching and consultation, staff performance assessment, and decision-support data systems (Fixsen et al., 2009).

But the program as it is implemented is also influenced by a variety of other factors, as shown in the model in Figure 1.1. In Durlak and DuPre's (2008) review of interventions conducted by community-based providers, the authors identified five categories of factors influencing program implementation: community, provider, intervention, delivery system, and support system characteristics. We include these same elements in our model, but organize them into three overarching domains: program context, intervention, and implementation process. Schoenwald and Hoagwood (2001) note that client characteristics can also affect the ability to take an intervention and implement it in a different community. Family-level characteristics also influence mental health program implementation in community-based

**Figure 1.1**
**Framework for Program Implementation**

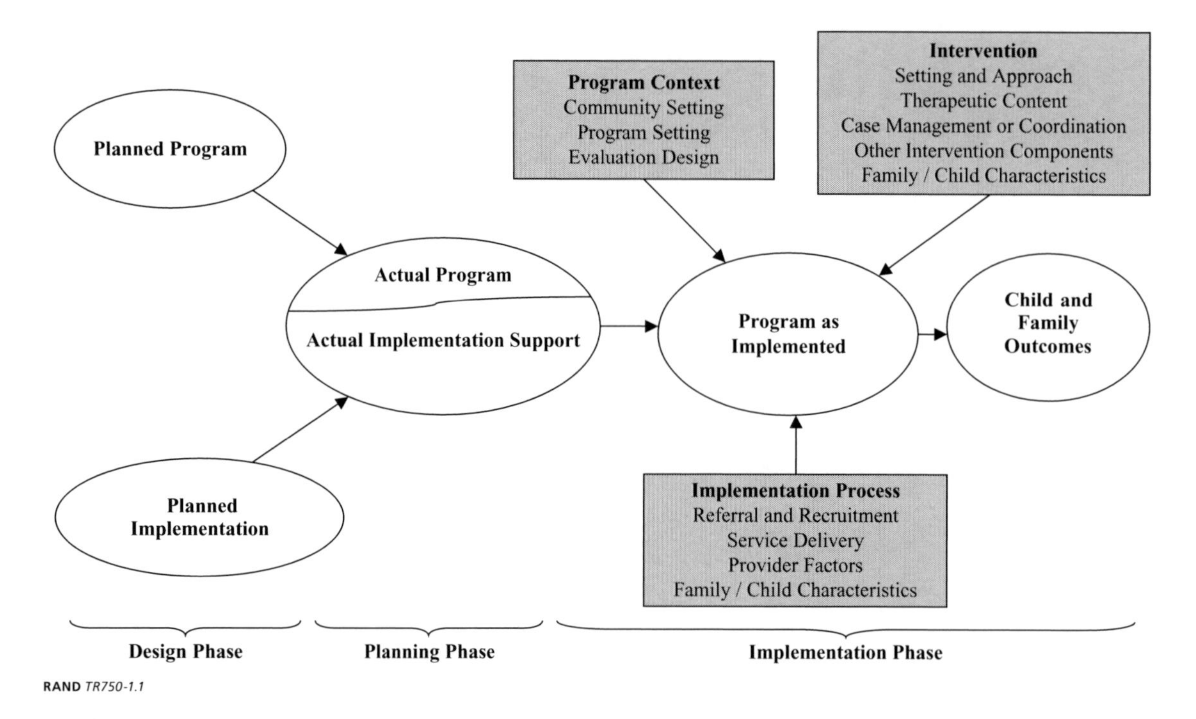


RAND *TR750-1.1*

settings. These include cultural factors, such as stigma, attitudes toward mental health services, and access to culturally appropriate services, as well as sociodemographic factors, such as insurance status and economic resources (McLoyd, 1990; McKay et al., 2001). These factors are included within the intervention and implementation process domains.

The **program context** domain includes community setting, program setting, and evaluation design. This domain encompasses factors such as community support and readiness for a program and the fit between the program and the community that influence the implementation of community-based violence prevention programs (Stith et al., 2006). Program-level characteristics that have been found to be related to implementation have included leadership, with supportive leadership positively influencing implementation (Durlak and DuPre, 2008). The **intervention** domain includes the intervention setting and approach, therapeutic content, case management or coordination, and other intervention components. Durlak and DuPre (2008) found that such characteristics of the intervention as a program's adaptability or fit with the provider and setting are likely to influence implementation. Finally, the **implementation process** includes referral and recruitment into the program and service delivery in addition to the family/child characteristics and provider characteristics. Provider-level factors include staff selection, facilitative administration, and financial, organizational, and human resources systems (Fixsen et al., 2009). Other studies have found that implementation was influenced by providers who saw the need for the program, recognized the potential benefits the program, had the skills to provide the services, and felt confident in delivering the services (Durak and DuPre, 2008). Factors such as family and child characteristics overlap across domains since they have an impact on the intervention itself as well as the implementation process.

Our evaluation of the SSPA programs assessed the impact of the program context, intervention, and implementation processes on the programs that were implemented.

Work in the earlier phase of the Safe Start Initiative provides some additional support for the importance of these factors in implementation. As mentioned, the first phase of the Safe Start Initiative was designed to create a continuum of services across the full spectrum of prevention, intervention, treatment, and response for children exposed to violence and to improve understanding of how communities can successfully develop and implement innovative policy and practice interventions. As part of their efforts, Phase One sites worked to improve referrals to services, provide clinical assessments, and deliver an array of therapeutic interventions for children and their families. A process evaluation of the Phase One demonstration sites found that implementation was facilitated by several factors included in our conceptual model: collaboration prior to Safe Start, diverse sectors represented, formal operating structure, capacity of leaders to influence community partners and lead collaborative, and participation or "buy-in" at high levels within organizations. In contrast, other factors were found to hinder implementation: limited support from community leadership, inadequate relationships with trusted and credible community agencies or leaders, philosophical differences among partners, and staff turnover in partner agencies (ASDC, 2005).

## Guide to This Report

The rest of this report presents the data gathered within the SSPA process evaluation. Chapter Two provides background information on the 15 sites across the United States that implemented SSPA programs. Chapter Three discusses the various program contexts and how factors associated with these contexts affected the interventions; Chapter Four examines the interventions themselves; and Chapter Five examines how the programs were implemented. Chapter Six discusses additional components of the programs that influenced the implementation of the programs. Chapter Seven presents our conclusions and draws implications for communities and other organizations that are considering developing and implementing similar interventions. Appendix A describes the process and training evaluation methodologies. In Appendix B, we provide a detailed program description for each of the SSPA sites. Appendix C presents the results of the training evaluation.

CHAPTER TWO

# SSPA Program Background

## Overview of the SSPA Program Sites

In 2005, OJJDP selected 15 program sites for Phase Two. Sites were chosen based on the strength of the evidence and theory base of their designs as well as the feasibility of the interventions. The 15 sites selected were diverse in their populations served, types of violence exposure, intervention strategies, implementation settings, and geographic location. The program locations were as follows:

- The Bronx, New York
- Broward County, Florida
- Chelsea, Massachusetts
- Dallas, Texas
- Dayton, Ohio
- Erie, Pennsylvania
- Kalamazoo, Michigan
- Miami, Florida
- Multnomah County, Oregon
- Oakland, California
- Providence, Rhode Island
- San Diego County, California
- San Mateo County, California
- Toledo, Ohio
- Washington Heights/Inwood, New York

The sites were originally funded for four years of program implementation, starting in October 2005 and ending in September 2009. However, this period was extended in some cases because sites took part in a planning period called the Green Light process to prepare them for the project prior to implementation. The Green Light process involved sites working with the national evaluation team to specify and document their plans in five areas (described below) and to align the study design with each program's goals. This alignment involved using a wait-list control design at some sites and randomizing at the classroom level, rather than the individual level, at a school-based site. The length of this extra time varied between six and twelve months, depending on each site's degree of readiness to implement its program services and to execute the evaluation plan.

Currently, timelines have been staggered such that one site has completed its services under the grant as expected in September 2009, 13 will complete services during 2010, and one site will extend into 2011. Sites were asked to avoid changing components of their intervention during the entire implementation period, although some changes to eligibility for the program, program setting, referrals, and similar aspects were sometimes approved. Any changes are noted in the detailed description of each program (Appendix B of this report). The findings in this report represent information gathered between 2006 and 2009, covering the Green Light period and two years of implementation at each site.

## The Green Light Process

Prior to using program funds, hiring staff, or conducting other implementation activities, each site participated in the Green Light process, as part of the "planned implementation support" portion of the framework. The purpose of the process was to make sure that sites were (1) ready to start implementation and (2) ready to be part of the evaluation. No formal evaluation data were collected until after the Green Light process was completed.

This process consisted of a review by the national evaluation team of a checklist of criteria. The checklist was developed by RAND researchers in consultation with the rest of the evaluation team to ensure that each site had the key components in place for implementation of its program and for participation in the national evaluation. As shown in the text box, the Green Light criteria included 27 items focusing on five areas: (1) program design, (2) control/comparison groups, (3) data collection, (4) RAND and local Institutional Review Board (IRB) approval, and (5) stakeholder agreements. Each site was asked to document its specific capabilities and plans in each area through an iterative process with the national evaluation team, culminating in receipt of Green Light approval from OJJDP and RAND for each site to begin implementation and evaluation activities. The process also provided an opportunity for sites to receive technical assistance in areas of need related to their intervention or evaluation, which in some cases resulted in changes to sites' original implementation plans.

For some sites, the evaluation component was completely new, and leaders at the site needed a good deal of guidance regarding the data collection and evaluation issues. The Green Light process provided an opportunity to explain the research component, randomization procedures, and IRB requirements and approvals that were necessary to participate in a research project. Given the variation in the Green Light process across the 15 sites, it is difficult to discern whether differences in implementation across the sites may have been related to the Green Light process.

### Green Light Process Checklist

***Program Design***

- ✓ Intervention is theory- and evidence-based and appropriate to the defined target population.
- ✓ Project logic model reflects theory base for implementation.
- ✓ Case flow is projected for both the intervention and comparison/control groups.
- ✓ Site has clearly defined:
  - Target population
  - Key elements of the intervention that distinguish it from usual services
  - Referral sources to the program
  - Entrance and inclusion/exclusion criteria
  - Starting point of the intervention
  - Criteria for ending the intervention
  - Criteria for when to count a case as a "dropout."
- ✓ Staff has been trained in the intervention.
- ✓ Where applicable, sites have a plan for:
  - Determining the duration for different elements of the intervention
  - Determining how cases will be assigned to each level or type of intervention.

***Control/Comparison Group***

- ✓ Relationships are established that ensure referrals into both intervention and comparison groups.
- ✓ Sites can create a control group within the program (e.g., randomizing) that is:
  - Feasible (no "spill-over" of intervention services to the control group)
  - Ethical (all families receive some services, stakeholder buy-in).
- ✓ If a control group is not feasible, a site has access to a comparison group that is:
  - Not exposed to the key elements of the program
  - Identified in the same way as the intervention group
  - Similar to the intervention group
  - Feasible (no "spill-over" of services, selected before services begin)

***Data Collection***

- A data collection person is identified who can oversee data collection for all participants (comparison/control as well as intervention).
- Training has been received from RAND on data collection and submission procedures.

***IRB Approval: RAND and Local***

- ✓ The IRB application:
  - Defines RAND's role.
  - Contains RAND's consent language.
  - The local IRB approval has been obtained and sent to RAND

***Stakeholder Agreement***

- ✓ All partners have agreed to participate in:
  - Finalized service delivery/implementation plans
  - Evaluation plans, including plans for comparison/control group and data collection

In some cases, the programs needed to educate their own staff and their community partners on the initiative overall, the specific program, and the importance of the research. Some sites took additional time (up to four months) between the green light date and their actual start date to begin implementation. Six of the sites received more intensive technical assistance during the Green Light process to help complete the checklist. The technical assistance was provided by the national evaluation team and involved conference calls, in-person meetings, and review of materials as necessary. The focus of technical assistance included the program design, implementation strategy, and target population.

In sum, the Green Light process enabled the sites and OJJDP to define the interventions in more detail, coordinate the intervention design with the evaluation, and receive technical assistance in areas of need and ensure readiness for implementation and evaluation.

CHAPTER THREE

# Assessment of the SSPA Program Contexts

## Community Setting

The 15 SSPA program sites represented communities that are geographically dispersed across the country. There were six SSPA sites in the East or Southeast (Bronx, New York; Chelsea, Massachusetts; Washington Heights/Inwood, New York; Providence, Rhode Island; Miami, Florida; Broward County, Florida). The Midwest had four SSPA sites (Dayton, Ohio; Erie, Pennsylvania; Kalamazoo, Michigan; Toledo, Ohio). The remaining five sites were in the west (Oakland, California; Multnomah County, Oregon; San Diego County; San Mateo County) and southwest (Dallas, TX).

As shown in Table 3.1, the communities served by the SSPA programs ranged from small cities with populations of less than 100,000 (Chelsea and Kalamazoo) to medium-sized cities, counties, or communities with populations between 100,000 and 500,000 (Dayton, Erie, Washington Heights/Inwood, Oakland, Providence, Toledo). Seven of the SSPA sites were located in large counties or boroughs of more than 500,000 people (Bronx, Dallas, Broward County, Miami, Multnomah County, San Diego, and San Mateo), with several of these serving catchment areas with more than 1 million people. Across all of the SSPA sites, children younger than age 5 represented 6 to 8 percent of the total population.

The SSPA sites were also racially and ethnically diverse. The white population ranged from 14 percent in the Washington Heights/Inwood section of New York City to 81 percent in Erie County. The black population was highest in Dayton, at 43 percent, and lowest in San Mateo, at 4 percent. The Hispanic population ranged from less than 5 percent in some of the Midwestern communities to 74 percent in the Washington Heights/Inwood section of New York City.

### Need for Services

In their original proposals to OJJDP, the selected sites described the degree of CEV in their communities. The sites reported a number of different indicators of exposure, depending on the specific focus of their proposed program:

- **Child Abuse and Neglect.** In the Bronx, for example, there were more than 14,000 children reported to child protective services for suspected maltreatment in 2003 (St. Barnabas Hospital, 2004). In Erie, Pennsylvania, the Office of Children and Youth received about 625 reports of child abuse and neglect annually (Children's Advocacy Center of Erie County, 2004).

**Table 3.1**
**Demographic Characteristics of the SSPA Sites[a]**

| Site | Catchment Area | Total Population (2000) | % of Total Pop Younger than Age 5 (2000) | Racial/Ethnic Distribution | | | | 1999 Per Capita Income (2005 $) | % Below Poverty Line |
|---|---|---|---|---|---|---|---|---|---|
| | | | | % White | % Black | % Other | % Hispanic | | |
| Bronx, NY | Borough of the Bronx | 1,332,700 | 8 | 30 | 36 | 29 | 48 | $16,344 | 31 |
| Broward County, FL | Broward County | 1,623,000 | 6 | 71 | 21 | 6 | 17 | $27,129 | 12 |
| Chelsea, MA | City of Chelsea | 35,100 | 8 | 58 | 7 | 28 | 48 | $17,127 | 23 |
| Dallas, TX | Dallas County | 2,218,900 | 8 | 58 | 20 | 19 | 30 | $26,465 | 13 |
| Dayton, OH | Montgomery County | 166,200 | 7 | 53 | 43 | 2 | 2 | $18,203 | 23 |
| Erie, PA | Erie County | 103,700 | 7 | 81 | 14 | 3 | 4 | $17,530 | 19 |
| Kalamazoo, MI | Kalamazoo County | 238,600 | 7 | 85 | 10 | 3 | 3 | $25,454 | 12 |
| Miami, FL | Miami-Dade County | 2,253,000 | 7 | 70 | 20 | 3 | 57 | $21,658 | 18 |
| Multnomah County, OR | Multnomah County | 660,500 | 6 | 79 | 6 | 11 | 8 | $24,468 | 13 |
| Oakland, CA | City of Oakland | 399,500 | 7 | 31 | 36 | 28 | 22 | $25,687 | 19 |
| Providence, RI | City of Providence | 173,600 | 7 | 55 | 15 | 25 | 30 | $18,177 | 29 |
| San Diego, CA | San Diego County | 2,813,800 | 7 | 67 | 6 | 23 | 27 | $26,843 | 12 |
| San Mateo, CA | San Mateo County | 707,200 | 6 | 60 | 4 | 32 | 22 | $42,204 | 6 |
| Toledo, OH | City of Toledo | 313,600 | 7 | 70 | 24 | 4 | 6 | $20,359 | 18 |
| Washington Heights/ Inwood | Community District 12 of Northern Manhattan | 208,400 | 7 | 14 | 8 | 3 | 74 | NA | 30 |

*SOURCE:* Based on information from the 2000 Census.
[a]Percentages may not sum to 100 because of rounding and multiple races/ethnicities.
NA = Data not available at the community district level.

- **Domestic Violence.** In Dallas, there were approximately 1,200 children who were provided services in residential domestic violence shelters in 2003 (Southern Methodist University, 2004). In Rhode Island, the Providence Police Department estimated that since 2001 there had been approximately 400 domestic violence incidents per year for which children were living in the home (Family Service of Rhode Island, 2004).
- **Community Violence.** The 2003 homicide rate in the city of Oakland was 27 per 100,000, compared with slightly more than 9 for Alameda County and about 7 for California as a whole (Safe Passages, 2004).

Prior to SSPA, the sites reported that available services for children exposed to violence varied quite a bit across the communities; however, as described in their original proposals, there were some commonalities in terms of gaps and barriers to services for children exposed to violence:

- limited identification of CEV by professionals in certain sectors
- limited outreach by service providers to engage at-risk families in services

- lack of follow-up and coordination of care for high-risk families
- inadequate array of age- and developmentally-appropriate services for children exposed to violence
- poor coordination of service providers and services
- lack of social supports for high-risk families.

To address these reported deficiencies, a lead agency in each site prepared a proposal to OJJDP in response to the SSPA solicitation.

### Program Focus

Across all of the communities, SSPA offered an opportunity to increase capacity, coordinate services, and address gaps in the array of services in the community for children exposed to violence. Many of the communities had very limited resources for serving this population (i.e., children younger than 18 years of age), particularly for children younger than 6 years of age. For these communities, the lead agencies that submitted proposals viewed the SSPA solicitation as an opportunity to build capacity for supporting services for children exposed to violence within their communities. Some of these took the form of building capacity in a particular service sector or group of residents, while others targeted the community in general. For example, in Dayton, the partner agencies involved in developing the proposal had started to educate themselves about infant mental health. They had participated in some training sessions and were beginning to think about how to proceed to address needs in their community. Dayton's partner agencies viewed SSPA as a way to take the next step and develop a means of delivering mental health services to very young children who had been exposed to violence.

For other communities, the lead agencies were already providing some services to help children and families stabilize after violence exposure, but these services were limited or fragmented. With SSPA, these communities were able to work toward more coordination of services for children exposed to violence. For example, in the Bronx, the SSPA program was designed to improve the physical, social, and mental well-being of children using the Medical Home for Children Exposed to Violence best practices model, which focuses on delivering primary care that is accessible, continuous, comprehensive, family-centered, coordinated, compassionate, and culturally effective (St. Barnabas Hospital, 2004).

A few of the communities aimed to both develop capacity and create an expanded and coordinated multiagency service delivery approach with their SSPA programs. For example, the Washington Heights/Inwood program proposed to develop a more coordinated community approach to children exposed to domestic violence by increasing identification and access to interventions and by implementing evidence-based interventions for these children and their mothers. In San Diego, the SSPA program was designed to raise awareness about the needs of children exposed to violence, improve system-level coordination, and increase capacity to provide evidence-based mental health services to this population.

## Program Setting

### Lead Agency/Organization

Within their communities, the SSPA programs were situated within or overseen by a variety of different lead agencies or organizations. As shown in Table 3.2, four of the SSPA programs were

**Table 3.2**
**Lead Agency/Organization and Partner Agencies/Organizations of the SSPA Sites**

| Site | Lead Agency/ Organization | Type of Agency/ Organization | Partner Agencies/Organizations |
|---|---|---|---|
| Bronx, NY | St. Barnabas Hospital's Children's Advocacy Center | Health clinic/ hospital | St. Barnabas Hospital Child Advocacy Center<br>St. Barnabas Hospital Pediatricians<br>Jewish Board of Family and Children's Services |
| Broward County, FL | Institute for Family Centered Services, Inc. | Human services agency | Henderson Mental Health Center<br>Women in Distress<br>ChildNet<br>Broward County Sheriff's Office |
| Chelsea, MA | Massachusetts General Hospital's Chelsea Health Care Center | Health clinic/ hospital | Chelsea Police Department<br>Harbor Area Department of Social Services |
| Dallas, TX | Department of Psychology, Southern Methodist University | University | The Family Place Domestic Violence Shelter<br>Genesis Women's Shelter<br>Salvation Army Family Violence Program Shelter |
| Dayton, OH | Artemis Center for Alternatives to Domestic Violence | Domestic violence agency | Young Children's Assessment and Treatment Services, Samaritan Behavioral Health<br>Brighter Futures |
| Erie, PA | Children's Advocacy Center of Erie County | Children's Advocacy Center | Crime Victim Center<br>The Achievement Center |
| Kalamazoo, MI | Child Trauma Assessment Center, Western Michigan University | University | Kalamazoo County Head Start |
| Miami, FL | Linda Ray Center, Department of Psychology, University of Miami | University | Miami-Dade County Homeless Trust/Community Partnership for Homeless<br>Miami-Dade County Human Services Violence Intervention and Prevention Services<br>11th Judicial Circuit of Florida, Administrative Office of the Courts |
| Multnomah County, OR | Multnomah County Domestic Violence Coordinator's Office | County-level government office | Gresham Child Welfare Office, Oregon Department of Human Services<br>Listen to Kids<br>Catholic Charities' El Programa Hispano<br>Volunteers of America Home Free Program |
| Oakland, CA | Safe Passages | Human services agency | Oakland Department of Human Services<br>Jewish Family and Children Services of East Bay<br>Asian Community Mental Health Services<br>Family Paths, Inc. |
| Providence, RI | Family Service of Rhode Island (FSRI) | Human services agency | Women's Center of Rhode Island<br>Providence Police Department<br>Rhode Island Department of Children, Youth and Families |
| San Diego, CA | Office of Violence Prevention, San Diego County Health and Human Services Agency | County-level government office | Child Welfare Services<br>Center for Community Solutions<br>Child and Adolescent Services Research Center<br>Chadwick Center For Children and Families |
| San Mateo, CA | Edgewood Center for Children and Families | Human services agency | Kinship Support Network |
| Toledo, OH | Toledo Children's Hospital's Cullen Center | Health clinic/ hospital | Help Me Grow<br>Family and Child Abuse Prevention Center |
| Washington Heights/ Inwood, NY | New York Presbyterian Hospital's Ambulatory Care Network | Health clinic/ hospital | Domestic and Other Violence Emergencies<br>The Mayor's Office to Combat Domestic Violence<br>Northern Manhattan Improvement Corporation |

within health clinics or hospitals. These sites were the Bronx, Chelsea, Toledo, and Washington Heights/Inwood. Another four of the SSPA programs were large human services agencies that provided an array of services to children and families in the community. These sites were Oakland, Broward County, Providence, and San Mateo. For three of the programs (Dallas, Kalamazoo, and Miami), the lead agency was an organizational unit (i.e., department or center) within a university. The lead agency for the Dayton SSPA program was a domestic violence services agency. In Erie, the lead agency was a Children's Advocacy Center that provided forensic interviews for children being investigated for child maltreatment. Lead agencies for two of the SSPA programs (Multnomah County and San Diego) were county-level government offices.

Results of the process evaluation showed that certain aspects of the lead agencies or organizations facilitated implementation of the SSPA interventions. The strength of individual leadership at the agencies appeared to be related to implementation success. Some sites had strong leaders who were able to develop relationships and institutionalize processes during implementation. For example, Erie hired a new Safe Start project director and lead agency head partway through the project, bringing renewed energy and commitment to the project. The new leadership worked to educate both new and existing referral sources on the program and its value. In Multnomah County, the strong commitment of the leadership of the Child Welfare Office hosting the SSPA program was seen as instrumental by the staff to the formation of a productive collaboration between the child welfare workers and domestic violence advocates. At the SSPA programs situated within a university setting (Kalamazoo, Miami, and Dallas), the lead agencies provided virtually all of the staff and resources to implement the interventions. Because the lead agencies were able to shoulder the bulk of the responsibility for implementation, the partner agencies were not burdened with SSPA responsibilities.

#### Partner Agencies/Organizations

In developing their program plans and proposals, the lead agencies partnered with a variety of agencies and organizations within their communities (see Table 3.2). These included law enforcement agencies, child protective services agencies, human services agencies, behavioral health organizations, and other community nonprofit agencies working with the target population. In some cases, the partnership developed because the agency would be providing referrals to the SSPA program. For others, the partner agencies would be delivering services, training staff, or conducting data collection in coordination with the SSPA program.

Results of the process evaluation show that the level of community support and the degree of involvement by participating agencies and organizations were related to how successfully sites implemented their programs. For example, Kalamazoo's program had buy-in from key staff and leadership at Head Start, which facilitated the classroom selection, assignment of children, and transportation arrangements for the program's implementation. In Dallas, the researchers who oversaw the program's implementation had prior experience implementing programs in the domestic violence shelters involved with Safe Start. This prior experience and established relationship meant that Dallas had a strong collaborative base to work from in implementing its SSPA intervention. Washington Heights/Inwood had success with enrolling families in part because of partnerships that existed prior to Safe Start that allowed its community partners to trust the program staff who would be implementing Safe Start. These types of established relationships between the SSPA programs and partner agencies and strong initial buy-in from the partner agencies contributed to successful implementation, particularly among sites in which partner agencies were referral sources for the SSPA program.

### Target Ages, Populations, and Referral Sources

Table 3.3 shows the age ranges, target population, and primary referral sources for the 15 SSPA programs. Six of the SSPA sites focused on very young children. Dayton, Oakland, and Toledo served children ages 0–5. While the Bronx expanded to serve children from birth through 6 years of age, San Diego included children up to age 7 and Broward County through age 8. Three SSPA sites served children from birth through age 12 (Erie, Miami, and Washington Heights/Inwood). Another three of the SSPA sites served children beginning at age 3: Kalamazoo served children ages 3–5, Dallas ages 3–9, and San Diego ages 3–12. Finally, Chelsea and Providence served children from birth through ages 17 and 18, respectively.

In terms of target populations, seven of the SSPA sites focused on children who had been exposed to domestic violence or community violence or who had experienced abuse or neglect (Broward County, Chelsea, Erie, Kalamazoo, Miami, Oakland, and San Mateo). Another six of the sites narrowed the focus to children who had been exposed to domestic violence (Dallas, Dayton, Multnomah County, San Diego, Toledo, and Washington Heights/Inwood). Providence targeted children exposed to domestic or community violence. The target population for the Bronx included children who had been exposed to community violence and family violence. The latter includes domestic violence as well as violence between siblings, elder abuse, and violence by children against parents.

The SSPA programs received their referrals from a variety of sources. The primary referral sources were sometimes closely tied to the program setting. For example, two of the SSPA programs within health clinics or hospitals received most of their referrals from within the clinic or hospital system (the Bronx and Chelsea). These types of internal referrals appeared to be facilitated by the existing strong relationships and close ties between the Safe Start program staff and other parts of the clinic or hospital system. The two programs led by county-level violence-related government agencies, Multnomah County and San Diego County, received referrals from and exclusively served a child welfare population. Two of the SSPA programs recruited participants directly from domestic violence shelters (Dallas and Miami). Two of the SSPA programs located within human services agencies received mostly internal referrals (Providence and San Mateo).

Other SSPA programs forged relationships with programs during the process of preparing the proposal to OJJDP for SSPA funding, and it was expected that these programs would provide most of the referrals. For example, Kalamazoo partnered with Head Start and provided services within Head Start classrooms, so the program recruited directly from the classrooms and did not have a referral process per se. This facilitated participation because the families did not have to do anything to participate other than to attend Head Start. For other programs, relying on a single referral source made it difficult to maintain the number of referrals needed to keep the program at full capacity. For example, Dayton and Toledo initially relied on one referral source to provide all of their referrals. When the pace of referrals did not meet expectations, the programs had to work with the existing referral source and simultaneously develop new partnerships in an effort to increase referrals.

Other SSPA programs had several main referral sources. For Erie, most of its referrals came from the Office of Children and Youth and internally from the Children's Advocacy Center. Broward County received most referrals from a local mental health agency, but also from the Sheriff's Office and child welfare. Oakland's program involved the development of a citywide referral process that targeted a host of public and private agencies that may encounter children exposed to violence. Oakland's program initially sought referrals from the specific agencies shown in Table 3.3.

**Table 3.3**
**Age Range, Target Population, and Primary Referral Sources for the SSPA Programs**

| Site | Age Range | Target Population | Primary Referral Sources |
|---|---|---|---|
| Bronx, NY | 0–6 | Children who have been exposed to, experienced, or witnessed family or community violence. | Saint Barnabas Hospital pediatricians, Children's Advocacy Center, and emergency department; local mental health and domestic violence agencies |
| Broward County, FL | 0–8 | Children who have been exposed to all types of violence, with a focus on exposure to domestic violence. | Henderson Mental Health Center's Family Resource Team, ChildNet, Broward County Sheriff's Office |
| Chelsea, MA | 0–17 | Children who have been exposed to violence. | Chelsea Health Care Center mental health and pediatric units, Chelsea Police Department's Police Action Counseling Team, Harbor Area Department of Social Services, and schools |
| Dallas, TX | 3–9 | Children exiting domestic violence shelters with their mothers who have been exposed to domestic violence. | Domestic violence shelters |
| Dayton, OH | 0–5 | Children who have been exposed to domestic violence. | Nurse home visiting program |
| Erie, PA | 0–12 | Children who have been physically or sexually abused, witnessed domestic violence, been a victim of any violent crime, or witnessed a violent crime. | Children's Advocacy Center, Office of Children and Youth |
| Kalamazoo, MI | 3–6 | Children who have been exposed to violence. | Head Start classrooms |
| Miami, FL | 0–12 | Children residing in specific shelters who have been exposed to domestic violence, community violence, and/or experienced abuse or neglect; or court-referred children for clinic-based treatment. | Domestic violence shelters, homeless shelters, juvenile court |
| Multnomah County, OR | 0–6 | Children within a county child welfare population who have been exposed to domestic violence | Gresham Branch Office of Multnomah County Child Welfare Services |
| Oakland, CA | 0–5 | Children who have been exposed to domestic violence, community violence, and/or experienced abuse or neglect. | Oakland Police Department, Family Violence Law Center, shelters, community-based organizations, Oakland Unified School District, Head Start, Family Justice Center, self-referrals, Department of Human Services, Children's Hospital |
| Providence, RI | 0–18 | Children who have been exposed to domestic or community violence. | FSRI, domestic violence shelter, Providence Police Department |
| San Diego, CA | 3–12 years | Children within a county child welfare population who have been exposed to domestic violence. | San Diego County Child Welfare Services |
| San Mateo, CA | 0–7 | Children in kinship care who have been exposed to domestic violence, community violence, and/or experienced abuse or neglect | San Mateo County Edgewood's Kinship Support Network |
| Toledo, OH | 0–5 | Children exposed to domestic violence | Help Me Grow |
| Washington Heights/ Inwood, NY | 0–12 | Children exposed to domestic violence | Domestic and Other Violence Emergencies (DOVE), Administration for Children's Services (ACS), Mayor's Office to Combat Domestic Violence, New York District Attorney's Office of Family Violence and Child Abuse Bureau, CONNECT's Family Violence Prevention Program, Harlem Legal Services, Dominican Women's Development Center, Northern Manhattan Improvement Corporation, Head Start, pediatricians, resident psychologist |

## Evaluation Design

At all of the sites, the interventions were implemented in the context of a rigorous evaluation, as required by OJJDP. Each site implemented an experimental or quasi-experimental research design, in collaboration with the national evaluation team. Eleven of the 15 sites had an experimental design in which eligible families were randomized to the SSPA intervention or a control group (usual services, enhanced usual services, or a wait-list for SSPA services). Three sites utilized a comparison group, in which different groups of families were recruited from a similar setting (e.g., another domestic violence shelter, clinic, or child welfare office) to participate in the comparison group. One of the sites used both approaches (control and comparison groups) for different types of services within their SSPA program. At all 15 sites, the treatment group received the SSPA intervention as well as any services and supports from the referring agency. At some of the sites, the control or comparison groups received only the usual services and supports from the referring or other agency in the community. At other sites, such as Dallas, usual services were supplemented by monthly phone contact, limited case management, developmental screenings, or drop-in support groups.

Longitudinal data were collected on each family for both treatment and control/comparison groups. Measures included four types of child-level data (demographic, violence exposure, child outcomes [behavioral, emotional, developmental, functional adjustment], and resilience) as well as information on the caregivers, custody arrangements, and services received.

Results of the process evaluation showed that the research requirements associated with the SSPA programs directly affected implementation, particularly referral and recruitment into the SSPA programs. At some sites (such as San Diego, San Mateo, Toledo), referral sources were particularly reluctant to refer because of the experimental design of the research, especially when there was random assignment to the intervention or a control group of some sort. For example, in Broward County, the primary referral source was initially reluctant to refer because of concerns about whether having families assigned to a control group would mean that they would not be able to fulfill their obligations to the family. In Dayton, the nurses from the home visiting program that made referrals had developed close relationships with the families. This made the nurses reluctant to refer because they did not want their families to be assigned to the control group and not get any services. In Washington Heights/Inwood, staff did not always adhere to the control group assignment, sometimes providing intervention services to families while they were on the waiting list. At other sites, the families were reportedly unsure about signing up for a program without knowing what it would entail.

## Summary

Looking across the 15 SSPA interventions, certain aspects of the communities, program settings, and evaluation design appeared to affect implementation of some of the SSPA interventions. Some factors facilitated implementation, while others hindered implementation of the SSPA programs. These factors included the following:

- **Widespread recognition of need.** Many of the communities involved in the SSPA initiative recognized the need for programs for children exposed to violence and identified gaps in the services available in the community. When there was widespread recognition among community agencies and service providers of the need to increase capacity and coordinate services, the lead agencies/organizations were better able to develop an intervention that addressed the gaps in the array of services for children exposed to violence.

- **Strong individual leadership at the lead agency.** Strong individual leaders at some SSPA programs served as program advocates in the community and within the lead agency/organization. These leaders were able to increase the program's visibility both externally and internally and provide support and direction for program implementation.
- **Clear division of responsibility for program implementation.** The structure of some of the lead agencies/organizations meant that they could take responsibility for providing the staff and resources for program implementation. In turn, partners/agencies were not burdened with responsibilities related to implementing the programs.
- **Close working relationships among partner agencies and referral sources.** Some SSPA programs took advantage of existing relationships and trust developed through prior experiences with partner agencies or organizations to smooth the way for implementing a new program in the community. These types of relationships were evidenced by strong buy-in from partner organizations, demonstrated by up-front support and understanding of the potential program benefits.
- **Burden of research requirements.** SSPA's research component posed challenges for program implementation. The reluctance of referral sources and families to participate when the program involved a control or comparison group negatively influenced the referral and recruitment processes, even though the services being offered were not otherwise available in the community.

CHAPTER FOUR

# Assessment of the SSPA Interventions

The 15 Safe Start programs comprised a range of intervention components that integrated or expanded evidence-based interventions (e.g., Child Parent Psychotherapy [CPP] or trauma-focused psychotherapy) or that have demonstrated promise during previous implementation and utilize recommended practices (e.g., Heroes or Head Start School Intervention Project). All of the sites had a therapeutic component, with about two-thirds focusing on dyadic therapy (a therapy for a parent/caregiver-child dyad together) or family therapy, while others used individual or group therapy approaches. In some cases, the modality varied by age, with dyadic or family therapy for younger children and group therapy for older children. Many of the sites also had some form of case management or case coordination, either along with the therapeutic component or as a more primary part of their intervention. Some of the sites had other intervention components, such as advocacy, parent groups, or other services (e.g., multidisciplinary evaluation of family needs, an in-home safety assessment, etc.).

Table 4.1 shows the intervention components and the length and setting for each of the SSPA sites. The interventions varied in length: two SSPA sites offered services for three months, seven provided services for six months, three offered services for up to one year, and one provided the intervention for one year or more. Two of the sites were flexible in their intervention length depending on the needs of the family.

The intervention setting also varied across the SSPA programs. Five of the interventions were offered in the families' homes, while three were conducted in a clinic setting. Another five sites provided services both in the families' homes and at the clinic. In Miami, the intervention was provided either at the shelter or in the child center. Kalamazoo's intervention was conducted in the Head Start classrooms, but parent meetings were held at a central Head Start administration building.

Each of these interventions is described in detail in Appendix B of this report. The remainder of this chapter describes the therapy, case management or case coordination, and other service components of the Safe Start programs.

**Table 4.1**
**SSPA Intervention Components, Length, and Settings**

| Site | Intervention Components | Intervention Length | Intervention Settings |
|---|---|---|---|
| Bronx, NY | Medical Home for Children Exposed to Violence, including multidisciplinary assessment, CPP, and case management | 1 year or more | Clinic |
| Broward County, FL | Family-Centered Treatment® | 6 months | In-home |
| Chelsea, MA | Group therapy, home visits, and case coordination | 3 months | Clinic and in-home |
| Dallas, TX | Project SUPPORT, including therapy, case management, and child mentorship | 6 months | In-home |
| Dayton, OH | CPP and case management/coordination | CPP: 6–12 months<br>Case management: up to 2 years | In-home |
| Erie, PA | Individualized therapy, case coordination, and parent education groups | 6 months | In-home or clinic depending on client's preference |
| Kalamazoo, MI | Head Start School Intervention Project, teacher training, and parent training program | 6 months | Head Start classrooms |
| Miami, FL | PREVENT assessment, Infant Mental Health (CPP) for children 6 months to 5, Heroes group therapy, and enhanced case management for children 6 through 11 | Infant Mental Health: 6 months<br>Heroes: 10 weeks | Domestic violence shelters, homeless shelters, and clinic |
| Multnomah County, OR | Domestic violence advocacy, CPP, and case coordination and consultation | Flexible | In-home and office-based |
| Oakland, CA | Case management integrated with dyadic caregiver/child psychotherapy | 6 months | In-home, community or office-based |
| Providence, RI | | | |
| Tier 1 | Crisis intervention | Initial contact and one follow-up contact | In-home |
| Tier 2 | Case management | 2 years | Shelter and in-home post-shelter discharge |
| Tier 3 | CPP and case management | 3 months | Clinic |
| San Diego, CA | Trauma-Focused Cognitive-Behavioral Therapy, child advocacy, and case coordination | Trauma-Focused Cognitive-Behavioral Therapy: 6 months<br>Advocacy: 6 months or more<br>Case coordination: 6 months or more | In-home |
| San Mateo, CA | CPP | 12 months | In-home |
| Toledo, OH | CPP | Flexible | Clinic |
| Washington Heights/Inwood, NY | CPP for children 0–5, Kid's Club and Reflective Parent Group for children 6–12. | CPP: 1 year<br>Kids' Club and Reflective Parent Group: 12 weeks | Clinic |

## Therapy Component

All of the SSPA sites had at least one therapeutic component to their interventions. Several sites offered different therapy approaches (dyadic or family, individual, or group) depending on the child's age. Eleven of the sites provided dyadic or family therapy. San Diego implemented an individual therapy. Four of the sites developed or modified group therapies as all or a portion of the therapy component of their Safe Start intervention (Chelsea, Kalamazoo, Miami Heroes, and Washington Heights/Inwood Kid's Club). Erie's therapy approach was individually tailored to the child's situation, so it could include any of the above modalities. Each therapeutic approach and any therapeutic models within the approach are described briefly below. More-complete descriptions of each site's therapy component can be found in the site-specific program descriptions in Appendix B of this report.

### Dyadic or Family Therapy

#### *Child-Parent Psychotherapy*

Eight of the 15 sites selected CPP as the therapy component of their intervention, although there was considerable variation in the mix of support services offered to families, the settings in which the sites delivered the therapy, and the types of families served. The sites offering CPP included the Bronx, Dayton, Miami's Infant Mental Health program, Multnomah County, Providence Tier 3, San Mateo, Toledo, and Washington Heights/Inwood.

CPP is a relationship-based intervention designed for use with children up to age 6. It can be used with any child whose relationship to his or her parent or other primary caregiver is impacted by negative circumstances, including family violence. CPP integrates psychodynamic, attachment, trauma, cognitive-behavioral, and social learning theories (NCTSN, 2008). The approach is designed to restore the parent-child relationship, the child's mental health, and the child's development following the negative impact of exposure to violence.

CPP has two components: assessment and treatment. The assessment is based on observing the child's relationship and behavior with the parent (caregiver) as well as the child's behavior in a number of different environments, such as engaging in play, interacting with the therapist, interacting at home, and so forth. The information gained during the assessment is used to inform the treatment component. This component makes use of six major intervention modalities: (1) promoting developmental progress through play, physical contact, and language to encourage healthy exploration, contain overwhelming emotions, clarify feelings, and correct misperceptions between the caregiver and child; (2) therapists' reflective guidance on child development through commenting on the child behavior observed during the session; (3) the therapist modeling appropriate protective behaviors for the parent (e.g., how to soothe a child in distress); (4) interpreting parent's and/or child's observed feelings, actions, and dynamics based on psychological theories; (5) providing emotional support/empathetic communication of the parent with the child (e.g., how to use supportive and nurturing words with the child during play or other interactions); and (6) offering crisis intervention, case management, and concrete assistance with basic needs of life, such as food, clothing, and housing (Lieberman and Van Horn, 2005). Generally, the entire intervention was designed to last about 12 months and consists of one-hour weekly sessions.

The overarching goals of CPP include increasing the child's and the caregiver's age-appropriate capacity to be emotionally attuned to each other's needs and changing negative patterns of interaction into positive and nurturing ones. More specifically, goals include encouraging normal child development through communication, play, and other activities; maintaining appropriate emotional responses (e.g., reducing the stress response); display of appropriate types and levels of emotions in given circumstances; achieving a sense of intimacy in the parent-child relationship for both the parent and the child; increasing the capacity of the parent and child to respond realistically to stressors; differentiation between reliving and remembering traumatic events; understanding common reactions to trauma; and placing the traumatic experience in a healthy perspective (Lieberman and Van Horn, 2008).

As shown Table 5.1 in Chapter Five, the sites varied in whether they offered only CPP or CPP in combination with other intervention components. For two of the sites (San Mateo and Toledo), their Safe Start intervention involved implementing CPP with the therapist providing the therapy and any necessary case management. Two of the sites (Dayton and Providence Tier 3) had a therapist and a separate case manager who worked with the family to provide supports. In Washington Heights/Inwood, the portion of the Safe Start program for birth through age 5 involved CPP. At three of the sites, CPP was one part of a comprehensive approach to serving children exposed to violence. The therapeutic component of Miami's Infant Mental Health program was developed by the CPP model developers and then refined for an earlier project. While the CPP portion is similar to that being implemented by the other sites, Miami's Infant Mental Health program was unique in its extensive assessments before and after treatment as well as its interaction with the dependency courts throughout treatment for cases that were court-referred. Similarly, the Bronx's Medical Home model involved multidisciplinary evaluations and intensive case management in addition to CPP. In Multnomah County, domestic violence advocacy and case coordination were the primary intervention components offered to all clients, with CPP provided depending on the client's needs and interest.

All of the sites offered CPP either weekly or bi-weekly in one-hour sessions with some variation in intervention length. In Providence, their Tier 3 CPP program provided 12 CPP sessions over three months. Miami's Infant Mental Health program offered CPP for six months. Following the standard practice described in the CPP manual, four of the sites provided CPP for up to one year (the Bronx, Dayton, San Mateo, Washington Heights/Inwood) (Lieberman and Van Horn, 2005). Both Multnomah County and Toledo were flexible in the intervention length, allowing the clinicians to deliver CPP over whatever time period they judged it to be needed.

Sites implementing CPP also introduced some adaptations to the intervention setting. While four of the SSPA sites provided CPP in the more traditional clinic setting (the Bronx, Providence Tier 3, Toledo, Washington Heights/Inwood), the other sites moved the therapy out of the clinic setting and into the client's home or the community. Dayton, Multnomah County, and San Mateo all worked exclusively out of the client's home to deliver CPP. For the Miami Infant Mental Health program, the clinicians provided CPP at domestic violence or homeless shelters for part of their project, and in the clinic for court-referred cases that involved substantiated child maltreatment. San Mateo's Safe Start program focused on kinship families. Since CPP was designed for a parent-child dyad, San Mateo worked with one of the model developers to provide initial training for the clinical staff to deliver the model in the kinship context and ongoing, in-person weekly clinical supervision. In particular, San Mateo incorporated some flexibility in which the caregiver was included in the dyadic therapy, drawing different family members into the therapy as care for the child shifted over time.

Some of the sites also received initial training and ongoing consultation or supervision on CPP from the model developers, funded through OJJDP's training and technical assistance resources, including the Bronx, San Mateo, Toledo, and Washington Heights/Inwood. All of these sites participated in the full CPP training with the model developers and then received weekly, bi-weekly, or monthly supervision or consultation from the model developers. Some sites, including Dayton, Multnomah County, and Providence Tier 3, trained and supervised their clinicians in the CPP model locally. Providence Tier 3 received extensive clinical training, education, and monthly consultation from a representative from one of the National Child Traumatic Stress Network sites that was implementing CPP.

### *Broward County's Family-Centered Treatment®*

In Broward County, the lead agency developed Family-Centered Treatment® more than 20 years ago. This intensive family-centered service model was designed to foster strong healthy attachment to parents and a sense of belonging, competence, independence, and value in children (Institute for Family-Centered Services, Inc., 2004). Family-Centered Treatment® involves five procedures, including safety assessment, crisis intervention, individual and family counseling, education about child development and appropriate expectations, and wraparound services 24 hours a day, seven days a week, for the duration of the service period. All services are provided in the family's own home and environment.

Generally, the first month of treatment was considered the Assessment and Joining phase, with the therapist gathering information in structured ways and using it to help the family formulate goals. Once goals were set, the second phase, Therapy with Families and Individuals, would begin, usually lasting for two to three months. This therapy would center on such issues as improving parenting, setting limits, continued safety planning, loss and separation, specific behavioral or emotional problems in the parent or child, and healing from the effects of trauma. The last phase of treatment, typically lasting about six weeks, was the Termination or Generalization phase, during which the therapist would observe and monitor the family to ensure that they are able to continue to maintain the things they learned during treatment.

Core concepts that were central to the model include the strength-based perspective, using experiential techniques rather than "talk" therapy, focusing on the power of peers and natural supports to the family, the value placed on practical services, and taking a holistic approach to work with the family to improve spiritual, emotional, physical, mental, and social functioning. During the sessions, the therapists worked toward helping to stabilize the family and to help the family access natural supports and to advocate for themselves, so they engaged "collaterals" (other community agencies) early on in treatment. Monthly team meetings brought all the players (e.g., social service agencies and family) together face-to-face to work toward common goals. Over time and under ideal circumstances, the family would lead those meetings and would set the agenda themselves.

### *Dallas's Project SUPPORT*

Dallas's Project SUPPORT was designed for use with children who exhibit clinical levels of conduct problems upon exit from domestic violence shelters with their mothers. The intervention was developed to address children's mental health problems related to domestic violence exposure, particularly conduct problems and symptoms of depression and trauma (McDonald, Jouriles, and Skopp, 2006). The intervention sessions delivered by the therapist combine case management (referred to in the model as "social and instrumental support") and training for mothers in nurturing and child behavior management skills. The nurturing and child behavior management components of the intervention sessions employ a behavior training model that involves assessing mothers' current knowledge and skills and providing education and training to enhance a specific skill set. The skill training involves therapist and parent role-play and therapist coaching of parents during observed parent-child interaction. Targeted skills are introduced progressively, and work on each skill continues until parents demonstrate its mastery. During Safe Start, both of these components were provided by a single therapist within the context of weekly home-based treatment sessions of 60 to 90 minutes in length over a six-month period.

#### *Oakland's Caregiver-Child/Infant Psychotherapy*

In Oakland, the Safe Start dyadic therapy was referred to as "caregiver-child/infant psychotherapy." This approach was described as a flexible, dyadic approach, targeted toward improving child social functioning, establishing or reestablishing positive parent/caregiver-child interaction and attachment, and identifying the root causes of maladaptive child behavior (such as anxiety, depression, or impulse control). The therapists who provided this therapy were trained in early child mental health and trauma and in the caregiver-child/infant psychotherapy approach used by the program. The dyadic therapy was delivered in the client's home during weekly sessions over a six-month period and sometimes involved additional family members.

### Individual Therapy

#### *Trauma-Focused Cognitive-Behavioral Therapy*

San Diego selected Trauma-Focused Cognitive-Behavioral Therapy as its therapy for the Safe Start intervention. Trauma-Focused Cognitive-Behavioral Therapy is a psychotherapeutic intervention used for children and adolescents who have developed clinical levels of PTSD resulting from various traumatic events, including child sexual or physical abuse, loss of a loved one, and domestic, school, or community violence (Cohen, Mannarino, and Deblinger, 2003). The program can be provided to children ages 3 to 18 by trained mental health professionals. It targets symptoms of PTSD that often co-occur with depression, anxiety, and behavior problems. The program seeks to teach children skills to cope with the difficulties this disorder creates. Trauma-Focused Cognitive-Behavioral Therapy involves individualized therapy sessions in which children are given emotional skills training; later, with the help of trained therapists, children begin to confront the traumatic experience associated with their PTSD symptoms. The individual sessions with the child are accompanied by meetings with the parents to provide education on trauma, parenting problems, behavior problems, and strategies. For Safe Start, San Diego coupled Trauma-Focused Cognitive-Behavioral Therapy with an extensive pre-treatment assessment using the Trauma Assessment Pathway model. The Trauma Assessment Pathway model used a multifaceted assessment process to assist clinicians in gaining a more in-depth understanding of the child, his or her developmental level and traumatic experience, and the family, community, and cultural system in which the child lives. The Trauma Assessment Pathway assessment process itself took several sessions to complete. Following that, the Trauma-Focused Cognitive-Behavioral Therapy intervention would begin and consist of approximately 20 sessions, delivered weekly in a clinic setting for a six-month period.

### Group Therapy

#### *Chelsea's ARC Group Therapies*

Chelsea's therapy component primarily involved group therapy models designed for different age groups. Each of the group therapy programs focused on attachment, regulation, and competency using trauma-informed interventions, techniques, and methods.

- **Rainbow Dance.** For children ages 0 to 3, Chelsea used Macy's curriculum to work on parent-child development as well as mind-body connections though the use of music, movement, and storytelling (Macy, 2007; Macy et al., 2003). The sessions were held weekly and there were no maximum or minimum numbers of sessions.

- **Kids Club[1].** For children ages 4 to 6, Chelsea used a group curriculum developed for the Massachusetts Department of Social Services using best practices gathered from the literature (Cohen, Rodriguez, and Green, 2005). The 12-session curriculum focused on feelings, safety, personal space, family structure, use of kind words, and problem-solving.
- **Cool Youth.** This group therapy for 8-to-11-year-olds used a 12-week interactive group therapy curriculum developed for the Massachusetts Department of Social Services (Northnode, 2007). The children and parents met at the same time but in separate groups. The curriculum for the children focused on violence exposure, with sessions on feelings, abuse, safety planning, family changes, substance abuse, solving conflicts, sexual abuse, and children's rights. The curriculum for the parent group focused on helping parents understand the children's experiences and symptoms.
- **Teen Group.** This group therapy for adolescents 12–17 years old was loosely based on the ARC (attachment, self-regulation, and competency) framework (Kinniburgh, Blaustein, and Spinnazola, 2005). With this model, the group worked toward improving affect and regulation by focusing on helping the teens identify the things that drive their feelings and then understand their choices for handling them.

#### *Kalamazoo's Head Start School Intervention Project*

Kalamazoo program leaders developed their Head Start School Intervention Project based on their own earlier work for school-aged children, which was funded by the National Child Traumatic Stress Network. The curriculum consisted of six core elements: feeling safe, making and keeping friends, calming my mind and body, feeling good about learning, making meaning of my experiences, and literacy. Within the general framework provided by the six core elements, there were specific "units," or topic areas, for teachers that describe in detail structured activities for teachers to engage in with the students in the classroom (Kiracofe et al., 2005). Within each unit, the structured activities address both social/emotional skills and literacy. The manual provides one to five activities for each week of the 26-week curriculum. Also included in the curriculum are professional development worksheets that allow staff members to develop their own intervention plans for the classroom that tie into the structured activity. The manual for the Head Start School Intervention Project was developed during Kalamazoo's pilot testing period and is detailed with goals, activity length, materials needed, instructional procedures, key points, and literacy tips to ease implementation. Along with the Head Start School Intervention Project curriculum, teachers and aides attended consultation meetings to review behavior problems and issues in the classroom and to get expert consultation on the possible role of trauma and violence in that behavior as well as possible strategies for managing the behavior.

#### *Miami's Heroes Group Therapy*

The Heroes program is an arts-based group approach to explore underlying distress related to exposure to violence developed by the Miami Safe Start program for children ages 5 and 12 who were not eligible for their Infant Mental Health program. Each of the 10 group sessions began with a clip from a children's animated film, to help engage the children. Then various processing questions were asked of the group, followed by an expressive art activity (music,

[1] Chelsea's Kids Club group has the same name as Washington Heights/Inwood's group therapy for 6-to-12 year olds, but these are different group therapy models.

drawing, role plays, etc.) and a closure activity. At the proposal stage of the project, the Heroes manual existed only in outline form, but the Safe Start program team developed it into a more comprehensive manual during the course of the funded Safe Start project.

#### *Washington Heights/Inwood's Kid's Club*

Washington Heights/Inwood used the Kid's Club program for children ages 6 through 12.[2] This program is a group treatment for children exposed to domestic violence that was designed to reduce the impact of domestic violence on children as well as to reduce the risk of repeated violence (Graham-Bermann, 2000). The program includes 12 group sessions based on three theoretical frameworks: social learning theory, attachment theory, and trauma theory (Graham-Bermann, 2000). The sessions target children's knowledge about domestic violence; their attitudes and beliefs about families, relationships and family violence; their emotional adjustment; and their social behavior. During Safe Start, the Kids' Club sessions took place once per week for 90 minutes over 12 weeks. This approach was bolstered by Parent Reflective Learning group for parents, and a psycho-educational group for teen siblings.

### Other Therapeutic Approaches

The therapy component of Erie's integrated treatment program was relatively unstructured and largely driven by the needs of the parent and child. The assigned therapist conducted an initial home visit guided by a written protocol designed to gather information about the child's developmental history, the family situation, and the home environment through questions and observations by the therapist. The therapist then used all the information gathered from the developmental screening conducted at intake and the home visit to develop an integrated treatment plan for the family, with flexibility in how the treatment was delivered and the amount of effort spent in any area. The types of therapy might include dyadic therapy, play therapy, or family therapy.

## Case Management or Case Coordination Component

Many of the sites also had some form of case management or case coordination. Recognizing that families are less likely to benefit from therapy when their basic needs are not met, the case management typically involved a case manager who was responsible for addressing the families' basic needs, such as food, housing, and transportation. The case management also involved linking families to other services or supports through referrals. The sites with case coordination as part of their intervention used a team approach to supporting the families. In addition to providing for the family's basic needs, the care coordination involved team meetings with different service providers and agency staff involved with the families. The purpose of these meetings was generally to coordinate services and communicate with one another about the family's needs and progress.

### Case Management

Six of the sites integrated case management with the therapeutic component of their intervention to address the families' basic needs and to refer families for additional services and supports.

[2] Washington Heights/Inwood's Kids Club group has the same name as Chelsea's group therapy for 4-to-6-year–olds, but these are different group therapy models.

Three of the sites had separate case managers to directly provide support, help with access to other supports and services, and make referrals. The Bronx Safe Start intervention involved a social work assistant to help the social worker coordinate services and support the family in getting their needs met. In the Bronx, the case management also involved advocacy work on behalf of the families to ensure that they received the supports and followed through with referrals. Dayton's intervention used an advocate to provide case management to the Safe Start families. The advocate accompanied the therapist on home visits and used a portion of the session to assist families with such concrete needs as housing, employment, and transportation. The advocate also incorporated domestic violence education into the case management when meeting with the family. In Providence, Tier 2 intervention in the domestic violence shelter involved only case management. The Safe Start advocate completed a general needs assessment with each mother while she was in the shelter to assess her needs and the needs of her child(ren) and then met weekly with the mother to discuss goals, progress, and other issues that may have arisen during her shelter stay. After the shelter stay, the advocate would maintain weekly or monthly contact. Providence's Tier 3 CPP intervention also had a separate case manager to make home visits to assist with housing, educational, and employment needs as needed. The case managers would also help the parent obtain individual mental health services as needed.

At three of the sites, the clinicians who provided the therapy component of the intervention were also responsible for case management. For Dallas's Project SUPPORT, the therapists devoted a portion of each session to case management-type activities. These may have involved assisting with obtaining food, clothing, rental assistance, child care, transportation, employment assistance, and health care. The therapists were trained to both make referrals and assist clients with accessing these services to whatever extent they were needed by the client. For Miami's Infant Mental Health program, the therapist who completed the PREVENT (Prevention and Evaluation of Early Neglect and Trauma) assessment conveyed the results to the shelter's case manager to improve planning for the family and to ensure that the basic needs were met. Oakland's Safe Start intervention consisted of intensive case management and the therapy described above. The case management activities included assistance to families in securing needed public and community services (such as legal aid, food, transportation, emergency financial assistance, medical care, housing support, childcare, and employment) as well as collateral contact with other agencies to facilitate families' access to necessary services.

### Case Coordination Meetings

Four of the sites used a case coordination approach that combined case management with team meetings and joint planning between service providers and agency staff involved with the families. Chelsea's case coordination was conducted through a multidisciplinary team that met weekly to discuss and review each family's progress. These meetings were attended by social workers, a pediatrician from the health care center, a representative of a domestic violence advocacy group, and a psychologist. The multidisciplinary team worked together to develop a treatment plan for each family. The case coordination also involved coordination among resource providers in areas such as mental and physical health, education, food and clothing, transportation, job training, and safety. Erie also convened an integrated treatment team each week to discuss and review each family's progress. The Safe Start case manager and therapists as well as someone from the child protective services agency and a community-based organization for crime victims attended these treatment team meetings.

In Multnomah County, the case coordination meetings involved discussions and joint case planning between child welfare workers and domestic violence advocates to coordinate efforts and discuss services to families. Case coordination involved both formal case review meetings (which might include multiple other service providers, such as the parent-child specialist providing therapy services) and informal conversations between child welfare workers and advocates about a particular family.

The San Diego Safe Start program also held regular case coordination meetings between the child welfare case manager, the Safe Start therapist, and the Safe Start child advocate. The monthly case coordination meetings were designed to allow the service providers to discuss their individual perspectives of the child and the family's status, needs, and progress. The meetings served as a forum for the three key service providers to jointly discuss any case difficulties, resolve any disagreements in service needs or provision, and jointly develop plans to help families achieve success in meeting goals in each of the three service domains: child welfare, advocacy, and therapy.

## Other Intervention Components

Some of the sites had other intervention components, such as advocacy, parent education, or other services.

### Advocacy

The two sites working out of child protective service offices provided direct domestic violence advocacy services within the child welfare setting as a primary component of their Safe Start intervention. In Multnomah County, domestic violence advocacy services were offered to all mothers with young children referred to child welfare for which a new or recent domestic violence incident had occurred. The domestic violence advocacy services for families involved conducting an initial safety assessment and assessing the family's basic needs. The advocate would then work with the mother to develop a safety plan and assist her to meet the basic needs. The advocates also offered domestic violence victim support groups and provided individual social support, such as accompanying mothers to court hearings. The length of the advocacy services was not predetermined and would continue based on individual need.

In San Diego, the Safe Start advocacy services were provided in a client's home or other location, depending on the needs of the child and family. The advocacy services were specifically focused on the child and family's domestic violence-related needs. For example, the child advocates would assist the family in finding community resources available to victims of domestic violence and their children, such as support groups, housing assistance, and legal aid. They also provided emotional support and accompanied the family to court and appointments with agency service providers. The advocacy component varied in length depending on the level of family need but was expected to extend approximately six months.

### Parent Education

Three of the sites implemented a parent education group as part of the intervention. Erie's parent education group was offered to families involved with their individualized therapy program and case management services. The curriculum was developed to expand parent knowledge, improve parent-child bonding, and provide child management and protection skills.

There was a standard curriculum for the 12 weekly 90-minute sessions, with materials and a participant workbook for each session; eight sessions were conducted with parents only and four were conducted with parents and children together. The first four sessions focused on psychoeducation, the next four—with the parents and children together—focused on parent-child attachment and bonding, and the final four focused on the parents' role as leaders of the family.

Kalamazoo's parent training program involved optional bimonthly parent group sessions. Each of the 12 group sessions was 90 minutes long, with transportation, child care, and dinner provided to those who attended. The groups were designed to provide specific and age-appropriate information about psychological, emotional, behavioral, social, and academic problems associated with exposure to violence and to help foster the development of the child in three domains: trust, autonomy, and initiative. The parent training was not manualized; it consisted of a series of agendas and parent materials. For example, one group's agenda began with a check-in procedure (ratings of parents' stress levels and control levels); followed by teaching some specific coping skills, included an activity that they could also do with their children afterward; and closed with a centering activity to teach parents how to calm themselves and focus on an external object rather than their own thoughts and worries. These parent groups were co-facilitated by two parent interventionists and organized in collaboration with Kalamazoo Head Start staff.

In Washington Heights/Inwood, the mothers of children attending their Kids' Club group therapy program were offered a parent group called the Reflective Functioning Parenting Group. The group's primary goal was to help parents understand and respect their children's independence and point of view and to guide parents to understand their children's behavior as a response to underlying feelings, thoughts, and attitudes. The group goals were tailored to better fit the domestic violence context, so that the mothers in the group would share their personal stories, discuss their own children's exposure to domestic violence, and attempt to understand the child's feelings and relationship to the other parent. Another goal of the group was to teach parents to attend to safety for themselves and their children to enhance the child's sense of safety. These group sessions were held at the same time, on the same schedule as the Kids' Club sessions, and also consisted of 12 weekly 90-minute sessions.

### Other Services

A few of the sites had additional services as part of their Safe Start intervention. In the Bronx, the Safe Start intervention began with a preliminary multidisciplinary evaluation to determine the needs of each child and family. The evaluation included a developmental, behavioral, psychosocial, and medical evaluation. The assessment team consisted of two pediatricians (one who conducted a neurodevelopmental pediatric assessment and another who conducted a pediatric exam), one psychologist, and one social worker. The neurodevelopmental pediatric assessment included standard developmental screenings to assess motor skills, language skills, and achievement for older children. The psychologist and social worker conducted a psychosocial evaluation of the family that included behavioral observations and administration of a standard behavioral checklist. After completion of the evaluation, the team met to develop a provisional diagnosis, develop the individualized treatment plan, and produce a report. The CPP and case management components of the Bronx's intervention then followed from this evaluation.

In addition to group therapy and care coordination, Chelsea conducted an in-home safety assessment with children ages birth to 7. The home visitor used a checklist with sections on child supervision, environment/safety, and media, computer, and video games. The purpose of the assessment was to observe these areas and then to provide supports such as advocacy, education, resources, and case management.

Dallas's Project SUPPORT included child mentors who went with therapists to each home-based session and worked with any children present in the home during the session. In advance of the home visit, child mentors were expected to plan and prepare interesting and appropriate activities that the mentor would engage in with the children. Also, mentors were charged with establishing positive, supportive relationships with the children by using praise and providing positive attention, and generally entertaining them while their mother was engaged with the therapist. This served the function of reducing the sources of parental distraction that can be problematic within a home-based setting.

The Tier 1 portion of Providence's Safe Start intervention involved an existing crisis-intervention program for families with children exposed to violence. In Tier 1, eligible children/families were identified by the police department when they responded to the scene. A police officer would contact the clinician on-call to come to the scene. The clinician provided crisis services, referrals, and follow-up care. The timing of the follow-up contact varied depending on the family's circumstances. With Tier 1, FSRI aimed to improve the care coordination of families who enter the larger system.

## Summary

Looking across the 15 SSPA interventions, it appears that certain aspects of the intervention approaches affected implementation.

Some SSPA programs faced challenges with service delivery because of a potential mismatch between the intervention components and the families' priorities and needs at the time. Because most of the information in this report about the implementation of the SSPA programs came from program staff, it is difficult to assess whether the intervention components were appropriate from families' perspectives. At most sites, the primary intervention component was mental health therapy aimed at detecting and treating violence exposure. However, this service-delivery approach may not have been aligned with the families' needs and issues at the time they were identified for services. The intervention approaches were in many cases not specifically tailored for the population to be served in terms of the symptoms or needs they were designed to address, making it possible that they were not culturally relevant or appropriate for the families who were identified for treatment. Specifically, many families required help with concrete needs at the time of entry, before they could turn to the therapy itself. San Diego found that its families had lower than expected levels of trauma exposure, so they had difficulty fitting the trauma-focused intervention to the population at hand.

The intervention approaches also raised challenges in terms of outcome evaluation, since the initiative as a whole was focused on assessing outcomes at the level of the individual child. Some of the interventions aimed to change the environment for the child, rather than affecting the child directly. For example, Kalamazoo's classroom intervention aimed to improve teachers' skills in working with the children who had been exposed to violence, as well as working directly with the children via curricular activities rather than direct intervention or therapy. Other SSPA interventions focused primarily on delivering services to the caregiver to improve safety and parenting, with the assumption that the benefits would trickle down to the child. These intervention approaches may not translate into observable child-level outcomes immediately.

The intervention setting also affected implementation, with advantages and disadvantages to the different intervention settings. With clinic-based services, attendance was an issue, since families had to come to the clinic to participate. While the clinic setting sometimes made it difficult for families to make and keep appointments, it did provide a safe and quiet environment for families to receive services. Some SSPA programs found home-based services to be advantageous because many families had transportation or child care issues that made it difficult to get to a clinic or agency for appointments. In Multnomah County, the home-based delivery of their therapy component made participation manageable and consistent for the families. In Broward County, the delivery of intervention within the home is an important part of the model, with lengthy sessions in the home setting used to help the family modify patterns of behavior in order to meet their treatment goals. In Oakland, the home-based setting was critical for engagement and helped staff better understand the case management needs of families. However, with in-home services there were also distractions from the home environment during service delivery. In Dayton, the therapists found that the homes were often busy, with many different people coming and going, which meant that it took time to learn the family's story and understand its circumstances. For Oakland and San Mateo, the in-home setting created challenges because it made travel time and service delivery time-consuming.

Despite differing priorities about the intervention components, once therapy started there were benefits to having flexibility within the therapy component. Several factors related to the therapeutic component also affected implementation. For those delivering CPP, the model itself offered flexibility in approach. In Multnomah County, CPP's flexibility allowed the team to modify strategies for use with a larger family context. San Mateo also appreciated the broad flexibility of the CPP model that allowed them to draw from a variety of therapeutic techniques and approaches. Oakland also found success in providing dyadic therapy services, in part because of the flexibility in the clinical model, which allowed them to tailor existing services more directly for families with children exposed to violence. Chelsea and Washington Heights/Inwood both found that the flexibility in the group therapy curricula allowed them to make adjustments to accommodate and meet the needs of the group.

Within the therapeutic component, some SSPA interventions had a flexible service delivery approach that allowed them to adapt to family needs and circumstances when providing therapy. For example, Chelsea's open-ended approach to therapy allowed families to cycle in and out as needed depending on what was happening in their lives. Similarly, Erie's integrated treatment model, with its flexible therapy options, meant that their SSPA intervention services were tailored, depending on family needs.

The flexibility in the array of therapy options also brought challenges, particularly related to how to monitor fidelity over time. Although each site had different ways to assess quality assurance and model fidelity, most of the monitoring was not at the level necessary to assess adherence per se. Instead, most programs relied on supervision and consultation for quality control, without direct observation, ratings, or monitoring of therapy itself. As a result, it is difficult to determine how well the sites adhered to the models in the therapy component of their interventions.

The case management or coordination component of the SSPA interventions was related to program implementation. For many SSPA programs, the case management or case coordination component of the interventions provided a way for the program staff to connect with families to address their basic needs. Doing so helped families who were unfamiliar with mental health treatment to begin to trust the program staff.

Finally, those sites that conducted needs assessment or developmental screenings found that this approach helped them engage families. Families and referral sources received detailed feedback from these screenings, and there was a period of time in which the families and therapists could get to know one another prior to initiating the therapy. For example, Erie and Bronx followed up with families after the developmental screening to discuss the results and make a plan for services. The assessments also helped the SSPA programs identify needs early in service delivery. Similarly, Broward County's lengthy assessment was considered to be the first phase of therapy, during which the therapist and family would "join" together and the family would identify goals for treatment.

In sum, certain characteristics of the intervention approaches appeared to affect implementation across the 15 SSPA sites.

- **Differences between the intervention approach and the families' needs and priorities.** While the intervention approaches were developed to fill a gap in mental health services in the community as perceived by community partners, the focus on mental health services did not necessarily fit with families' own priorities, which were often directed toward addressing safety and basic needs before turning to mental health. This issue with the sequencing of services created challenges with service delivery, as families had other priorities at the time of their referral into the programs.
- **Convenience of intervention setting.** The convenience of the intervention setting for the program's target population affected implementation. Many of the SSPA programs delivered the services in families' homes, which enabled them to address some of the logistical challenges related to successful engagement of families in treatment and provide a safe environment for families to receive services. Other programs were successful in a clinic setting by providing an array of services in a location that was familiar and convenient for families.
- **Use of needs assessment or developmental screenings.** SSPA programs that included a needs assessment or development screening as one of their intervention components found that this approach helped them engage families.
- **Ability to provide for families' immediate and basic needs.** The case management or coordination component enabled the SSPA programs to connect with families and address their basic needs. Doing so helped providers engage with families who were unfamiliar with mental health and begin to establish trust and increase comfort with the intervention.
- **Wide array of therapy options.** By offering a wide range of therapy options, some SSPA programs were able to tailor the therapeutic component to the families' needs and circumstances. This flexible approach helped these programs be responsive to the unique needs of families.
- **Adaptable components of the therapy models.** Some therapy models provided guidelines rather than manuals. This enabled the clinicians to tailor the therapeutic strategies and techniques to the families' circumstances.
- **Inability to monitor adherence to the therapy model.** Because of resource constraints, many SSPA programs were unable to systematically ascertain whether individual project staff were following the therapeutic guidelines or standards when delivering the intervention services. This made it difficult to assess whether the therapy was delivered as intended by the model developers.

CHAPTER FIVE

# Assessment of the SSPA Implementation Processes

The SSPA sites began implementation after completing the OJJDP Green Light process. The first site received approval to begin enrolling families into the program in March 2006, and the last site received approval in November 2006. Partway through implementation, OJJDP extended the timelines such that all but one of the sites would complete implementation during 2010. Kalamazoo completed implementation in the summer of 2009, according to the plan they worked out with OJJDP during Green Light. The present report covers the first two years of implementation.

Figure 5.1 shows the implementation of the SSPA interventions. Implementation began with referrals or recruitment to the program of families with children in the target age range that had been exposed to violence. At some SSPA sites, there were training activities related to referrals into the SSPA programs or to the intervention services that occurred in parallel with the referral process and service delivery. Once families were referred into the program, those assigned to the treatment group received each site's specific intervention services (described in Chapter Four). Outcomes from the SSPA interventions varied by site and were expected at the individual, family, and system levels. At the individual level, some of the SSPA programs were focused on improving child well-being and functioning or parent stress levels or coping skills. At the family level, some of the SSPA programs worked to improve the parent-child relationship, increase safety, and reduce violence exposure. At the system level, a few SSPA programs targeted changes within or across agencies responsible for responding to CEV.

Specific and detailed descriptions of the implementation of the Safe Start Program at each site can be found in Appendix B of this report. In this chapter, we identify general themes and implementation issues that we observed across the 15 sites.

**Figure 5.1.**
**Model of the SSPA Interventions**

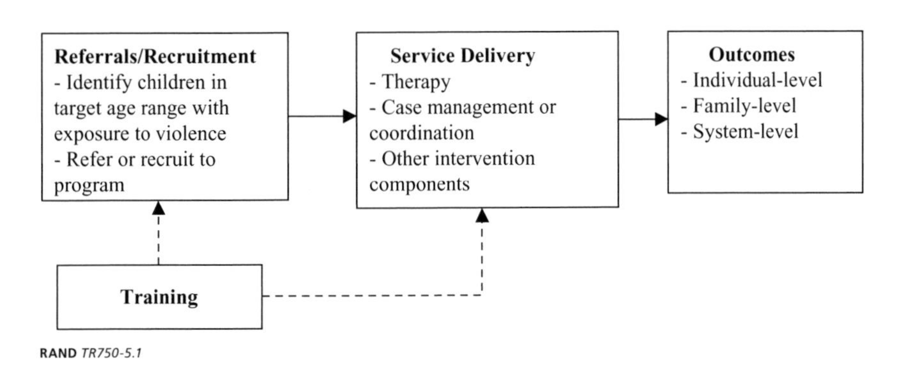


RAND *TR750-5.1*

## Referral or Recruitment Process

### Overall Assessment

As noted in Chapter Two, the SSPA programs received referrals from a variety of sources. These referral sources used different methods to identify families.

Sometimes, the referral source would screen the children for violence exposure during a scheduled appointment with the family. For example, in the Bronx and Chelsea, pediatricians identified families using screening tools or checklists that were routinely administered during well-child visits to the health care clinic. These tools or checklists included items related to violence exposure that enabled the pediatrician to identify families for SSPA. In Dayton, the protocol for the nurse home-visiting program included questionnaire items on domestic violence to be administered during certain visits. When the nurse detected domestic violence based on responses to these items, a referral would be made.

For other sites, the referral sources did not use a specific tool or questionnaire to identify families. Rather, the violence exposure was detected during the course of their interaction with the families. For example, in Multnomah County and San Diego, child welfare agencies referred families during their investigation of new reports of child abuse or neglect, and Miami's program linked with the dependency court for referrals of children with substantiated abuse or neglect.

Other SSPA programs identified and recruited families themselves. For example, Dallas's SSPA program staff reviewed lists of shelter admissions to find families who met the eligibility criteria, and Miami's program recruited families directly from domestic violence and homeless shelters. In Kalamazoo, the Head Start teachers in the intervention classrooms distributed information and a consent form about Safe Start to families at the beginning of the school year, and interested families were screened for exposure to violence.

Finally, some sites received referrals from other agencies that were already working with families with exposure to violence. For example, Broward County and Washington Heights/Inwood both received referrals directly from agencies working with families exposed to domestic violence.

The detailed procedures for referring families who had been identified as potentially eligible for the SSPA interventions also varied. Most of the SSPA programs used a centralized intake procedure so that all of the referrals came into a single place. Some of the sites had referring parties complete fax forms with relevant information, while others conducted intakes via telephone or in person.

Once a referral was made or a family expressed interest in the program, the next step was to determine whether the family met the eligibility criteria. Some of the sites confirmed eligibility with the referring party at the time of the referral. Other sites conducted screening directly with the family during the intake process to determine whether the family met the eligibility criteria. Usually the intake or screening procedures gathered very basic information about exposure to violence, the age of the child, custody of the child, and any other eligibility criteria (e.g., location of the household in the catchment area), leaving the more detailed assessments for a subsequent assessment.

Overall, the SSPA programs had varying degrees of success with the referral and recruitment process. Despite a high degree of perceived need in the community, as articulated in the applications to OJJDP for funding and various stakeholder meetings and committees, most sites experienced lower-than-expected referrals. The remainder of this section describes some of the factors that facilitated the referral process, challenges faced in the referral process, and the strategies the sites used to increase referrals into their programs.

#### Factors Facilitating the Referral Process

Looking across the 15 SSPA programs, some factors appeared to facilitate the referral or recruitment process.

- **Physical proximity of referral sources to the program staff or location.** The physical proximity of the referral source to the SSPA program location appeared to help some sites maintain a steady flow of referrals. Some of the SSPA programs that received referrals internally and employed strategies to keep the referral source engaged had success in terms of their ability to keep referrals coming into the program at a steady pace. For example, the Bronx program received most of its referrals internally from the hospital clinics. This reliance on internal referrals was successful in part because they used strategies such as trainings and email reminders to keep the pediatricians and residents engaged in the referral process. Other SSPA programs were successful by co-locating program staff at the referral source or maintaining regular contact with the referring agency. In Multnomah County, the Safe Start advocates were co-located at the child welfare office that provided the referrals, which helped streamline the referral process and make the program accessible. Similarly, the Erie SSPA program was housed with the Children's Advocacy Center, which served as a primary referral source. In Washington Heights/Inwood and Broward County, program staff maintained regular contact with the partner agencies that made referrals to help ensure a steady flow of referrals into the program.
- **Recognition of program benefits among referral sources.** When those making referrals were able to recognize the benefits of the program, it helped cultivate referral sources that then provided a steady stream of referrals. For example, the Chelsea program involved on its multidisciplinary team a pediatrician from the pediatric unit that provided many of the program's referrals. By working closely with the program, the pediatrician was able to share information about the program and its potential for benefiting specific families with the rest of the pediatric unit. Once the unit saw the benefits of the increased communication and coordination, it continued referring at a steady pace. In Multnomah County, Safe Start program staff engaged in training for and consultation with child welfare workers to help demonstrate the ways that Safe Start services could assist child welfare workers with their own responsibilities, in the course of serving families on their shared caseloads.
- **Mechanics of the referral process.** The mechanics of the referral process appeared to help some sites maintain a steady flow of referrals. In Dallas, the Safe Start staff regularly visited the participating domestic violence shelters to identify and approach families to participate in the program. This freed shelter staff from having responsibility for the referral process. Similarly, the Miami program's referral process involved having program staff attended weekly shelter meetings to meet families and arrange appointments for those interested. Kalamazoo staff screened students within Head Start themselves, after families expressed interest in participating. These referral methods ensured that most families within the system could be approached, but referrals were limited by the capacity of those systems. For instance, Miami staff worked in one transitional housing setting that housed only about 20 families, many of whom stayed in the shelter for more than a year.

### Challenges with Referrals and Recruitment

While some sites were able to establish and maintain a steady flow of referrals, most sites struggled with referrals and recruitment into their SSPA programs. Some of the challenges related to the referral process itself, but many of the barriers to identifying and recruiting families revolved around issues faced by the families and how to work with them.

- **Developing trusting relationships with families.** At some of the sites, it was necessary for staff at the referring agencies to build relationships and establish trust with families before starting a discussion about violence exposure and its potential impact on children. For example, in Dayton the nurses at the referring agency reported needing time to build relationships with families to the point where they felt safe and comfortable discussing domestic violence and the effect it might be having on children. In Toledo, staff at the referring agency were not experienced in recognizing or assessing families for domestic violence, which made them hesitant to broach the topic with their clients. While developing trusting relationships is clearly essential when working with vulnerable populations, this is a time-intensive activity that sometimes precluded or delayed the referring agencies from making referrals to the SSPA program.
- **Recruiting for the research project as well as for services.** The research context of the SSPA interventions presented an additional challenge at many sites. Some referral sources were hesitant to refer to the programs because they were uncertain whether families would be assigned to the treatment or control group. Recruitment of individual referred families was sometimes also complicated by the research context. For example, the San Mateo program staff reported that the often-older caregivers in their kinship care service population were particularly suspicious of the research context and expressed concern about being "experimented on."
- **Ability to enroll families in the program.** Families were sometimes difficult to find. For example, Dallas recruited from domestic violence shelters with short lengths of stay, which meant that there was a narrow window of opportunity to identify and recruit an eligible family. Even after being identified and referred or recruited, many of the SSPA programs had difficulty contacting families by phone or mail to schedule appointments to complete the intake process and/or determine eligibility. Many families changed housing often, and missed appointments were common.
- **Addressing the stigma related to mental health services.** Several sites faced issues with families' willingness to accept a referral for mental health services, particularly when the services were being provided at a mental health clinic or agency. For example, in Oakland, SSPA program staff reported that the stigma associated with receiving mental health services was a barrier to recruiting families to the program. Chelsea staff also struggled with cultural issues around the stigma of mental health, reporting that many of their clients were racial/ethnic minorities who were concerned about seeking mental health services and thought it was a sign of weakness or brought shame to the family.
- **Handling turnover issues at referral agencies.** Several of the SSPA programs experienced challenges due to staff turnover at the referring agencies, which made it difficult to maintain the flow of referrals. In some cases, referring agencies lined up in the planning stage of the project changed leadership, and the partnership changed or ended under the new leadership. In Dayton, the referral agency experienced a lot of turnover among the nurses who referred families. The new staff had to learn how to identify and assess

domestic violence in addition to the required components of the nurse home-visiting program. In San Mateo, turnover among the community workers who made referrals was also an issue because it required program staff to train new staff on the referral and screening process.

- **New or cumbersome referral processes.** For some SSPA programs, the referral process itself was either new or cumbersome, making it difficult to develop a steady pace of referrals. In Oakland, referrals to the SSPA program came through a newly implemented process that took some time to take hold with the referring agencies. In San Diego's child welfare setting, agency requirements necessitated a two-stage procedure for referring and recruiting families. First, child welfare workers would contact potentially eligible families and ask them whether they were interested in being contacted to hear about a research-related service their family could choose to participate in. When families voluntarily agreed, child welfare workers were then authorized to provide the family's contact information to staff in a research organization for recruiting purposes.

### Strategies to Increase Referrals

Together, the SSPA programs tried a variety of strategies to increase the number and pace of referrals. Many of the strategies to increase referrals were aimed at helping referral agencies identify families with children exposed to violence who were eligible for the SSPA intervention. In addition, recognizing the importance of facilitating mutual exchange between the SSPA programs and the referral agencies, some strategies sought to provide benefits to the referring agencies to incentivize them to make referrals.

- **Providing training and conducting outreach with staff and community.** In response to the slow pace of referrals, some of the SSPA programs provided training to current and potential referral agencies to incentivize them to refer families to the programs. In addition, the programs conducted outreach with staff and community partners to raise awareness about the problem of CEV and to present the potential benefits of SSPA interventions to families who were referred and participated in the programs. Many programs also developed materials to distribute to partners and staff. For example, the Bronx program conducted training with the pediatricians and residents who performed the screening and made referrals to Safe Start. In Multnomah County, Safe Start brought in a nationally known expert on collaborations between domestic violence and child welfare organizations for an on-site training on the roles and functions of child welfare workers and domestic violence service providers. In San Diego, Safe Start participated in a Safe Futures training (about domestic violence issues) and employed a train-the-trainer model whereby training participants were asked to share the information with others in the community or at their agency. Oakland's program staff undertook a variety of training and outreach efforts to increase the referrals coming from the community agencies involved in the collaboration. The Providence program had an agency-wide training to increase referrals coming internally from FSRI staff. San Mateo, Broward County, and Washington Heights/Inwood conducted ongoing trainings and informal discussions with the community workers who made referrals to increase their familiarity and comfort with the intervention. Broward County also revamped their initial program materials to make them more appealing to referring agencies and potential families. In San Mateo, Safe Start staff worked to refine the manner in which the program was presented to families during recruitment. They identified language that would minimize caregiver concerns about the stigma associated with mental health services and the research component.

- **Maintaining regular contact with referral sources.** To encourage referrals and help referral sources identify families, some SSPA programs set up routine meetings or contacts with some of the community agencies that made referrals. For example, Dayton's Safe Start program staff met regularly with the nurses at the referring agency to build rapport and trust with them. San Diego program leadership met monthly with the child welfare workers who provided referrals to train them on the referral process and identify potentially eligible families. San Mateo staff regularly checked with the community service workers who made referrals to discuss the recruitment process and the identification of potentially eligible families. Other sites attended standing meetings or workgroups focused on violence, such as Broward County. Kalamazoo created its own workgroup for this purpose, convening it for the first 18 months of the project until the relationships were well established.
- **Expanding referral sources.** Many of the sites expanded the number and variety of referral sources in an attempt to increase the number of referrals and to reach families across multiple systems of care. The Bronx program added local domestic violence and mental health agencies that were eager to provide referrals because they did not offer services for very young children. Dallas added an additional domestic violence shelter to provide referrals and expanded to allow referrals from families receiving nonresidential services at one of the shelters, and Miami expanded from domestic violence shelters to homeless shelters. Dayton expanded to include referrals from an early intervention program, Head Start, and a teen parenting program. San Diego added another child welfare office. Toledo also added a few referral agencies, such as the county child protective services agency, the hospital system, and a domestic violence shelter. Washington Heights/Inwood expanded its referral sources to include other community agencies working with the target population, such as a legal services agency.
- **Streamlining the intake process.** Several SSPA programs streamlined their intake process to make the referral process more efficient. Chelsea centralized its process so that all of the referrals for children's violence exposure flowed through the mental health unit's intake coordinator for eligibility screening. Erie developed processes with the county child welfare agency so the intake and ongoing caseworkers could easily make referrals to the program. Providence switched from telephone intake to in-person intake for the Tier 3 part of their program in order to connect with families when they were already at the clinic.
- **Changing eligibility criteria.** Another common approach to addressing the slow pace of referrals was to broaden the eligibility criteria. The changes included expanding the age range of children served (e.g., Dallas, San Diego, and San Mateo) or the geographic region served (e.g., Providence). The Washington Heights/Inwood program also expanded its criteria for admission to focus on safety and potential need for mental health services rather than specific forms of violence exposure.
- **Conducting initial case management with families.** To address the sometimes immediate basic needs of the families referred, some of the SSPA programs provided some up-front services at the time of the referral. For example, the Bronx program provided some initial case management in the form of referrals to community resources prior to enrolling the family in Safe Start. In Oakland, before enrollment into the Safe Start program, an intake coordinator assessed a referred family's basic needs for things such as food,

housing, and clothing and provided short-term case management services for those families whose needs were immediate and pressing.

- **Providing some services to families in the control group.** All families assigned to the SSPA control groups were, at a minimum, eligible to receive whatever community or agency services would have been available to them before the advent of the Safe Start program. To address some of the concerns raised by referral agencies or other staff related to the research component, some sites provided enhanced services to families assigned to the control group. For example, Broward County developed a detailed protocol for providing referrals and support to families assigned to the control group. This helped increase referrals because the referral source reported feeling more confident that even control group families were receiving some meaningful benefit. In the Bronx and Broward County, SSPA program staff developed protocols for working with control group families. The Miami program developed a protocol for sharing assessment information to shelter staff to enhance case management in the shelters that did not provide its two interventions. Washington Heights/Inwood staff did not always adhere to the stated protocol, providing services earlier to families than described in the protocol.

## Service Delivery

After receiving a referral or recruiting a family to participate in the program, the sites moved to service delivery, implementing a variety of intervention components. Depending on their intervention components, the sites employed a mix of therapists, case managers, advocates, and other staff to deliver the SSPA interventions. The remainder of this section describes the aspects of service delivery that were observed to have worked well for sites, some of the challenges sites reportedly faced in delivering services, and the strategies they implemented or modified to improve service delivery.

### Factors Facilitating Service Delivery

Despite the sometimes low enrollment, many of the SSPA program staff reported that they were able to engage families in service delivery. Some of the factors that appeared to facilitate service delivery are described here.

- **Close connections with families.** Several of the SSPA programs reported using strategies that helped them connect with families and helped them recognize the potential benefits of services aimed at children with behavioral issues related to their violence exposure. In Broward County, SSPA program staff found that their ability to connect with families and to develop trusting relationship helped families understand the potential value of services and keep them engaged throughout service delivery. This process of "joining" with the family through an extended assessment period is an integral part of the program's therapeutic model. Chelsea found that staff were able to connect with families because of their presence in the community and their long-standing relationships with many of the families who came to the clinic for health care and social service needs. By capitalizing on its presence and standing in the community, the Chelsea program was able to create buy-in among the families referred for services. Dayton's program staff were able to build independence, develop rapport, and establish trust during the first few in-home sessions with families. The therapist and advocate were able to maintain engagement by following through with clients, clarifying roles of the advocate and therapist, and allowing the family to take the lead on the pace or intensity of services.

- **Communication and coordination between program staff and other service providers.** The multidisciplinary or case coordination meetings that many SSPA programs convened helped to improve communication and coordination between program staff and other service providers. At several sites, the meetings facilitated understanding and communication and provided a forum for troubleshooting for certain processes or families. For example, Erie's case coordination meetings gave staff from several agencies involved with the families the opportunity to discuss the family's status, ask questions, and plan next steps. In Miami, program staff were able to share assessment information with the referral source to help them with their work with the family and to allow them to integrate the information into their case plans. Multnomah County's co-location efforts meant that the child welfare workers and domestic violence advocates became familiar with one another and developed trusting and collaborative relationships. Their case coordination meetings helped partners understand responsibility and roles and diffuse distrust.
- **Flexibility for program staff in delivering services.** Several of the SSPA programs used flexibility within the service delivery model to make adjustments based on the families enrolled in the program. Such adjustments were made to help the staff better manage their time and caseloads. For example, Miami and Washington Heights/Inwood staff were able to adjust workload and roles as implementation progressed in order to ensure manageable caseloads for the therapists (e.g., by removing assessment duties so they could focus on therapy). For a similar reason, San Mateo shifted from exclusively home-based service delivery to serving some clients in the office. This flexibility made it possible to serve more cases than in a home-based-only approach. The Bronx program adjusted its staffing several times, increasing hours for part-time clinicians, to increase capacity, and decreasing time for administrators on the project once the logistical details had been worked out. Providence staff found that having both a case manager and therapist available helped build relationships with families.

### Challenges with Service Delivery

Service delivery to families with children exposed to violence also brought challenges. Some of the challenges related to how the SSPA programs engaged with families to deliver services, while other derived from the service delivery process.

- **Multiple stressors and competing priorities among families.** Once enrolled, the sites often found that the families were facing multiple stressors and were overwhelmed dealing with day-to-day problems. Common difficulties were homelessness or housing instability, food insecurity, unemployment, lack of access to medical care, no or limited child care, and other difficulties associated with poverty. These sorts of immediate needs often took priority for individual families and preempted the delivery of the therapy component of the SSPA interventions. For example, most of Dayton's families were in chronically difficult living situations. The challenges of their daily lives meant that their immediate and basic needs took precedence over the CPP therapy component of the Dayton program's intervention. Dayton's advocate found that she needed to address the concrete needs during the first few sessions before the family was able to start working with the therapist. The Dayton therapist needed to spend time helping families understand the role that therapy could play in helping them cope with their family's difficult circumstances, both in the short and the long term. In San Mateo and Miami, the therapists found that they needed to spend time attending to the case management needs before attempting to deliver the therapy component. In Dallas, the therapists found it difficult to transition from the case management part of their service delivery model to therapy. Early on in the program implementation, Dallas altered its program delivery in response to this challenge. It explicitly divided its sessions into two time-limited portions. One portion focused on the delivery of case management services to help address basic needs, and the other session was reserved for the therapeutic component.

- **Complex treatment needs.** Families also had complex treatment needs that went beyond the services offered directly through the Safe Start program. Many families were impoverished and involved with multiple sectors of the social service system. Their treatment needs were related not just to violence but also to developmental delays, substance abuse, court involvement, and parental mental health. For instance, Bronx staff found that they needed to work more closely with children with developmental delays, to share information with schools, and provide follow-up appointments over time. In San Diego, clinicians reported that it was difficult to implement their therapeutic approach in families where the primary caregiver needed individual therapy. Miami developed a close relationship with the court for one of their programs, while Erie collaborated with a crime victim organization for some of their families.
- **Consistent engagement in services.** Several of the sites found it difficult to consistently engage and retain families in services. Families tended to fade in and out of treatment, reportedly returning to reengage in services when their needs intensified. For example, Chelsea's families moved in and out of treatment as they returned to the health care center and Safe Start when they were in need of services. Oakland and Washington Heights/Inwood also faced difficulties with families tending to stop and start services depending on their immediate needs. In fact, in Washington Heights/Inwood, staff members did not always adhere to the control group assignment and instead provided services more immediately to families. Some programs also had difficulty tracking and locating families over time. The mobility and transience of the population made completing therapy sessions difficult. Without consistent attendance, the sites found it difficulty to delivery the therapy component of their interventions with fidelity to the models.
- **Termination of service delivery.** During the Green Light process, all SSPA programs established criteria for terminating services. Typically, programs planned to end services after a predetermined number of sessions or a specified period of time, or by mutual agreement between the service providers and the families. When they were able to successfully engage families in the therapeutic component, some SSPA programs found it difficult to terminate services. For example, the Dayton and Multnomah County programs both struggled with closing a case because the therapists or advocates had developed close relationships with the family and the families continued to have some level of need for or interest in services. In Chelsea, therapists found that families often wanted to stay in treatment once they had started, and the therapists themselves found it difficult to end services. The clinicians felt that the families had become attached to them and the

services and the families were reluctant to end that relationship due to ongoing concerns about the stability of the family.

- **Staffing issues.** The SSPA programs also faced a variety of staffing issues, including turnover, retraining, quality, and burnout. For example, Washington Heights/Inwood experienced staff turnover among the direct service providers, which required that new providers be trained in the service delivery model and program; this made it difficult to track procedures over time. Several sites used contracted service providers who were not fully integrated with the lead agency. At times, this led to quality issues with the service providers, since there was less oversight and contact with the contractors and it was more difficult to systematically monitor adherence to the therapy models. In Kalamazoo, the Head Start teachers and aides faced many competing demands and were not always able to deliver the intervention as planned. Several sites had concerns about burnout among those delivering services. In Dallas, the supervisors of the therapists providing the therapy needed to be very attentive to the issue of therapist burnout because of the intensity of the service delivery, and thus the supervisors deliberately planned low caseloads. They monitored staff morale and looked for signs of "compassion fatigue."
- **Balancing and clarifying roles.** Several of the SSPA programs had issues related to helping families understand and distinguish among the different service providers. For example, Multnomah County's co-location meant the advocates sometimes faced difficulty helping mothers see a distinction between themselves and the role of the child welfare worker. The Oakland service providers had difficulties balancing the dual roles of the case manager and mental health provider. Oftentimes, the staff emphasized the role with which they had more experience. Providence's Tier 2 also found that there was confusion about roles and responsibilities, resulting in coordination difficulties between the Safe Start advocate and the shelter staff.
- **Cultural aspect of service delivery.** Some of the SSPA programs also struggled with cultural consistency related to race/ethnicity, neighborhood, experience, and other demographic characteristics between those providing services and the families being served. For example, Dallas staff found that the racial and cultural differences between the therapists and the families they served sometimes represented challenges in service delivery. Early in implementation, Kalamazoo also noted that cultural differences in expectations about parenting and child behavior between program staff and families created some difficulties in determining the goals for the intervention for some students. Oakland's staff anticipated challenges because of the language and cultural barriers, so they partnered with two agencies with different cultural and language competencies to increase the diversity of clients it was able to serve. Even so, some referred clients could not be matched with a provider proficient in their culture or primary language.
- **Navigating the relationship between child welfare and domestic violence agencies.** Historically, collaboration between child welfare and domestic violence agencies has been difficult because of divergent perspectives on family needs. Traditionally, child welfare agencies have focused on the needs and safety of the child, whereas domestic violence agencies have focused on the adult female victim and her needs. Some of the SSPA programs found it challenging to navigate these divergent perspectives and integrate the different approaches to families. For example, San Diego advocates reported experiencing some difficulty in getting used to working with adult victims of domestic violence in a child welfare setting.

### Strategies to Improve Service Delivery

The sites employed a variety of strategies to address service delivery challenges.

- **Providing upfront case management and support.** Some SSPA programs focused on the families' immediate basic needs during their early work with families. In Dayton, the case management activities that occurred early in treatment helped to provide safety and stability and allow the families to move to the next level of need. Multnomah County and Oakland staff worked to assist families by providing immediately needed resources. By sequencing service delivery to be responsive to the families' immediate and basic needs, they were able to establish trust with families and prepare them for the other intervention components.
- **Allocating time spent on different intervention components.** To help balance the intervention components, some SSPA programs more clearly articulated and enforced service mix. In Dallas, staff decided to divide the session time more strictly between case management and therapy so the case management component would not dominate the treatment sessions and the therapists would have time for the therapy.
- **Supporting families' access to services.** Many of the SSPA programs provided resources to help families access services. For example, the Erie program provided child care and transportation assistance so families could attend the parent education group sessions. Chelsea's efforts to retain families in services involved hosting dinners and open houses so families could meet and connect in an informal setting. The Providence program sponsored a monthly family night to help retain families in the therapy component of the intervention. Several other sites offered to provide services at home, to ease the burden on families.

## Summary

As shown in Table 5.1, certain factors related to the referral and service delivery processes affected program implementation for the SSPA interventions.

**Table 5.1**
**Factors Affecting Program Implementation**

| Factor | Description |
|---|---|
| *Referral or Recruitment Process* | |
| **Close physical proximity of referral sources and program staff** | Some SSPA programs were structured so that referral sources were located at the program office or program staff regularly went on-site to the referral agency to identify referrals. Referrals from internal or co-located staff at the referral source made it easier for program staff and referral sources to communicate and resulted in a steadier flow of referrals. |
| **Provision of incentives (e.g., training) to the referral sources** | Some referral sources had been trained by program staff about the issues of CEV and the program's benefits and understood the potential positive impact of the program on families. These referral sources were better positioned to maintain a steady flow of referrals. |
| **Stable referral sources** | Some SSPA referral agencies experienced frequent staff turnover, making it difficult to maintain a steady flow of referrals and necessitating efforts to re-educate new staff. |
| **Cumbersome referral processes** | The referral processes for some SSPA programs were complicated and new. This meant that the referring agencies were sometimes slow to start making referrals or were reluctant to refer into the program. |

**Table 5.1—Continued**

| Factor | Description |
|---|---|
| **Highly mobile families** | After initial referral, some families were difficult to enroll because of their residential mobility. Some of this mobility was undoubtedly related to their violence exposure. This prevented the programs from completing the intake process and/or determining eligibility for referred families. The mobility of some families also made completing therapy sessions difficult. |
| **Families' negative views and experiences with mental health services referrals** | Some referral sources faced problems with families' negative experiences or perceptions about mental health services, and sometimes around issues of mandatory reporting of child abuse and a desire to keep violence exposure private. These factors affected families' willingness to accept a referral for mental health services. |
| *Service Delivery* | |
| **Complexity of families' treatment needs** | Many SSPA programs found that the families had multiple and complex situations and difficulties meeting day-to-day needs, including safety issues. These immediate needs often took precedence for families and made it difficult for service providers to deliver the therapy component of the program. |
| **Close relationships with families** | The referral sources and program staff at some SSPA programs invested time and resources into building close relationships with families. These close relationships helped the referral sources engage families in discussions about violence exposure and the SSPA program. The program staff felt the closer relationships helped engage families in the intervention. |
| **Culturally inconsistent services** | Some of the SSPA programs struggled with a lack of cultural consistency related to race/ethnicity, socioeconomic status, and other demographic characteristics between those providing services and the families being served. These differences posed challenges in service delivery if families could not be served by providers proficient in their culture or primary language. |
| **Clearly defined program parameters** | Some SSPA programs had problems clarifying the roles and responsibilities of different program staff and determining when to end services for individual families. This confusion within the program sometimes made if difficult for the program to engage and retain families in the program. |
| **Flexible service delivery model** | Some SSPA programs had flexibility within the service delivery model that allowed them to adjust caseloads, the intervention setting, or program staff roles. This flexibility helped the programs be responsive to the families' circumstances. |
| **Staffing issues among service providers** | Some of the service providers experienced issues with staff turnover, ongoing training needs, and staff burnout. These types of staffing issues made it challenging to maintain consistent, quality services. |
| **Close communication and coordination between program staff and other service provider(s)** | Some SSPA programs worked to establish and maintain clear lines of communication between program staff and other service providers working with the families. Coordination strategies such as multidisciplinary or case coordination meetings provided opportunities for sharing information, coordinating services and supports, and planning next steps. |
| **Strained relationships between child welfare and domestic violence agencies** | Historically, collaboration between child welfare and domestic violence agencies has been difficult because of different priorities. Traditionally, child welfare agencies focus on the needs and safety of the child, whereas domestic violence agencies focus on the battered woman and her needs. Some of the SSPA programs found it challenging to navigate these divergent perspectives and integrate the different approaches to families. |

CHAPTER SIX

# Assessment of Other Aspects of the SSPA Programs

At each of the SSPA sites, there were other components of the intervention that helped shape implementation, including training activities, program outreach efforts, and development of policies and programs. Each SSPA site completed QARs with sections on training, program outreach, and policy development activities. Each site began completing the quarterly reports once they received Green Light approval to begin implementation. As a result, training, program outreach, and policy development activities that occurred before Green Light approval are not included. Quarterly reports were collected through March 2009 and are summarized here. We also gathered information from sites on program costs, including how grant resources were allocated and what in-kind support was leveraged, if any, in order to describe where programs started in terms of resources and where more or less resources were needed to implement the program. We provide a brief description of these findings in the final section of this chapter.

## Training

For training activities, the sites were asked to record information on training for staff and/or community partners related to the needs of children exposed to violence. This included training conducted by the Safe Start program and training attended by Safe Start program staff or partner agency staff.

In total, 954 training sessions were conducted across the 15 sites from 2006 through the first quarter of 2009. This total does not include trainings that were conducted prior to Green Light approval. Most of the trainings occurred early in the implementation of the program, with 22 percent of trainings occurring during the first year of the initiative and 56 percent during the second year.

Table 6.1 summarizes the content of the sessions, which were coded based on the title or content description provided by sites (coding was reviewed by two RAND research team members for agreement). Overall, the clinical intervention that sites were implementing as part of Safe Start, such as child parent psychotherapy (21%) and domestic violence (19%), were the main topics of sessions, but sites also focused on understanding child welfare system issues (13%). Sixteen percent of trainings covered Safe Start program processes or general service provision issues, such as how to enhance communication among agencies serving youth. Seven percent of trainings covered child health or mental health issues, but were not specifically related to violence or trauma; for example, a few sites conducted sessions on cultural competency and mental health service delivery.

**Table 6.1**
**Training Topics across SSPA Sites**

| | Number | Percentage |
|---|---|---|
| Safe Start selected mental health intervention | 197 | 21% |
| Domestic violence | 181 | 19% |
| Mental health interventions (other than main Safe Start intervention) | 167 | 18% |
| Safe Start service delivery and coordination | 155 | 16% |
| Child welfare | 120 | 13% |
| Mental health or child health topics (not trauma or violence related) | 63 | 7% |
| Other training topics | 29 | 3% |
| Referral processes | 22 | 2% |
| Engaging families | 20 | 2% |

*NOTE:* The table percentages sum to more than 100 because of rounding.

Some of the training sessions related to the referral process (2%) and engaging families in the Safe Start intervention (2%). Three percent of the trainings reported on the QAR were on other topics.

Figure 6.1 shows three of the training types by site: domestic violence, child welfare, and clinical. These training types were most directly related to implementing the SSPA interventions and the most frequently implemented as part of the interventions. Overall, Washington Heights/Inwood Safe Start focused the most on domestic violence trainings (57%), while Erie Safe Start reported the most child welfare (41%) trainings. Trainings on Safe Start mental

**Figure 6.1**
**Safe Start Training Topics by Site (n = 498 trainings in three categories)**

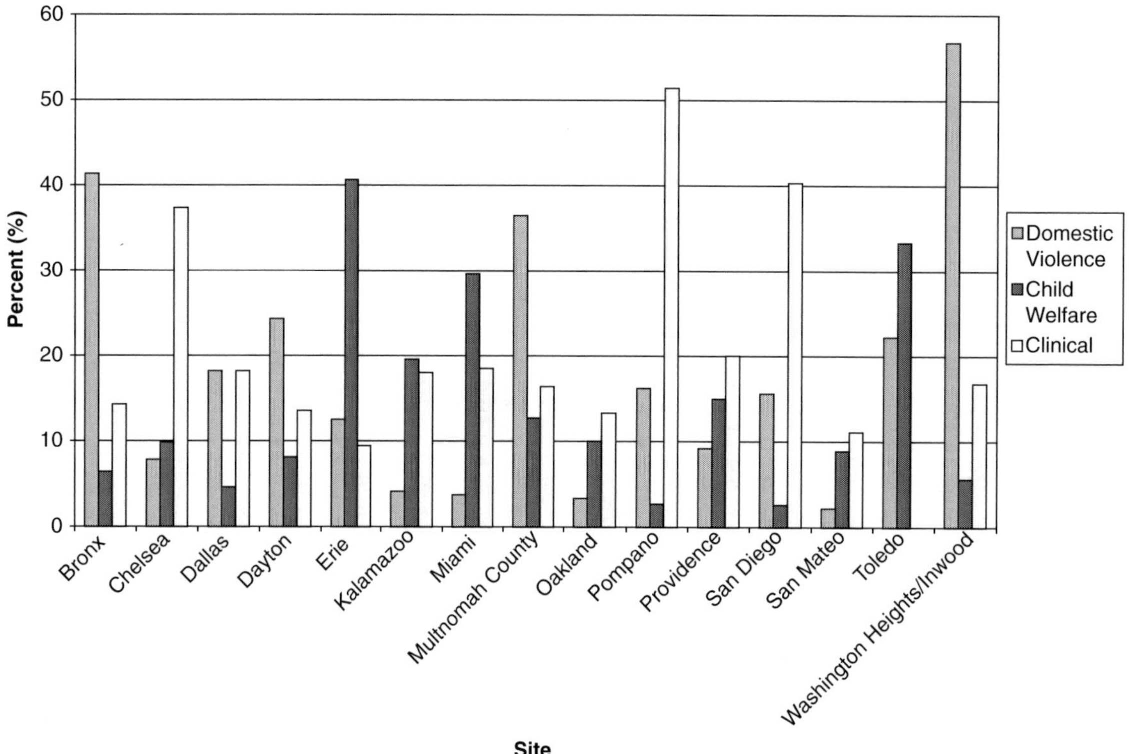


RAND *TR750-6.1*

**Table 6.2**
**Average Length of Training Sessions, by Topic**

| | Length of Session (hours) |
|---|---|
| Domestic violence | 5 |
| Other mental health interventions | 4.4 |
| Safe Start selected intervention (clinical/treatment) | 4.8 |
| Child welfare | 4.3 |
| Safe Start service delivery and coordination | 2.5 |
| Mental health or child health topics (not trauma- or violence-related) | 7.4 |
| Referral processes | 3.7 |
| Engaging families | 5.3 |

health interventions made up the majority of trainings that Chelsea (37%) and San Diego (40%) reported, and most of these centered on the ARC framework and Trauma-Focused Cognitive-Behavioral Training, respectively (described further in Appendix C of this report).

Training sessions varied in length and type of attendees, depending on content. For example, Safe Start sessions on service delivery, coordination, or procedures were shorter in length relative to the sessions focused on clinical interventions (Table 6.2).

Most of the trainings were conducted by staff participating in the Safe Start program (66%), and the rest were conducted by a partner organization but attended by Safe Start program staff. Most of the trainings reported by sites did not use Safe Start funds (76%), instead leveraging resources of the participating organization(s). The majority of trainings that used Safe Start funds were on domestic violence (24%) and Safe Start service delivery and process (23%). In general, sites split the funds used for clinical trainings between Safe Start grant funds and other funding sources, and trainings about the child welfare system were almost exclusively funded with other resources.

## Program Outreach

The SSPA sites were also asked to report quarterly on their efforts to conduct program outreach and advocate within their communities on behalf of the Safe Start program. This included efforts to increase funding, educate the community about CEV, develop collaborative relationships with other agencies, and advocate for policy changes. The sites took different approaches to conducting these outreach and advocacy efforts, including conducting intra- and interagency presentations and/or meetings, conducting training or education sessions, and disseminating print materials. Additional details on each program's outreach efforts are provided in Appendix B of this report.

Some Safe Start sites also worked to supplement program funding with additional local dollars to strengthen programming and sustainability. For example, the San Diego Safe Start project manager wrote a proposal for programming related to domestic violence, children, and youth, with an emphasis on young parents. Representatives of the Washington Heights/Inwood site met with potential funders for resources to better link Safe Start with early childhood education programs for the 0-to-3-year-old population, to provide funds for a part-time psychologist to deliver the CPP component of the intervention, and to expand services to youths ages 13–18 years old.

The SSPA sites also conducted outreach and advocacy to educate different community partners on issues around CEV. This included such efforts as training pediatricians to identify CEV in the Bronx and Washington Heights/Inwood sites. The Miami, Oakland, and Providence sites developed and/or implemented trainings for law enforcement personnel on identification and the impact of violence and maltreatment of children. As part of its program outreach efforts, Miami provided training to child care providers on the impact of CEV.

Other program outreach and advocacy efforts involved building or improving collaborative relationships or partnerships. For example, in Dayton, Safe Start program staff met with the leadership of the Children's Advocacy Center to enhance collaboration between the agencies. In Broward County, the Safe Start program worked to develop relationships with a few key judges at domestic violence court-sponsored events. Chelsea met with multiple community groups, such as a local Boys and Girls Club, the police department, the Department of Social Services, a local Home Depot, and a local health center to initiate collaborations or partnerships to support their program activities. Finally, some of the outreach efforts involved program expansion. For example, in Dallas, San Mateo, Oakland, and many other sites, outreach efforts targeted expanding the eligible population and/or sources of referrals to the program.

Some sites' efforts involved advocating for statewide policy changes related to children exposed to violence. For example, in Erie, the project director and 50 other invited individuals from throughout the state participated in a meeting convened by the Department of Health to discuss improving the agency and service provider responses for maltreated children. Also at the state level, Multnomah County advocated to the Oregon legislature for placement of domestic violence advocates in child welfare offices statewide. Multnomah County's efforts contributed to the proposal and passage of Oregon House Bill 3273, which encourages child welfare agencies to contract with domestic violence victim services to provide services to the victims with child welfare cases.

## Policies and Protocols

The SSPA sites also reported quarterly information on policies, protocols, or procedures that were newly developed, changed, or expanded to address issues related to children exposed to violence and/or their Safe Start programs. Innovations and reform efforts addressed operations within the Safe Start program or the broader community of services for children and families exposed to violence. Many of the new or modified policies, protocols, or procedures related to the following:

1. administrative processes
2. program expansion/replication
3. service delivery
4. information sharing/communication
5. education/training.

The majority of the new or modified policies, protocols, or procedures addressed administrative processes within the Safe Start programs (e.g., on-site logistics and procedures for the project) or their affiliated agencies. In addition, programs found it necessary to create new policies, protocols, or procedures when there were not existing policies, protocols, or procedures in the areas of expanding the program, delivering services, sharing information, and educating the local agencies or providers. Specific examples of the SSPA sites efforts to develop, change, or expand policies in these areas are provided below.

#### Administrative Processes

Several of the policies developed, changed, or expanded by the SSPA programs related to administrative processes, such as referral processing, screening, and reporting of families. For example, in an effort to expedite referrals from Erie's primary referral source, the site leaders modified their recruitment procedure whereby the Safe Start case manager met briefly with all families whose child had completed a forensic interview regarding child abuse at the Children's Advocacy Center. To increase referrals to the program and improve access to community services, the Oakland site collaborated with the Oakland Police Department to develop protocols for the police to refer children and families involved in family violence situations to community-based service providers, including referring to the Oakland Safe Start program. In the Bronx, St. Barnabas Hospital changed a protocol to expand screening for child abuse and domestic violence to every child seen in the pediatric clinic or emergency room or admitted to the hospital. This revised protocol institutionalized screening for children exposed to violence within the hospital system. Another example of reformation of administrative processes was the San Diego site's involvement in updating a protocol used by law enforcement agencies throughout San Diego County. This protocol provided guidelines on handling domestic violence and CEV cases, including standardized reporting of domestic violence and CEV. Finally, as part of Miami's efforts to address issues of the juvenile court, the program developed a template for making court reports to the court on family and child progress for use by the staff of an early education program.

#### Program Expansion/Replication

Increased awareness of the need for services offered by the Safe Start programs for children and families exposed to violence and the motivation to serve a greater number of families resulted in the development, expansion, or modification of policies, protocols, or procedures to expand the reach or to allow replication of the Safe Start programs. For example, during interactions between a clinician and the police department in the eastern region of Providence, it was determined that there was need for Safe Start services in this area. As a result, the Providence program expanded program eligibility to include families who were residents of the eastern portion of the city and added the police department in this region as a referral source. Miami extended services to families who were involved with the court system. Several sites expanded the program's reach by extending their upper age limit to serve older children exposed to violence.

#### Service Delivery

Another target of policy, protocol, and procedure development and reform was the delivery of services or the mix of services offered to children exposed to violence. For instance, the Chelsea program worked with the state child welfare department to develop a procedure to reduce the wait-time for medical evaluations of children who were removed from their homes. Prior to the creation of this procedure, children had to wait extended periods of times for medical evaluation, which was required before they could be placed in another home. An example of a program site's efforts to improve engagement of families in services is the Washington Heights/Inwood site's modification of their services to include more telephone contact with families and additional family events, such as for Mother's Day. Similarly, the Providence site created a monthly "family night" event for Safe Start families and increased phone and in-person contacts to ensure participation in the Safe Start program. Finally, the Broward County program developed a policy for increasing engagement through monthly phone calls to the families in the control group while they were on the wait-list, to help them address safety issues.

### Information Sharing and Communication

The SSPA sites also developed, changed, or expanded policies, protocols, or procedures related to information sharing and communication among the agencies or organizations involved with children exposed to violence. For example, Chelsea created an email distribution list for Safe Start clinical team members and Department of Social Services staff and supervisors so that everyone could be notified when a new child abuse or neglect report was filed. The notification system also included Massachusetts General Hospital/Chelsea security in case there were any concerns that the situation might warrant their involvement. In Multnomah County, to encourage collaboration in addressing the co-occurrence of domestic violence and child abuse, the Safe Start program developed a new protocol that provided guidelines for information sharing and communication between the District Attorney and Child Welfare Offices. This protocol was developed to ensure timely communication of information across both agencies and to clarify expectations for staff.

### Education and Training

Many Safe Start programs established or altered policies, protocols, or procedures for education or training community agency staff concerning the needs of children exposed to violence. For example, the Kalamazoo Safe Start program and community partners identified a need for more capacity to deliver evidence-based care for children exposed to violence within the community. Together, they arranged for a training in Parent-Child Interactive Therapy, an evidence-based intervention for children exposed to violence between the ages of 2 and 7 and their caregivers. Following training, the 16 trained therapists began regular weekly conference calls, as well as feedback and discussions on written reports from supervisors, to further support and enhance this capacity. Also, the Dayton Safe Start program helped the county-level criminal justice subcommittee on domestic violence add a section related to CEV to an existing criminal justice protocol on domestic violence. The new educational section of the protocol included suggestions to police officers on interacting with children as well as information about symptoms that children may exhibit after exposure.

## Resources and Costs

### Background

The SSPA process evaluation included a description of the resources that each site used to implement its program, to provide information about program resources and costs and some of the budgeting issues that arose during implementation. Ideally, a cost analysis would include information about program effectiveness so as to provide an understanding of the tradeoffs in selecting certain treatment approaches and preparing budgets. For example, a cost-outcome analysis helps elucidate whether a program is of value to society from a monetary and social perspective (e.g., costs of program X result in Y reduction in children who have long-term mental health service needs). Since we did not have the benefit of information on effectiveness for this description, this type of analysis was not possible. However, we were able to categorize the types of costs that sites budgeted for and incurred as part of their program implementation. Given the relative lack of information about mental health service costs, particularly for a range of community-based programs targeting violence exposure, these cost data provide a critical first snapshot of program expenditures in the context of a grant-funded research project.

### Methods

The SSPA sites prepared budgets for OJJDP prior to their initial two-year grant award, and again in Year 2 for an additional two-year grant period. Funding was set at $210,000 per year, with no more than $10,000 to be used for evaluation activities. The OJJDP grant, however, required that grantees allocate their spending according to particular requirements, largely tied to the budget allocations outlined in their original funding proposals. These categories were personnel (including fringe benefits), travel, equipment, supplies, construction, indirect costs, and subcontracts. Grantees had the flexibility to move up to 10 percent of their funding between categories, but greater percentages required direct OJJDP approval.

For our cost analysis, 12 SSPA sites submitted their Year 1 and 2 budgets, and three sites submitted their Year 3 and 4 budgets. Because so few sites provided their Year 3–4 budgets, we only report the Year 1 and 2 budget allocations in this section. While we repeatedly sought budget information from all sites, some sites ultimately did not provide it, for unknown reasons.

In order to organize the cost data in meaningful ways that are appropriately comparable to other mental health service studies, we followed the model provided by Chatterji (2004), which assessed the costs of school-based mental health services. In that study, authors organized cost data into the following categories: (1) labor costs (salary and fringe); (2) operating costs (materials and resources); and (3) indirect costs. We included new categories relevant to Safe Start, such as travel to attend conferences and conduct trainings, and rent for those sites that reported those expenses. We also identified which costs were covered directly by OJJDP and those that were in-kind.

In addition to this descriptive analysis, we interviewed leaders at five sites (out of all 12 sites we attempted to interview) in order to discuss the cost issues. We primarily focused on the expenditures that facilitated program implementation and those resources that were needed but unavailable.

### Key Findings

In the next sections, we describe trends in how sites used their budgets across the categories described earlier. These data represent information provided by the 12 (out of 15) sites that shared their data for this cost analysis. Note that this analysis is based on projected spending in the first two years. Further, sites shared this information for analysis only, and it should not be considered for any auditing purposes.

#### *Personnel/Salaries*

Sites used the majority of their SSPA budgets for supporting salaries (Figure 6.2), with the average percentage of budgets devoted to personnel costs at 79 percent. This allocation ranged from 51 percent to nearly 97 percent and includes cost equivalents for in-kind personnel. However, one site separately reported that half of its personnel resources were in-kind. Only five of the 12 sites used some of their salary budget for a program director. All of the sites used their salary budgets for clinicians, who in some cases provided data collection support, but only one site used salary dollars for a position to specifically support intervention recruitment/

**Figure 6.2**
**Percentage of Safe Start Budgets For Personnel (n = 12 sites sharing cost data)**

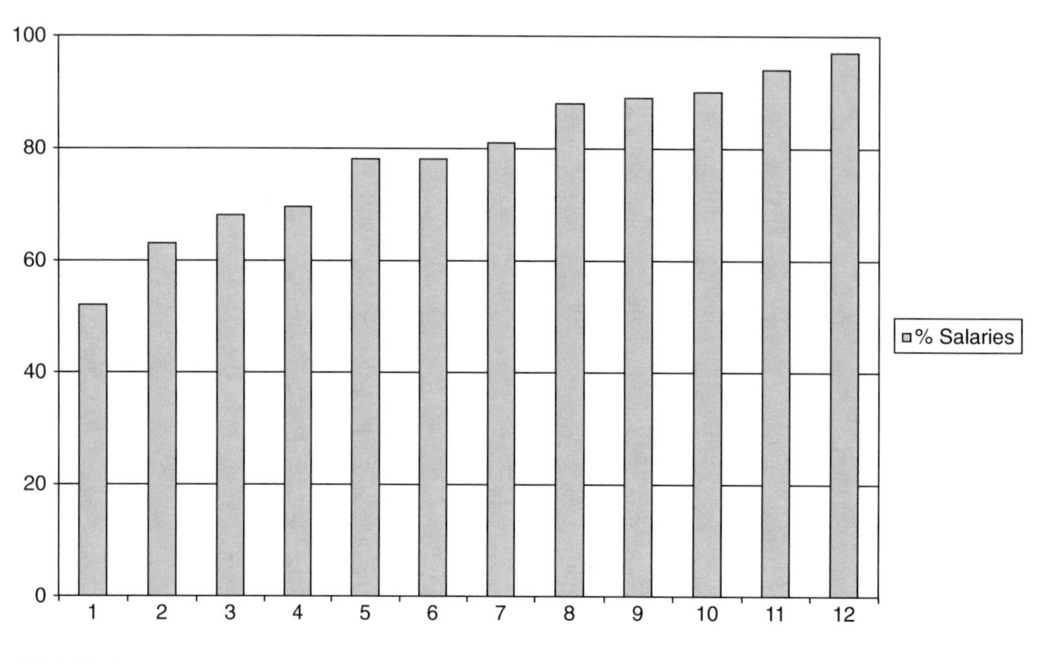


RAND *TR750-6.2*

retention (e.g., recruitment/retention specialist), and three sites used funds to support devoted data collection staff.

Salaries included a mix of staff dedicated full-time to Safe Start (e.g., 1 FTE) and those with partial salaries supported. Among the 12 sites that provided data for this analysis, five reported that at least one of their staff members was fully dedicated to the project and worked full-time. Of these five sites, three had one full-time person and two had two full-time staff members, primarily for project management and data collection.

#### *Resources/Materials*

On average, sites spent only about 4 percent of their budgets on resources or materials (range 2–9%) (Figure 6.3). These resources included computers, cell phones, assessment tools, and participant incentives. Four of 12 sites used these funds for participants incentives, three of 12 sites used funds for vouchers (bus passes, tokens), and all sites used resources for computer costs (e.g., printers). In addition, three sites used more than 50 percent of their resource budget on clinical tools, including purchasing screening instruments and child toys to implement CPP.

#### *Travel*

Nine of 12 sites spent Safe Start dollars on travel for additional staff to attend meetings (beyond what OJJDP covered), but most of these expenses were related to sending staff members to annual OJJDP meetings. On average, sites spent 1.8 percent of their total budgets on travel. There were few travel expenses incurred outside of these trips.

#### *Training*

While most sites conducted training sessions for their staff members and/or community partners, only two of the 12 sites in this analysis reported using their budgets for training sessions. These sites only spent 1 or 2 percent of their total budgets on training costs.

**Figure 6.3**
**Percentage of Safe Start Budgets for Resources/Materials**

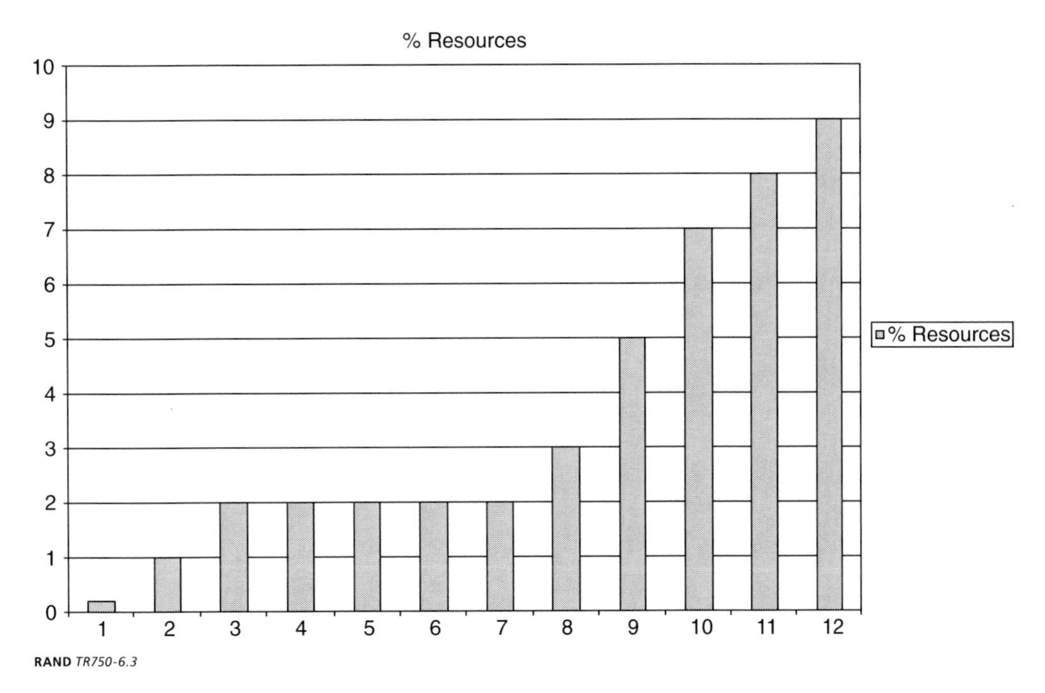


RAND *TR750-6.3*

### *Rent*

Five of the 12 sites used some of their Safe Start budget for rent costs. The other sites had this covered from either other grant sources or as part of their general operating costs of providing usual services. On average, these sites only used 2 percent of their budgets on rent.

### *Other Services*

Three sites used Safe Start funds for other services. The percentage of funds used for these other services ranged from 3 to 41 percent. For the site that used nearly half of its funds for other services, these resources went to direct client assistance from the agency as well as services supported by a partner organization.

### *Indirect Costs*

Some of the funds were used by a subgroup of sites (n = 8) to support their indirect costs/overhead. These rates were on average 8 percent but ranged from 2 to 31 percent.

### *In-Kind Resources*

Only three sites reported in-kind resources. For two sites, these in-kind resources covered rent only. However, for one site, in-kind resources were a significant percentage of their Safe Start program, including salary time for two staff members, service provision by a partner organization, and rent.

## Perspectives on Cost

During brief interviews with a sample of five sites, Safe Start project leaders articulated successes and challenges with their resource allocations. Overall, these project leaders felt that funding was adequate to support the direct services provided within the Safe Start program. While they felt that additional funding would be welcomed, they felt that the funding provided is typical for these types of programs. In addition, they had relatively few concerns about whether they had properly allocated resources to service provision and related needs (e.g., materials).

Despite this general sentiment, program leaders described three main concerns about their budgets and resource allocations. First and foremost, the participants shared that there were not enough resources for data collection and adherence to human subject protections and data safeguarding procedures, even among those sites that had a designated staff member in charge of data collection. Second, they felt that the guidelines for budgeting and how to determine costs for each recruited family were unclear. For example, there was not consistency in what costs to include when determining costs per recruited family. Third, they felt that more time should have been built into the budget period to allow for adequate start-up. During the Green Light period described earlier in this report, sites were asked by OJJDP to not expend any funds on services and to conserve resources, but they reported that it would have been desirable to fund this period separately.

## Summary

The 15 SSPA sites supplemented the core program components with additional activities that influenced program implementation, including staff trainings; program outreach to community partners; the development of new or revised policies, procedures, and protocols to better address the needs of children exposed to violence; and program budgets and the allocation of resources.

Early in the implementation process, the SSPA sites conducted or attended several trainings that were mostly focused on the target intervention, domestic violence, or child welfare. Trainings were tailored to meet the needs of each program, so there was variation across content, length, and type of attendees. In addition, while the majority of the trainings were conducted by Safe Start personnel, more often than not the SSPA sites also leveraged resources from external organizations for training purposes.

The Safe Start programs also sought to increase program funding, educate the surrounding community about CEV, increase collaboration with other agencies, and promote changes to policies related to violence through outreach efforts. Each of the sites conducted outreach in different ways. This included conducting trainings with partners, assembling meetings with potential funders, presenting to community members, and sharing information through various mediums.

The SSPA sites developed or modified internal and external policies, protocols, and procedures in order to improve processes that serve children exposed to violence. New or reform efforts centered on administrative processes (e.g., processing referrals, and screenings and reporting procedures), program expansion/replication (e.g., increasing the target age range or program catchment area), service delivery or mix of services offered, information sharing/communication with partner agencies, and education/training of community agencies.

The data on costs highlight how sites allocated their resources for Safe Start program implementation. Most resources were used to cover staff salaries, primarily those of the clinicians, with comparatively less available for project management or data collection (as required under the grant mechanism). The amount of funds available for data collection may need to be revisited for future efforts to ensure that rigorous standards are met. For example, more attention may be needed to calculate the costs to complete initial and particularly follow-up assessments, and to adhere to human subjects and data safeguarding procedures. This information can inform decisionmakers about resource requirements for replicating these SSPA programs. However, using these data as a foundation, a subsequent study should consider more sophisticated cost savings or cost outcome analyses with data on intervention effectiveness.

CHAPTER SEVEN

# Conclusions and Implications for Similar Interventions

Our assessment of the 15 SSPA programs found that certain factors influenced implementation. These factors are described earlier in this report, at the end of each chapter. Here, we summarize the implications of these factors, provide a comparison of these results to those from Phase 1 of the overall Safe Start Initiative, and conclude with an overall summary and suggestion of possible next steps.

## Implications for Similar Interventions

In Table 7.1, we summarize factors related to the program's context that affected program implementation both positively and negatively and discuss the implications for community-based programs targeted at children exposed to violence. In the first column, we identify factors, as summarized earlier in the relevant chapter. In the second column, we present implications of these findings for future intervention efforts.

**Table 7.1**
**Findings and Implications for Program Context Domain**

| Factor | Implication |
|---|---|
| **Importance of widespread recognition of need** | **Provide opportunities to bring community agencies and service providers together to identify and address gaps and barriers to services for children exposed to violence.** For community agencies and service providers that have identified a need for services for children exposed to violence, a promising avenue for responding is collaboration to develop a program that addresses gaps in the existing network of services and supports and fits the needs of children exposed to violence. |
| **Importance of strong individual leadership at the lead agency** | **Dedicate a staff leader with power to make program-level decisions and adjustments.** A program leader with adequate time to lead the program can effectively develop collaborative relationships with community partners and implement the program. Ideally, the program lead person would have decisionmaking authority for program activities and modifications. |
| **Importance of a clear division of responsibility for program implementation** | **Design a program that places primary responsibility for implementation with a lead agency or organization.** It is important for the program to be structured with a clearly delineated lead agency/organization to take primary responsibility for program implementation. |

**Table 7.1—Continued**

| Factor | Implication |
|---|---|
| **Importance of close working relationships among partner agencies and referral sources** | **Capitalize on existing strong relationships with partner agencies and referral sources.** It is important for those involved in the program's design and planning phases to take advantage of existing collaborative efforts and relationships and prior experiences together. Trust between agencies appears to be particularly important for interventions for children exposed to violence. This can increase initial buy-in and ensure that the partner agencies understand why the supports and services are needed and how the planned program is expected to affect outcomes for participating families and children. |
| | **Select known or internal referral sources.** To the extent possible, take advantage of existing relationships with community agencies/organizations or internal referral sources. Structuring the program with referral sources that are known or internal to the lead agency/organization can also help ease program implementation. |
| **Problem with burden of research requirements** | **Assess the impact of the evaluation design on program staff, families, and referral sources.** If an evaluation component is included, a first step is to recognize and understand how the specific research plan affects different parties, including the program staff providing services and supports, the participating families, and the staff at the referral sources. |
| | **Develop tools to increase buy-in for the evaluation component and minimize the negative impact.** A next step is to educate all parties about the benefits of the research project, including its role in augmenting services available in the community and ensuring effective treatment for families. Education tools might include program brochures or fact sheets geared toward the intended audience that use nontechnical language to explain the research design and the importance of the research component to the overall program. |

## Interventions

In Table 7.2, we summarize the factors from the intervention domain that affected program implementation. For each factor, we discuss the implications for community-based agencies that may be developing similar intervention approaches for children exposed to violence.

**Table 7.2**
**Findings and Implications for Intervention Domain**

| Factor | Implication |
|---|---|
| **Problem with differences between the intervention approaches and the families' needs and priorities** | **Understand the priorities and needs of families in the program's target population.** When selecting the intervention components, it is important to align the overall intervention approach and the mix of services and supports offered with the needs and issues of the families with children exposed to violence. Despite the identified violence exposure, families may have more pressing basic needs that need to be addressed before addressing mental health issues related to the violence exposure. |
| **Importance of a convenient intervention setting** | **Consider the intervention setting.** The location of service delivery has implications for implementation. In an effort to help engage families and address some of the transportation and child care issues related to participating in a mental health program, it may be beneficial to offer the program in the home or in a school or day care setting. Particularly for families with small children, the location of service delivery can help ease the burden of participating in mental health treatment and increase the families' engagement. |
| **Importance of needs assessments and developmental screenings** | **Conduct needs assessments or developmental screening to engage families.** An intervention approach that includes a thorough assessment of the families' needs can help ensure that the overall intervention approach aligns with families' circumstances, including their safety issues related to violence. |
| **Importance of provision for families' immediate and basic needs** | **Ensure that families are provided with or connected to sources of assistance to meet their basic needs.** Many of the families with children exposed to violence have multiple stressors in their lives. The complexity of their situations may make it difficult to focus on and engage in mental health treatment. At the outset of the program, assess families' basic needs for services and supports and either provide them with case management or coordination as part of the program or refer them to an agency or organizations that can help address some of their immediate needs. |

**Table 7.2—Continued**

| Factor | Implication |
|---|---|
| **Importance of an array of therapy options** | **Offer more than one therapeutic approach to facilitate the matching of the services to individual family's needs and circumstances.** There is no one therapeutic approach that is appropriate for all families with children exposed to violence. By assessing the therapeutic needs of families and offering differing therapeutic options that can meet those needs, the program can better address the unique needs of different families. |
| **Importance of adaptable components of the therapy models** | **Modify the selected therapeutic model to offer activities or curriculum most suitable for the target population.** Certain therapeutic models offer flexibility in the guidelines for their use. If the therapeutic model allows, tailoring certain activities, examples, or techniques can help the program better meet the needs of families with children exposed to violence. It is important to consult with experts before making any modifications to make sure that the core components of the model are retained. |
| **Problem with monitoring adherence to the therapy models** | **Develop a process for monitoring adherence to the therapy model over time.** To maximize the effectiveness of the therapeutic models, it is important to integrate methods for monitoring how program staff who are providing the treatment are following the intervention guidelines or standards. By designating someone to take responsibility for adherence, the program can assess whether the clinicians delivering the intervention are adequately trained, demonstrate acceptable skills levels, and adhere to the intervention standards described in the site's model. |

## Implementation Processes

Our observations about the implementation process at each of the sites suggest several activities that would benefit program implementation. We present this information in Table 7.3.

**Table 7.3**
**Findings and Implications for Implementation Processes Domain**

| Factor | Implication |
|---|---|
| **Importance of close physical proximity of referral sources and program staff** | **Develop internal agency referral sources or co-locate program staff with the referral source.** Close physical proximity of the referring party to the program staff can help ensure a steady stream of referrals. For programs that receive some or all referrals internally, the staff can be educated about the program and the mechanics of the referral process. For programs that receive external referrals, consider placing program staff on-site with the referral agency or organization to facilitate referrals. |
| **Importance of incentivizing the referral sources** | **Provide training and outreach to referral sources.** The agencies and organizations that are providing referrals or conducting recruitment for the program need to understand how the planned program is expected to affect outcomes related to violence exposure for participating families and children and how it benefits their agency or organization. Education and outreach efforts can include program materials, training sessions, or one-on-one meetings with staff making referrals. |
| **Importance of stable referral sources** | **Prepare for staff turnover at referral agencies.** To plan for turnover, develop program materials and referral processes that can be transferred as referral agency staff turn over. The program materials, referral forms, contact information, and communication pathways need be clear, concise, and readily accessible and transferable for existing and new staff at the referral agency or organization. |
| **Importance of ongoing training of staff members** | **Plan for training over time rather than simply at the beginning.** Our training evaluation revealed that early gains in knowledge in serving children exposed to violence do not sustain over time; thus, booster sessions to maintain skills and comfort levels may be needed, particularly in the areas of family engagement. |
| **Problem of cumbersome referral processes** | **Streamline referral processes.** It is important to make the referral process as simple and straightforward as possible for the referring agencies, so as to bring interested families into the intervention as quickly as possible after referral for or detection of violence exposure. |

**Table 7.3—Continued**

| Factor | Implication |
|---|---|
| **Problem of highly mobile families** | **Recruit families from multiple systems of care and use multiple approaches to track and locate families.** High rates of family transience, partially related to violence exposure, can negatively impact program recruitment and retention. Recruitment from more than one system of care may broaden outreach to eligible families and increase the number of families served. Also, a "tracking and locating" form can help reach families who are referred to the program to complete the intake process and to maintain contact with them during service delivery. The form may contain standard contact information such as address, telephone numbers, and email addresses in addition to name and contact information for employers, family, or close friends and names of places that the person might be found, such as a church or community center. |
| **Problem of families' negative views or experiences with mental health services referrals** | **Work with referral agencies to address issues around the stigma of mental health services.** To reduce the stigma associated with mental health services and increase families' interest in accepting mental health services referrals, those who are making referrals or recruiting families to participate need to frame the program as something that will help their children. |
| **Problem of families' multiple and complex treatment needs** | **Develop a complete treatment plan to address all of the families' needs.** To address families' complex treatment needs, program staff and service providers should develop a comprehensive plan for services and supports with clearly defined responsibilities and lines of communication to coordinate among the different social service organizations involved with these families. It is also important to provide up-front case management and support to families to address the immediate and basic needs of families related to exposure to violence and other disadvantages. |
| **Importance of close relationships with families** | **Work with the referral sources and service providers on strategies to build relationships, establish trust, and help families understand the potential benefits of mental health services.** Those making referrals need to be educated on recognizing CEV and the symptoms of trauma so they feel comfortable discussing these issues with families. It is also important for the referral process to allow enough time for those making referrals to establish a trusting relationship with families. To help develop strong connections between families and the program's service providers, it is important to consider including an assessment and relationship-building component that enables families to become familiar with and accepting of the providers. |
| **Problem of culturally inconsistent services** | **Educate program staff about cultural differences and develop service delivery approaches that respect cultural issues.** To address the cultural aspects of service delivery for the target population, the lead agency or organization should employ staff and partner with agencies with different cultural and language competencies. |
| **Problem of unclear program parameters** | **Define the roles of different service providers for families.** The program can be structured such that those providing services to families have clearly defined roles and the criteria for ending services are clear. It is important that the families understand who is responsible for the different intervention components and the conditions under which the intervention will end. |
| **Importance of a flexible service delivery model** | **Adjust the service delivery processes to help program staff manage time and caseloads.** A flexible service delivery model can enable the program's service providers to change the setting, staff hours, staff roles, or caseloads to allow them to serve more families and better manage their time and caseloads. |
| **Problem of staffing issues among service providers** | **Maintain regular contact with program staff and provide routine refresher training and supervision.** Program management can improve service delivery by maintaining regular contact with those providing services and providing opportunities for refresher or supplemental training. The program's clinical supervisors should also monitor caseloads, staff morale and burnout, and the quality of the services being offered. |
| **Importance of close communication and coordination between program staff and service providers** | **Plan multidisciplinary or case coordination meetings.** To facilitate understanding and communication and provide a forum for troubleshooting, the program's staff and service providers can plan regular case management or coordination meetings that allow those involved with the family to share information, discuss the family's situation, ask questions of one another, and plan next steps. |
| **Problem of strained relationship among partner agencies** | **Recognize the different perspectives of partner agencies/organizations.** In planning the program, it is important to recognize that some partner agencies have differing perspectives and orientations about children exposed to violence. |

## Comparison with Findings from Phase 1 of the Safe Start Initiative

Findings from Phase 1 of the initiative were summarized in Chapter One. A comparison of findings from the 15 Phase 2 SSPA programs to the process evaluation findings from Phase 1 shows a good deal of similarity, despite a great diversity in sites and the types of interventions delivered in the two phases of the Safe Start initiative. It is perhaps not surprising that the sites in both phases faced similar challenges and generated similar responses to those challenges, because all sites were attempting to serve families of children exposed to violence.

Some of the common implementation challenges across the two phases included service providers finding the following:

- Families affected by violence are difficult to engage and retain in services, particularly mental health interventions.
- When engaged in services, families' basic needs often took priority and preempted the delivery of therapeutic interventions.
- A variety of staffing issues (including turnover, retraining, quality, and burnout) made it difficult for sites to provide services as planned.
- Mental health professionals who were proficient in the culture and primary language of families were difficult to find (ASDC, 2007).

Sites in both phases planned programs to engage and retain families in services. The engagement strategies included offering logistical supports to help with childcare and transportation and hosting social events (i.e., parent's nights, birthday parties, or community meetings). Such supports to promote families' comfort and sense of safety have been associated with engagement and retention in parenting programs and mental health interventions for children (Annie E. Casey Foundation, 2004; Dumka et al., 1997; Harachi, Catalano, and Hawkins, 1997; Simpson et al., 2001).

To promote retention with families initially engaged in services, sites in both phases attempted to sequence services in a way that prioritized basic needs of families, especially the safety and protection of children and their caregivers. Consistent with the published literature on promising practices for interventions with children exposed to violence, many of the sites allowed families to fully participate in decisions about what services and supports were most appropriate to meet their needs (Groves and Gewirtz, 2006). This approach is also consistent with the social service systems reform literature (Bruner, 2006) and children's mental health "system of care" principles (Stroul and Friedman, 1996) that suggest that integrated service delivery designed to be convenient for families facilitates participation in recommended interventions and treatment.

Finally, the rapid turnover of staff and limited pool of specialized professionals that work with this high-risk population is not unique to the sites that participated in both phases of the initiative (see Leiter and Harvie, 1996). OJJDP encouraged providers in both phases to seek peer support from other sites and to engage in self-care processes within each site (e.g., stress management and brief relaxation techniques), to help reduce provider burnout and minimize negative impacts on emotional health of care providers. Future initiatives may want to explore strategies to help mitigate the impact of these challenges on service delivery. For example, in the short-term, sites may want to explore the role of paraprofessionals in treating this population, and, in the long-term, sites may want to focus on recruiting and training for a wider diversity of providers.

## Conclusions

Our process evaluation of the 15 SSPA programs was designed to describe and assess the implementation of the interventions at each site. The 15 sites varied substantially in terms of their interventions, targets, settings, and strategies for implementation. While we were able to shed light on how different factors appeared to affect program implementation, this evaluation was not designed to test specific implementation strategies or to draw firm conclusions about the relationship between a specific factor and successful implementation. Moreover, this report does not contain information on implementation or perception of services from the perspective of participating families. Resources prohibited us from collecting these important data systematically. Further, we do not yet know the impact of the interventions on child and family outcomes. The outcome evaluation component of the national evaluation, to be published in a subsequent report, seeks to address those questions. Nonetheless, this process evaluation does identify some factors that were evident across more than one site or that offered a clear implication for future work with children exposed to violence.

In looking across the SSPA programs, the only true commonality was their focus on providing interventions for children exposed to violence. The communities shared an understanding of the clear need to address the consequences of CEV and recognized gaps in their existing service delivery system. Despite successes in launching programs and delivering needed services to children, most programs faced difficulties getting referrals, engaging families in treatment, and providing a program that aligned with the families' individual priorities.

For multiple reasons, most of the sites struggled with lower-than-expected referrals throughout implementation. Some programs experienced difficulties establishing or enhancing collaborative relationships with the partner agencies/organizations that were providing referrals into the program. In some cases, the agency's own services to the family took precedence over identifying and referring for violence exposure. In other situations, the research component of the intervention made referral sources reluctant to refer, knowing that some families would not receive the program. The structure of the referral process itself also provided challenges, with proximity and burden on referral sources playing a role in the flow of referrals into the program. These challenges suggest that, when designing programs for children exposed to violence, it is important to develop strategies for educating, collaborating, and maintaining strong relationships with referral sources.

The SSPA programs also struggled with engaging the families in the interventions being offered. The challenges arose for a variety of reasons, including the multitude of stressors faced by the family, perceived stigma of mental health treatment, cultural differences, and families' reluctance to participate in a research project. The experiences of the SSPA programs highlight the critical role that engagement and retention strategies play in providing community-based programs for children exposed to violence.

Finally, with multiple and complex treatment needs in addition to pressing basic needs, families of children exposed to violence often needed interventions with flexibility in the array of services and in the sequencing of components, focusing first on addressing basic needs. Among the diversity of program settings, populations, and intervention types, this may be the most consistent experience of the 15 SSPA interventions and therefore potentially the most central lesson for future undertakings focused on addressing the needs of children exposed to violence.

APPENDIX A

# Process and Training Evaluation Methodology

In this appendix, we provide detailed information about the process and training evaluation data sources and then discuss how we synthesized and analyzed the data collected from these sources.

## Data Sources and Collection

Data were collected for this report from a variety of sources:

- site visits
- QARs
- document review
- regular email and telephone communication
- evaluation of staff training.

### Site Visits

During the first two years of implementation, each site was visited twice by members of the RAND research team.[1] The site visits allowed the team to gather detailed qualitative information about the program's implementation from a variety of perspectives.

While each site visit was tailored to the specific program, the main questions the research team sought to answer through each visit were as follows:

- How were sites operating their Safe Start intervention in practice?
  - What were key challenges in implementation?
  - What were the facilitators to implementation?
  - What were the lessons learned?
- What were the staff perspectives on each components of the intervention?
  - What was necessary to implement the program?
  - What was working well?
  - What was not working well?

[1] The second Chelsea site visit was conducted through a series of telephone interviews. The second Toledo site visit was not conducted because the site experienced very low enrollment and thus there was not sufficient implementation of the program to observe during a visit.

The site visits involved (1) key informant interviews, (2) structured case reviews, (3) quality assurance checklists, and (4) observations. For each site visit, we summarized the salient issues in a brief summary report. This report highlighted how the program was operating and identified some specific technical assistance needs. The draft summary was shared with the site's project director before being sent to the national team, so that any technical assistance or troubleshooting needs could be addressed.

**Key Informant Interviews.** In preparing for the site visit, we worked with each site to develop a list of target respondents for the key informant interviews. The list was tailored to each site depending on their circumstances. Procedures were fully reviewed and approved by the RAND Institutional Review Board. The types of respondents at the sites included

- agency director
- project director/coordinator
- therapists
- case managers
- advocates
- other clinician(s) or service provider(s)
- data collection supervisors
- administrative staff involved in intake, referrals, or randomization
- community partners involved in the service provision (e.g., police, child protective services, domestic violence shelter, police department)
- financial staff.

As the list above indicates, family members were not interviewed. For both rounds of site visits, we followed a semi-structured interview protocol that outlined the key topics and questions to be asked. For each interview, the topic areas were selected based on the roles and responsibilities of the respondent. During the first annual site visit, the data collection focused on the following:

- Planning process
  - Components of the program
  - Working with OJJDP, technical assistance providers, and RAND
- Early implementation
  - Referrals
  - Enrollment
  - Collecting data
  - Providing services
  - Engaging families
  - Staffing
  - Training
  - Quality assurance monitoring
  - Policies and protocols
  - Costs
  - Relationships with community partners
- Next steps in the site's implementation plan.

In the second annual site visit, the protocol explored the implementation process, what lessons had been learned from the early experiences, and what mid-course adjustments were made. The questions focused on the following:

- Implementation
  - Receiving referrals
  - Engaging children and families
  - Providing services
  - Integrating and coordinating services
  - Monitoring quality assurance
- Safe Start collaboration and community setting
- Safe Start administration and other activities
  - Staffing
  - Documenting services
  - Training
- Relationship with national partners
  - Working with OJJDP, technical assistance providers, and RAND
- Next steps for the Safe Start intervention.

**Structured Case Reviews.** During the key informant interviews, a structured case review was conducted with therapists, case managers, advocates, or other program staff who were involved in providing services to Safe Start families. The purpose of the case review was to obtain more details on the process that the program staff used with families to deliver services and treat families. Prior to each site visit, we randomly selected the cases of two or three families enrolled in Safe Start services for the structured case review. At the second site visit, we also selected two or three cases from the control or comparison group. The latter was done so that we were able to document in more detail how the Safe Start services compared with those provided to similar families who were not enrolled in Safe Start. For each case review, we followed a structured case review protocol that asked specific questions on the following issues:

- How the family was referred to Safe Start (e.g., referral source, reason for referral)
- Family's living situation and presenting issues at time of referral
- Start and end dates of services
- Issues with and strategies for engaging families in services
- Issues retaining the family in services
- Intervention or treatment process for family
- For families receiving therapy:
  - Number of sessions with the family
  - Family (or individual member's) engagement in and response to therapy
  - Facilitators and challenges in providing therapy to the family
- For families receiving case management or advocacy
  - Number of and reasons for contacts with the family
  - Number and type of referrals to other agencies or providers
  - Number and type of collateral calls on behalf of the family
  - Number of times the family was discussed at service provider team meetings

  - Family's engagement in and response to case management or advocacy
  - Facilitators and challenges in providing services to the family
- Next steps in the services for the family.

**Quality Assurance Checklists.** During the site visit, we also completed a "quality assurance checklist" to document the quality assurance processes and procedures the sites used to assure quality implementation of the therapy component of their interventions. Specifically, this refers to strategies that the program used to assess whether the therapists followed the procedures or practices that the program intended them to follow in delivering treatment to families. The quality assurance checklist was completed with the person responsible for clinical supervision of the therapists providing the Safe Start services. The questions focused on the following:

- Whether there were standardized intervention and training materials available to the therapists
- What form of ongoing supervision and feedback was provided
- What specific procedures the agency has in place for quality assurance monitoring overall and for individual therapist's training and skills
- What degree of agency/organizational support there was for quality assurance monitoring in terms of the staff and budget resources provided.

**Observations.** When applicable and feasible, we also observed activities related to the Safe Start programs. These observations were meant to further our understanding of how the programs were implemented. The observations included the following:

- staff meetings related to the Safe Start program
- clinic flow or processes
- training sessions
- multidisciplinary team meetings or case review meetings
- group therapy sessions.

#### Quarterly Activity Reports

The QARs were designed to collect information on study enrollment, service delivery, training, policies and protocols, and advocacy. The forms were standard but customized for each site so that at each site and across sites we would be able to report on the amount and types of services delivered, trainings conducted or attended, and policies created or changed. The standard QAR included three forms:

1. Reporting Safe Start Referrals and Safe Start Services Delivered in Last Quarter. This form was used to record information from the program's referral log on the number of children referred and enrolled during the quarter. The form also contained sections to record information on the services that were delivered to children and families. The services section was tailored specifically for each site by listing and describing each type of service.
2. Logging Trainings on Children Exposed to Violence. This form was used to log any trainings related to the needs of children exposed to violence that the agency conducted or participated in during each quarter.

3. Documenting Policy and Advocacy Efforts Related to Safe Start. This form was used to document any policies that had been developed or changed by the agency or in the community that affects the way children exposed to violence were served. There was also space to list new partnerships that the site had developed and to describe advocacy that the site had conducted on behalf of children exposed to violence (e.g., to raise awareness, to increase funding).

Each site started completing the QARs for the quarter during which they completed the Green Light process (described in the next section). This meant that nine of the sites started completing the QARs for the second quarter of 2006, two started for the third quarter of 2006, and four started for the fourth quarter of 2006.

#### Document Review

We gathered a library of materials from the sites about their inputs and activities. These were things such as the original proposal, agency and program brochures and descriptions, training presentations, budgets, agency annual reports, and policy manuals.

#### Regular Email and Telephone Communication

The regular email and telephone communications we had with the sites were also part of the process evaluation data collection. From these, we learned more of the descriptive and contextual information about the inputs and activities.

#### Evaluation of Staff Training

Over the course of the Safe Start program, sites conducted or participated in trainings related to improving awareness, knowledge, and practice for children exposed to violence, and how to work with families to address these issues. In order to describe and track the impact of these trainings, the Safe Start evaluation included a component to assess how some of these trainings changed program staff perspectives in working with these children. There were two components to the training evaluation. First, we administered pre-, post-, and three-month follow-up surveys for a select number of trainings for which programs shared training information and we were able to survey the participants. Second, we also conducted short, key informant interviews of training participants to obtain their perspectives on the sessions. We include illustrative quotations from these interviews in Appendix C of this report, where appropriate.

In conducting the training evaluation, we attempted to capture trainings across sites within the first two years of Safe Start, to the extent that sites were willing to participate in this part the evaluation and could participate in the planning necessary to carry it out. We worked with trainers and their training materials to develop surveys collaboratively to ensure that survey content was appropriate to the planned training curriculum. While most training opportunities were site-specific and tailored to the needs of that program, all sites participated in the engaging families in mental health services training funded by the Safe Start Center.

For the training surveys, it should be noted that some sites started training sessions that were not fully completed, thus we only have three-month follow-up surveys on a subset of trainings (further described in the next sections). Further, we provided gift card incentives to improve retention at follow-up; however, in some cases, our retention rates were less than ideal.

## Data Synthesis and Analysis

The information collected from the process evaluation was used to develop the program descriptions that appear in Appendix B of this report and for the cross-site analyses in the main body of this report.

The program descriptions were developed to describe the development and implementation of the Safe Start program at each site. These descriptions synthesize the information gathered on the different aspects of the intervention from each source, including:

- Key informant interviews with key program staff and community partners
  - Lead agency director and financial staff person
  - Safe Start project directors and staff
  - Partner agency leaders and staff
  - Community representatives
- Case review of randomly selected treatment and comparison/control group cases
- Quality assurance checklist completed by the clinical supervisor
- Observation of partner agency meetings, multidisciplinary team meetings, and case consultation meetings
- Quarterly activity reports on services, training, policies, and advocacy
- Grant application
- Green Light process notes
- *Safe Start: Promising Approaches Communities Working Together to Help Children Exposed to Violence* (Safe Start Center, 2008).

Each program description was written by two members of the project team and reviewed by at least two other members. Any variations among the team members in describing the sites' activities were resolved by reviewing site visit notes or program materials or by collecting additional information directly from the site. The program descriptions followed a structured outline, with sections on the program and community setting, intervention, implementation, and a summary. Each site was given an opportunity to review its program description. Once drafted, the program description was sent to the site for review. After this review, we met with the site staff to discuss their comments. At most sites, the comments were clarifications or corrections to factual information.

The program descriptions also served to provide information for the cross-site analysis presented in the main body of this report. After completing all 15 program descriptions, we used them to synthesize information for the remaining sections in this part of the report. In developing Chapters Three, Four, and Five of the main report, we reviewed the corresponding sections of each program description to identify the factors that facilitated or hindered implementation. For example, in examining the referral processes for Chapter Five, we carefully reviewed the referral section of all 15 program descriptions. This analysis revealed the factors that facilitated the referral process, the challenges in the referral process, and the strategies used to address the challenges. If the finding was found for only a few of the sites, then examples were listed for each site. If the factor strategy was found in many of the sites, then a few examples were selected to illustrate the finding.

The results of the training evaluation are provided in Appendix C of this report. For these analyses, we describe the content of site-specific trainings, provide site-specific data on participant characteristics, and detail changes in knowledge and perspectives where appropriate. We also briefly summarize pooled data across sites, with attention to changes in attitudes and practice in working with CEV. For these analyses, the retention issues coupled with general problems of sample size precluded tests of statistical significance, but we report trends that highlight changes in knowledge and attitudes over time.

APPENDIX B

# SSPA Program Descriptions

## Contents

## 1. Bronx, NY, Safe Start Program Description

### Bronx Safe Start

- **Intervention type:** Medical Home for Children Exposed to Violence, including multidisciplinary assessment, Child-Parent Psychotherapy, and case management
- **Intervention length:** 1 year or longer
- **Intervention setting:** Hospital clinic-based services
- **Target population:** Children living in the Bronx who were exposed to, experienced, or witnessed family or community violence
- **Age range:** 0–6
- **Primary referral sources:** Saint Barnabas Hospital (SBH) pediatricians, SBH Children's Advocacy Center, SBH Emergency Department, mental health and domestic violence agencies

## Program and Community Setting

The Bronx Safe Start program is located in the borough of Bronx, New York, which, as of the 2000 Census, had a population near 1.33 million; more than 8 percent are younger than age 5. Thirty percent of the population is white, 36 percent black, 25 percent identify their race as "Other," and half are Hispanic. The per capita income is lower than in most other Safe Start programs: $16,344;[1] slightly more than 30 percent were living below the poverty line.[2] As a large population center bordering New York City, the Bronx has a large variety of existing social service agencies serving children in need.

In 2003, more than 14,000 children were referred for abuse or neglect to child protective services in the Bronx (St. Barnabas, 2004). In addition, rates of violent crime are elevated, with 1,124 violent crimes reported per 100,000 persons in 2001, as compared to the national rate of 504 per 100,000 (St. Barnabas, 2004).

In 2000, the St. Barnabas Hospital Children's Advocacy Center (CAC) was created in response to the "urgent need for comprehensive, coordinated, crisis intervention services for children victimized by abuse, neglect, and exposure to domestic violence" (St. Barnabas, 2004) (see below for a brief description of the CAC). However, after a few years of providing services to children exposed to violence and their families, the CAC identified three major gaps in services: (1) limited identification of children exposed to violence, (2) lack of short- and long-term intervention services for this population, and (3) poor coordination of intervention service providers and services (St. Barnabas, 2004).

To address these gaps, the CAC submitted a proposal to OJJDP for the development of the Bronx Safe Start program. As the lead agency, the CAC proposed a collaboration with the Jewish Board of Family and Children's Services' Bronx Domestic Violence Program (BDVP) (see below for a brief description of the BDVP). As members of the Bronx Consortium on Domestic Violence and Children—a group of community-based organizations, including substance abuse treatment, immigration rights, women's health care, and mental health providers—the CAC and BDVP had prior experience working together (St. Barnabas, 2004). The primary mission of the Bronx Safe Start program was to improve the physical, social,

---

[1] $16,344 is the 1999 per capita income in 2005 dollars. The 1999 per capita income was $13,959.

[2] All of the above information is from the 2000 Census and was gathered from Infoplease, 2009.

and mental well-being of children from birth to age 6, via engagement and participation of the family with the resources of the Medical Home for Children Exposed to Violence best practices model. This model would be created in the spirit of the American Academy of Pediatrics "medical home," a model of delivering primary care that is accessible, continuous, comprehensive, family-centered, coordinated, compassionate, and culturally effective (American Academy of Pediatrics, 2010). This model strives toward forging a personalized relationship between patients and a primary care provider, who then links the patient with other necessary services, with the overall care meeting the standards described above. Specifically, the goals of the program were to implement organizational changes necessary to create the medical home model, to improve identification of children exposed to violence by domestic violence advocates, pediatricians, and child protective service workers, and to increase access to developmentally appropriate services for children and their families.

Children enter the medical home from one of three points: (1) referral following the pediatric well-child visit within pediatricians' offices at St. Barnabas Hospital, (2) after being identified as a child witness to domestic violence by a BDVP Domestic Violence Victim Advocate, who would be housed at the program site, and (3) after being identified by a caseworker in the Child Protective Services Division of the Administration for Children's Services (ACS). As originally envisioned, the medical home would contain an individualized intervention plan, including child-focused intervention services (assessment, school advocacy, safety planning, pediatric care, psychotherapy, case management) as well as family-focused intervention services (advocacy, case management, referrals for substance abuse and mental health treatment, health care, safety planning). These referral sources were adjusted over time, as will be described below, and the ultimate partnering agencies are presented in the box titled "Bronx Safe Start Partner Agencies and Referral Sources."

The Bronx was selected as a Safe Start site just as its medical director, who had designed the original concept, left St. Barnabas Hospital. The assistant director then assumed the position. This staffing change led to some reconsideration of the design of the project. Specifically, during OJJDP's Green Light process to prepare for program implementation and evaluation, Bronx Safe Start focused on the type of psychotherapy that would be offered within the medical home—and chose CPP (Lieberman and Van Horn, 2005)—as well as specified the conditions under which therapy would be offered. Bronx Safe Start planned to offer the therapy component to children exposed to severe violence who had problematic symptoms or behaviors (e.g., acting out, school problems, hitting, and regression in toileting) that had persisted for at least three months or children whose parents were not attuned to their needs. Thus, a subset of children would be offered therapy, but the number of children who needed therapy was unknown when the program began.

In addition, after the grant award, there were staffing changes within the collaborative partner, BDVP, and one of the referral sources, ACS. In each case, the person who had collaborated on the proposal with the CAC left, and the established relationship suffered as a result. In addition, the constraints of the research component of the evaluation (e.g., consent forms, institutional review board approvals) impeded progress in collaborating with ACS. Thus, activities with the sites were mostly limited to cross-training, case coordination, and few referrals, rather than active partnership in the medical home. Ultimately, the primary sources of referrals to the Safe Start program were the CAC, SBH pediatricians, and medical staff who worked in the SBH Emergency Department (see below for a brief description of referral sources), plus some new community partners that began referring families midway through the project.

### Bronx Safe Start Partner Agencies and Referral Sources

**St. Barnabas Hospital.** The Bronx Safe Start program is located at the CAC within St. Barnabas Hospital, a large, private, nonprofit Level I trauma center and inpatient and outpatient facility, with a large network of primary care and community health sites. The hospital has more than 400 beds and admits about 25,000 patients each year.

***Child Advocacy Center.*** The CAC provides diagnostic evaluations and treatment for children who are suspected of being abused or neglected. Evaluations are conducted in a child-friendly setting designed to minimize trauma and maximize safety for the entire family. Each child receives a physical examination from a medical professional and a psychosocial evaluation from a bilingual social worker with special training in child abuse, crisis counseling, and forensic interviewing. When necessary, the program coordinates the evaluation with police, the district attorney, and ACS. Bilingual parenting and prenatal classes are also offered to young mothers and their children and are intended to prevent further abuse.

***Pediatricians.*** There are more than 50 pediatricians employed by SBH. The Pediatric Department addresses pediatric problems ranging from primary care to complex medical conditions. Department divisions include Inpatient Pediatrics, Pediatric Emergency Medicine, Normal Newborn Nursery and Neonatal Intensive Care, and Ambulatory Care.

***Emergency Department.*** A state-of-the-art Emergency Department operates 24/7, serves 95,000 patients annually, and offers pediatric emergency services. All physicians and pediatricians are board certified in Emergency Medicine.

**Sanctuary for Families.** This agency is a nonprofit organization in New York State that offers a range of services to domestic violence victims and their children. Services include clinical, legal, shelter, children's, and economic stability services, as well as outreach, education, and advocacy. Sanctuary for Families has two service sites in the Bronx: the Bronx Community Office and the Bronx Family Justice Center. This site began referring families with young children to Bronx Safe Start midway through the project.

**Violence Intervention Program, Inc.** VIP is a nationally recognized Latina organization dedicated to ending violence in the lives of women, by offering a full range of culturally competent services. VIP's Triborough Office began referring families with young children to Bronx Safe Start midway through the project.

**South Bronx Mental Health Council, Inc.** The South Bronx Mental Health Council is a large agency that provides outpatient mental health and substance abuse services. The Council began referring families with young children exposed to violence to Bronx Safe Start midway through the project.

## Intervention

The medical home included three components: multidisciplinary evaluations (MDEs), CPP, and intensive case management. The intervention period lasted approximately two years, but families were welcome to return to the medical home at any point to receive additional help. All services were provided in the clinic.

### Multidisciplinary Evaluation

The intervention began with a preliminary MDE to determine the needs of each child and family. The initial MDE included developmental and behavioral pediatrics, psychosocial, and medical evaluations, as well as assessment scores from the research evaluation. The assessment team comprised two pediatricians (one who conducted a neurodevelopmental pediatric assessment and another who conducted a pediatric exam), one psychologist, and one social worker. The neurodevelopmental pediatric assessment included standard developmental screenings to assess motor skills, language skills, and achievement for older children. The psychologist and social worker conducted a psychosocial evaluation of the family that included behavioral observations and administration of the Child Behavior Checklist.

After completion of the MDE, the team met to develop a provisional diagnosis, to develop the individualized treatment plan, and to produce a summary report. The social worker or therapist then met with the family to discuss recommendations for treatment. In all cases, the family was able to decline services or postpone them as desired. This report was also used to guide ongoing treatment and was reviewed quarterly by the assessment team.

### Child-Parent Psychotherapy

The therapy component involved parent-child dyadic therapy using the Lieberman model for CPP. CPP is a relationship-based intervention designed for use with children up to age 6. It can be used with any child whose relationship to the parent or other primary caregiver is impacted by negative circumstances, including family violence. CPP integrates psychodynamic, attachment, trauma, cognitive-behavioral, and social learning theories (NCTSN, 2008). There are two components to CPP: assessment and treatment, with information gained during the assessment used to inform the treatment component. In the intervention component, child-parent interactions are the focus of six intervention modalities aimed at restoring a sense of mastery, security, and growth and promoting congruence between bodily sensations, feelings, and thinking on the part of both child and parent and in their relationship with one another (NCTSN, 2008). This therapy was delivered on a weekly basis, for up to a year.

The Bronx Safe Start staff were trained by one of the model developers, Patricia Van Horn, in the summer of 2006. Following the initial training, Van Horn provided biweekly phone consultation/supervision; however, during the project, the staff felt that they could benefit from more clinical support, so the frequency of phone consultation increased to once weekly and continued at this rate for the remainder of the project. In addition, Susan Chinitz, director of the Early Childhood Center at the Children's Evaluation and Rehabilitation Center at the Albert Einstein College of Medicine at Yeshiva University, who is trained in CPP, provided an additional hour of clinical supervision once weekly, starting about two years after project implementation.

### Intensive Case Management

Bronx Safe Start planned to include intensive case management, in recognition that all families have different needs, face different barriers, and need different levels of support to access and engage in services. A family coordinator (social work assistant) was hired to assist with case management. Case management activities were performed to coordinate services, prevent duplication of services, and support families in getting their needs met. As the social worker, therapist, and family coordinator worked to build and maintain relationships with families, they planned to engage in ongoing assessment of the family's needs and provide support and referrals for services. The program regarded advocacy as an essential component of case management, intended to help troubleshoot barriers so that families could receive the services they need and learn to advocate for themselves. Bronx Safe Start specified particular activities within this approach, including pre-intake activities (e.g., calling to confirm appointment 1–2 days in advance) and post-intake activities (e.g., helping to arrange services, helping to maintain the family in services by checking on whether families were continuing in services).

### Other Direct Services

Other direct services were planned to be offered as needed to augment the core services. Examples included plans to establish a Safe Women and Girls Center domestic violence outreach program run by groups on parent education, literacy, and provision of medical care for undocumented or untreated medical conditions. A domestic violence consultant for the Jewish Board of Family Services was available one day per week in a small office in the lobby of the clinic building. This "Safe Women and Girls Center" had resources, handouts, and referrals available for interested patients.

The intervention was conducted in the context of a rigorous outcome evaluation, as required by OJJDP (see the box titled "Bronx Safe Start Evaluation" for a description).

**Bronx Safe Start Evaluation**

**Design.** This randomized control effectiveness trial was focused on child outcomes.

**Treatment vs. control group services.** Treatment consisted of being enrolled in the medical home and receiving MDEs, CPP, and intensive case management. Those who were assigned to the control group received usual services in the community along with phone calls every two months and limited case management and referral to community agencies.

**Data collection.** Data were collected through longitudinal assessments of child-level outcomes.

**Enrollment.** The site originally planned to enroll 25 families in the treatment and control groups in the first year and 30 in each group subsequent years, for a total of 115 per group. Funding for the National Evaluation ended prematurely. By the time it ended, enrollment had taken place over two years and nine months and resulted in 68 families in the treatment group and 56 in the control group.

## Implementation

Figure B.1 provides a diagram to show Bronx Safe Start's implementation of its intervention. The following description of the program implementation is the result of data collected for the national evaluation. See Appendix A for a full discussion of the data collection methodology employed at each of the Safe Start sites.

### Referrals

Bronx Safe Start originally expected to receive referrals from pediatricians within St. Barnabas Hospital and its satellite clinics as well as from the CAC itself, the Jewish Board of Family and Children's Services BDVP, and the ACS. As a way to increase referrals, pediatric residents and pediatricians were trained to understand the impact of violent exposure on children and to

**Figure B.1**
**Model of St. Barnabas Hospital Children's Advocacy Center Safe Start**

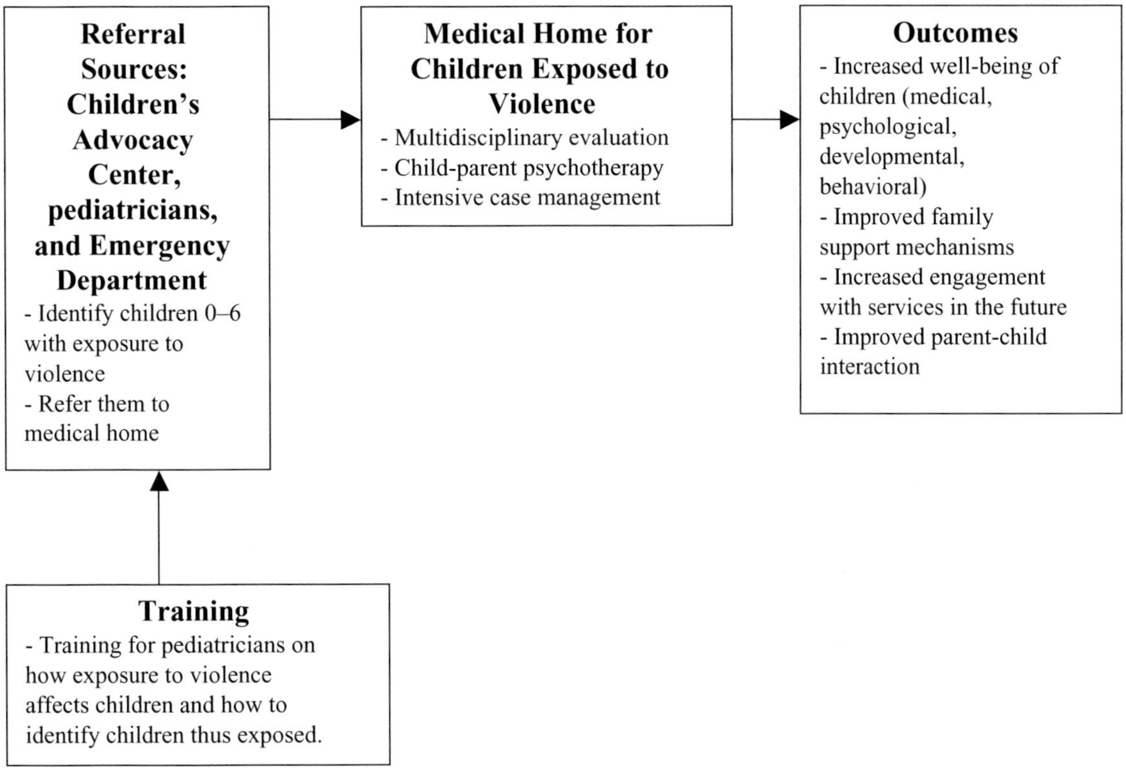

**Referral Sources: Children's Advocacy Center, pediatricians, and Emergency Department**
- Identify children 0–6 with exposure to violence
- Refer them to medical home

**Medical Home for Children Exposed to Violence**
- Multidisciplinary evaluation
- Child-parent psychotherapy
- Intensive case management

**Outcomes**
- Increased well-being of children (medical, psychological, developmental, behavioral)
- Improved family support mechanisms
- Increased engagement with services in the future
- Improved parent-child interaction

**Training**
- Training for pediatricians on how exposure to violence affects children and how to identify children thus exposed.

RAND *TR750-B.1*

identify children exposed to trauma. Periodic emails to the attending pediatricians and residents reminded them of the need to screen for domestic and community violence. This method was successful enough to generate the bulk of the referrals necessary for this project and was extended from one pediatric clinic (adjacent to the Safe Start program) to include four others.

Additional families were self-referred, referred by the CAC or Emergency Department, or occasionally by community partners. Later, Bronx Safe Start's participation in the Domestic Violence Action Network introduced the program to other local domestic violence and mental health agencies. Many of those agencies were able to provide services to parents and older children but had no services available for the young children. Specifically, Sanctuary for Families, the VIP, and the South Bronx Mental Health Center began to refer families with younger children to Bronx Safe Start, leading to an informal partnership over time. Safe Start estimated that about 60 percent of referrals came from these sources and 40 percent from pediatricians toward the end of the project.

Most families were referred via telephone, but there were also walk-ins that could have been served either by the CAC or by the Safe Start program. Referring agency staff and Safe Start staff found that the families were sometimes in a state of crisis and not ready to engage in the medical home services. These families had many concrete, immediate needs (safety, housing, need for food, public assistance) that needed to be addressed before the family was ready to commit to weekly psychotherapy sessions. Often, some initial case management (e.g., referrals to community resources) occurred prior to enrollment in the Safe Start program to address crisis issues, particularly for families that entered via the CAC. One of the main challenges was recruiting families into the program. Even after being identified and referred, families were difficult to contact by phone or mail. They moved frequently and did not keep appointments.

Once enrolled, all families took part in the research evaluation assessments and then were randomized into treatment or control groups. The treatment group began with the MDE. Services were provided in a satellite health center located a few blocks from the main hospital.

## Services

Table B.1 summarizes service delivery for those who received services through the Bronx Safe Start program over the first three years of implementation (through March 2009). The program had two (full- or part-time) therapists (the social worker and the psychologist) at any one time during the project. In addition, a family coordinator provided case management services and a second case manager was hired at the end of Year 2.

### *Multidisciplinary Evaluation*

The MDEs with the families typically occurred in two separate appointments (a psychosocial evaluation on one day, and the developmental and health assessment on a separate day). During the multidisciplinary team meetings, team members reported their assessment findings and impressions to the team. Preliminary diagnoses were documented as a team. Many of the children assessed had developmental delays. Copies of previous evaluations were requested (mostly from Early Intervention and the Committee of Special Education). Other children were referred for formal testing, particularly for use in obtaining special education services in school. An example of treatment goals developed via this assessment was to begin weekly CPP, to refer the child for a hearing evaluation, and to obtain school educational plans for the team to review. Staff members noted that some service referrals, such as those to domestic violence services, did not result in immediate visits because of long wait times at the relevant agencies.

During enrollment, the developmental pediatrician noted that some children needed follow-up after their initial pediatric developmental assessment. Many of the children enrolled were doing poorly in school, yet developmental delays were not identified or else not being treated in school. Some children had attention-deficit hyperactivity disorder or other conditions that would benefit from medication. So, several months after starting, the developmental pediatrician had a small cohort of children that needed follow-up visits to address these issues. This had not been anticipated during the planning phase.

**Table B.1**
**Service Delivery for Enrollees in the Bronx Safe Start Intervention**

| | Year 1 | Year 2 | Year 3 (9 months) |
|---|---|---|---|
| Average quarterly caseload per therapist | 4.4 | 12.4 | 19 |
| Total number of CPP sessions | 120 | 237 | 149 |
| Total number of MDEs | 41 | 46 | 42 |
| Total number of pediatric care visits | 8 | 1 | 0 |
| Total number of case coordination meetings | 44 | 36 | 21 |
| Total number of referrals and case management contacts with clients and service providers | 131 | 382 | 292 |
| Total number of follow-up developmental assessments | N/A | 39 | 9 |

### *Child-Parent Psychotherapy*

Almost all families were referred for CPP, and most parents were interested in the therapy because they were aware of behavioral issues that could benefit from the intervention. In the first two years of the project, CPP typically began one to two weeks after the multidisciplinary team meetings. As time elapsed and more families were enrolled, waits for therapy became longer, and a waiting list was needed. The program staff was not expecting the majority of families to be referred for CPP. During the interviews with program staff, it was reported that many more children than originally anticipated displayed behavioral problems warranting CPP, and most families that were eligible wanted the therapy to help them handle these problems. Bronx Safe Start had originally hired a psychologist for three days per week to implement the CPP intervention. As the demand for CPP increased, the social worker began providing CPP two days per week. Later in the project, the psychologist's workweek increased to four days and the social worker's to three days; however, the program still experienced capacity problems. Thus, some families had to wait for CPP up to two months or more after enrollment. Case management was in place at all times.

In terms of actual implementation of CPP, although most families were interested in therapy, a significant group had difficulties keeping the weekly therapy appointments.

### *Intensive Case Management*

The intensive case management included identifying concrete needs and providing intensive support in person or via telephone. After identifying the needs, the case manager provided referral links for services such as shelters, early intervention and special education services for children through the schools, and legal services. In some cases, the parent was referred for individual mental health services to address concerns such as depression. In many cases, the case management began with the first contact with the family, even prior to enrollment in the Safe Start project. Thus, both the control group and the treatment group families received some degree of case management. As the program evolved, Bronx Safe Start realized that the need for more concrete services (housing, immigration, public assistance, access to mental health) was a priority for the families enrolled, and this realization directly affected readiness to attend psychotherapy sessions. A second case manager was hired during Year 3 of the program.

### *Other Direct Services*

Bronx Safe Start expected to implement some other programs, focusing on domestic violence and child abuse prevention issues. During the partnership with the Jewish Board of Family and Children's Services BDVP in the first year of the project, the Safe Women and Girls Center was created. This center consisted of a domestic violence worker available in the clinic lobby one day per week, with resources and literature to hand out to women as they came in. However, the center did not attract much interest from patients, perhaps because of its location or part-time nature. Safe Start staff concluded that this method of reaching families was not productive, and they closed the center after about a year.

As part of the medical home model, staff also expected to deliver pediatric care for unmet medical conditions, especially for the families that were referred from ACS, the emergency room, or community agencies. But because most referrals came from pediatricians, most families entering the program were already receiving health care and continued to see their own providers, making health care delivery less frequent within the program.

There were other components of the Bronx Safe Start program that helped shape the implementation. These are described in the box titled "Bronx Safe Start Additional Program Components."

### Bronx Safe Start Additional Program Components

**Quality Assurance.** At the beginning of the program, the Bronx Safe Start staff participated in a three-day training on CPP with one of the model developers. Throughout the implementation, the service providers had access to materials that described the treatment model, the Safe Start program, and the implementation plans. The model developer initially provided biweekly phone consultation/supervision, which later increased to once weekly and continued at this rate for the remainder of the project, alternating between the developer and another expert. A licensed clinical social worker with the CAC provided an additional hour of on-site clinical supervision once weekly and reviewed all case notes, as well as participating in each multidisciplinary team meeting.

**Training.** The Safe Start program conducted and/or participated in 47 trainings over the first two years of implementation. Approximately 42 percent of these trainings focused on issues of domestic violence, 23 percent on the Safe Start program, 11 percent on child-parent psychotherapy or other clinical topics, and 9 percent on child welfare issues. Domestic violence trainings were on topics such as domestic violence and immigration, the intersection of domestic violence with child abuse, and the effects of violence on the developing brain. Trainings varied in size, attracting 8 to 35 participants on average.

**Policies and Protocols.** The Bronx Safe Start program developed new or changed existing policies to try to improve safety for children. Specifically, as an institution St. Barnabas Hospital changed the protocol to expand screening for child abuse and domestic violence to every child seen in the pediatric clinic or admitted to the emergency room or hospital. The hospital also initiated a special project that designated the hospital and its affiliates as a "No Hitting Zone" to promote a safe environment, and trained all staff on CEV and domestic violence. Also, as a part of this initiative, posters and brochures were distributed to parents on child discipline.

**Program Outreach.** Advocacy efforts were all aimed at increasing community awareness and support for the Safe Start program. They included presentations within the hospital and to community partners and meetings with key community stakeholders.

**Resources and Costs.** In the first two years of SSPA, Bronx Safe Start devoted most of its resources to labor costs, particularly for the project coordinator, data consultant, and child psychologist. Bronx SSPA used a significant amount of in-kind support, particularly donated time from the hospital medical director. Other expenses included therapeutic supplies, such as play therapy materials and assessment tools.

## Summary

The Medical Home for Children Exposed to Violence was a new concept at the beginning of this project, and thus many aspects of it were developed while the project got under way. The core elements and community partners were defined in advance, but the mix of services and the strength of the partnerships emerged over time as the program was implemented. Thus, a great deal of flexibility was required to accommodate changes over time. Staff turnover at partnering agencies as well as within the Bronx Safe Start project itself imposed additional need for flexibility. Fortunately, the pediatricians within this large hospital system proved to be good sources for identification and referral of families into the program, and they provided a steady of stream of referrals despite slower-than-anticipated referrals from community partners. It was not until the third year in the project that referrals came regularly from domestic violence and mental health community agencies.

A major challenge for this site involved not knowing exactly what to expect in terms of the types of services that would be needed within the Medical Home model. Once staff launched the program, they realized that nearly all families were eligible, which severely impacted their capacity to deliver CPP. On the other hand, fewer families needed medical treatment than expected, as most families continued to see their regular pediatricians for medical care. This resulted in the need to adjust the mix of services from what was planned, finding ways to adjust staffing to deliver more CPP and less medical care than expected.

One challenge was how to engage families in treatment. Families' readiness for services varied depending on the referral source. Referred families were seen by program staff as more often in crisis and therefore in need of safety planning, stabilization, and case management prior to beginning treatment, which had to be addressed prior to beginning CPP. In contrast, families referred by pediatricians were often seen as more ready for treatment. In addition, many families had greater immediate needs (e.g., housing, safety) than expected and experienced difficulty meeting the various demands of the project (e.g., completing the initial assessment, attending therapy sessions).

Another change to the menu of services offered was the elimination of pediatric care. According to the Safe Start program staff, this change was made because most families were already connected with medical care providers and were pleased with the pediatric services they were receiving.

The Bronx Safe Start leadership saw sustainability as a major challenge, as some of the services, particularly case management, were not easily reimbursed by their usual funders (e.g., insurance agencies, Medicaid). However, given that there were not any comparable programs in the community, the program leadership hoped to be able to secure grant funding to sustain the Bronx Safe Start program after the support form OJJDP ended.

**Data collection for this program summary included:**

- Key informant interviews with key program staff
  - Project director, project manager
  - Director, Child Advocacy Center/Clinical Supervisor
  - Therapists and social workers
  - Referring pediatricians
  - Developmental assessment pediatrician
  - Data collectors
- Case review of randomly selected treatment and control group cases
- Observation of multidisciplinary team meeting
- Quality assurance checklist completed by the clinical supervisor
- Quarterly activity reports on services, training, policies, and advocacy
- Grant application
- Green Light notes
- *Safe Start: Promising Approaches Communities Working Together to Help Children Exposed to Violence* (Safe Start Center, 2008).

## 2. Broward County, Florida, Program Description

### Broward County Safe Start

- **Intervention type:** Family-Centered Treatment® (FCT)® (intensive, home-based, family-centered therapy)
- **Intervention length:** Up to six months
- **Intervention setting:** In-home
- **Target population:** Children who were exposed to all types of violence, with a focus on exposure to domestic violence
- **Age range:** 0–8
- **Primary referral source:** Henderson Mental Health Center (Family Resource Team), ChildNet, Women in Distress, Broward County Sheriff's Office

### Program and Community Setting

The Broward County Safe Start program operates within Broward County, Florida. According to the 2000 Census, the population in the county was a little more than 1.6 million, with 6.3 percent of the population younger than age 5. The population was 71 percent white, 21 percent black, 17 percent Hispanic, a little more than 2 percent Asian, and about 3 percent reporting some other race. The income per capita was $27,129,[3] with 11.5 percent of the population living below the poverty line.[4]

In 2001, Broward County ranked 22nd among the 67 counties in Florida in crime rate; as of 2003, domestic violence offense rates in the county were high, with 8,000 domestic violence offenses. Child abuse and neglect rates are also high in Broward County: According to the Florida Abuse Hotline Information System (FAHIS), in the fiscal year 2001–2002 there were 16,488 reports received for Broward County child abuse and neglect. The most prevalent type of abuse was domestic violence (11.53%; Institute for Family Centered Services, Inc., 2004).

The Institute for Family Centered Services, Inc. (IFCS), the developers of Family Centered Treatment®, is a privately owned organization founded in 1988 in Virginia. The mission of IFCS is to enhance family strengths and resources through direct involvement with the family that preserves the dignity of all families within their community. Throughout 21 years of providing services to children and families, IFCS had earned a reputation for successfully engaging, intervening with, and treating the most challenging and resistant families. At the time of this project, IFCS was providing services to youth and families in four states: Virginia, Maryland, North Carolina, and Florida. In Florida, services were offered in English, Spanish, and Creole, the three most common languages in Broward County.

IFCS applied for Safe Start funding in order to evaluate its services, with Broward County as the location, and in collaboration with several county partners who serve children exposed to domestic violence and child abuse or neglect. IFCS had been working in Broward County for four years prior to its Safe Start submission, and was able to develop memoranda of understanding with several agencies in the county for the proposal, including

---

[3] This is the 1999 per capita income converted to 2005 dollars. The 1999 per capita income as originally reported was $23,170.

[4] All of the above information was taken from the 2000 Census and can be found on its website (U.S. Census Bureau, no date).

child welfare, juvenile justice, domestic violence, and mental health agencies (see the box titled "Broward County Safe Start Partner Agencies" for a brief description of the partner agencies). IFCS had existing contractual and informal referral relationships with several of these agencies as well. In many ways, the Safe Start work was an effort to examine the services already in place in Broward County to determine its impact on children, rather than to launch new services. However, IFCS also included plans for training parents and staff members at other agencies within Broward County on the impact of domestic violence on young children, and enhancing collaborations with their community partners by participating in a Task Force and developing cross-agency protocols and policies for working with young children and their families.

The core components of the model that distinguished it from other services in the county were its family-system approach (in contrast to a medical model or individually focused approach), home-based services, focus on family strengths, the family-driven approach in goal-setting and a "value change" focus (working with the family members to "own" and value changes in behavior), and the intensity of the approach (multiple hours, multiple meetings per week). The main goal was to stabilize the family by building on family strengths and supporting the family in taking up other relevant services (e.g., specialty mental health care).

### Broward County Safe Start Partner Agencies

**Institute for Family Centered Services.** IFCS is a privately owned organization founded in 1988 that provided services in four states in 2009: Virginia, Maryland, North Carolina, and Florida. In 2008, it received accreditation from the Council on Accreditation in Family Preservation Services for its FTC®. In 2009, IFCS employed more than 300 people throughout 21 regions of the company, actively serving more than 2,500 families annually.

**Henderson Mental Health Center** is a private, not-for-profit behavioral health care center providing comprehensive, recovery-focused services to more than 20,000 people of all ages. The center provides a continuum of community-based prevention, education, treatment, and rehabilitation services by utilizing best practice and evidence-based treatment models to maximize recovery in 16 facilities throughout South Florida. The center's **Family Resource Teams** provide case management to families referred by the Broward Sheriff's Office following an abuse or neglect allegation. The goal is to help families reduce parenting stress and prevent subsequent abuse or neglect.

**Women in Distress** has the mission of providing victims of domestic violence with safe shelter, crisis intervention, and resources and educating the community in order to Stop Abuse For Everyone (SAFE) through intervention, education, and advocacy. They strive to accomplish this mission by offering a 24-hour crisis hotline, emergency shelter, counseling, education, and professional trainings on domestic violence and related topics.

**Broward County Sheriff's Office:** The Broward Sheriff's Office is America's largest nationally accredited sheriff's department and provides full-time law enforcement services in 14 Broward cities and towns and in all of Broward's unincorporated areas, serving more than one-third of the county. The Department of Law Enforcement includes the Child Protective Investigations Section, which investigates allegations of abuse and neglect against Broward County's children. Their Special Victims and Family Crimes Section is available for help for domestic violence.

**Broward County Safe Start Partner Agencies (continued)**

**ChildNet:** In 1999, the state of Florida began a process to transfer care of abused and neglected children from the Department of Child and Family Services to community-based agencies. ChildNet is Broward's community-based care lead agency, selected by the state to manage the local system of services and supports for Broward's abused, abandoned, and neglected children and their caregivers. A network of community providers—including IFCS, as well as foster care and adoption services—managed by ChildNet deliver a wide variety of services (shelter and group care, foster home management, family strengthening, and adoption support services).

For Safe Start, the proposed target population included children (ages 0–6) residing in Broward County, Florida, who had been referred to the IFCS because of exposure to any type of domestic or community violence. Due to the nature of the referral sources, most children were referred for exposure to domestic violence, but some were referred for child abuse, and many had exposures to multiple forms of violence. Children and primary caregivers were also required to be proficient in English or Spanish to understand the informed consent process and the assessments.

IFCS originally planned to receive referrals from a number of sources within Broward County, including ChildNet, Women in Distress, the Broward County Sheriff's Office, and other partnering community agencies. These referral sources were adjusted over time, as will be described below, and the ultimate partnering agencies are presented in the box titled "Broward County Safe Start Partner Agencies."

The proposed program was FTC®, which comprised three different levels of intensity:

- Project Support, a short-term crisis intervention and stabilization program. (Note that this is not the same model as the one offered by Dallas Safe Start, despite the same name.)
- Project Foundation, a two to three month program for skill development and psychoeducation.
- Project Hope, a four to six month program designed to include the other services but also to change patterns of family interactions to reduce violence and improve family functioning.

However, these three tiers of services were not ultimately used, as we discuss later.

After being selected as a Safe Start site, IFCS participated in the Green Light process. During this process, IFCS worked to specify its plans for a control group, ultimately deciding to use a six-month wait-list control group. This Green Light process was seen as a challenging but important task by project leaders, since they were initially unsure how to create an ethical and feasible comparison group. They were concerned that, with a long-term control group, families would not have access to any intensive services, since those types of services were not offered at other agencies within Broward County. Safe Start staff also increased their age range to include children up to age 8, in an effort to ensure adequate referrals into the project. Finally, the Green Light process included detailed planning for assessing the safety and protocols for when to include the perpetrator in therapy to ensure that the families would be safe during the course of the intervention.

## Intervention

IFCS developed FCT® more than 20 years ago. The intensive, family-centered service model used in this project offered "practical, experiential ways to have families rediscover the components of effective parenting and communication skills" (IFCS, 2004). The goal was to foster strong, healthy attachment to parents and a sense of belonging, competence, independence, and value in children. FCT included five procedures:

- safety assessment
- crisis intervention
- individual and family counseling
- education about child development and appropriate expectations
- wraparound services, 24 hours a day, seven days a week for the duration of the service period.

The intervention generally started with five to six hours per week (at least two meetings per week) and then tapered off to once a week later on, as the therapy moved toward termination, for a period of roughly six months. All services were provided in the family's home. Prior to initiating the intervention, a thorough safety assessment was conducted to determine where the perpetrator of violence was located and how the family could be safe. Generally, the first month of treatment was considered the Assessment and Joining phase, with the therapist gathering information in structured ways and using it to help the family formulate goals. For instance, therapists generally began by developing an "eco map," a pictorial depiction of each family member and the people and relationships around him or her, including closeness and conflict in each relationship. These were developed individually with each family member and then shared with other family members.

Another assessment was the family life cycle exercise, in which the therapist works with the family to identify the families' stage in development and the key tasks related to this stage. For instance, a family might be in the "Family with Young Children" stage of the family life cycle, in which the key tasks are to adjust the marriage to make space for the children, child-rearing responsibilities and roles, and adjustment of the relationship with extended families and friends to accommodate children.

A key part of the assessment was the Structured Family Assessment, containing five parts: development of a genogram (a family tree including violent relationships and mental health issues), individual interviews, a "family fishbowl" activity in which the therapist observed the family discussing three questions and coming to a conclusion on a major issue facing the family, a "reverse fishbowl" activity in which the therapist fed back information gleaned from the family, and a closure activity in which the family developed its goals for treatment. Examples of treatment goals might be to heal from the effects of violence, to be safe, and for a particular child to reduce angry outbursts. For some families, goals might include finding ways to reintegrate the father into the family.

Another example planned was the development of a "gendergram" for each person to describe generational family patterns and roles, used to clarify the core elements of family gender models. This would allow family members to understand the implicit assumptions about gender roles that they brought from their family of origin into roles as parents. This proposed evaluation activity was not ultimately implemented, however, as will be discussed later.

Once goals were set, the second phase of "Therapy with Families and Individuals" began, usually lasting for two to three months. This therapy centered on such issues as improving parenting, setting limits, continued safety planning, loss and separation, specific behavioral or emotional problems in the parent or child, and healing from the effects of trauma. Typically, the tone would be directive, with therapists suggesting specific changes in patterns of behavior within the family to promote the family's goals (the "Restructuring Phase"). But toward the end, this tone would shift to the "Value Change Phase," in which the therapist would challenge family members to move past "conformity and compliance" to consider the changes suggested to them by the therapist and to come to their own conclusion about whether they wanted to embrace those changes or not.

The last phase of treatment, typically lasting about six weeks, was the Termination Phase, or Generalization Phase, during which the therapist would observe and monitor the family to ensure that they were able to continue to maintain the things they learned during treatment. This phase also helped the family members get ready to formulate their own goals and advocate for themselves with social service agencies. The treatment ended when most of the treatment goals were met and social workers were able to connect family members with the other need services in their community.

Core concepts that were central to the model included this strength-based perspective, using experiential techniques rather than "talk" therapy, focusing on the power of peers and natural supports to the family, the value placed on practical services, and taking a holistic approach to working with the family to improve spiritual, emotional, physical, mental, and social functioning. During the sessions, the therapists worked toward helping to stabilize the family, to help the family access natural supports, and to advocate for themselves, so they engaged "collaterals" (other community agencies) early on in treatment. Monthly team meetings brought all the players (e.g., social service agencies and family) together face-to-face to work toward common goals. Over time and under ideal circumstances, the family would lead those meetings and would set the agenda themselves.

The intervention was conducted in the context of a rigorous outcome evaluation as required by OJJDP (see the box titled "Broward County Safe Start Evaluation" for a description).

### Broward County Safe Start Evaluation

**Design.** This randomized control effectiveness trial was focused on child outcomes (wait-list control group).

**Treatment versus control group services.** Families assigned to the treatment condition received FTC® for up to six months. Families on the waiting list received enhanced usual care (extra support and referrals) during the waiting period and were eligible to begin FTC® after completion of the first follow-up assessment at six months.

**Data collection.** Data were collected through longitudinal assessments of child-level outcomes.

**Enrollment.** The site originally planned to enroll 190 families over a four-year period (95 in each group).

Funding for the national evaluation ended prematurely. By the time it ended, the total enrollment for Broward County Safe Start over two years and nine months was 102 families in the treatment group and 99 in the control group.

## Implementation

Figure B.2 provides a diagram of Broward County's implementation of its intervention. The following description of the program implementation is the result of data collected for the national evaluation. See Appendix A for a full discussion of the data collection methodology employed at each of the Safe Start sites.

### Referrals

Broward County Safe Start originally proposed to receive referrals from a number of community sources, including justice (Broward Sheriff's Office and juvenile justice), domestic violence (Women in Distress), and mental health (Henderson Mental Health Clinic) agencies.

During program implementation, the majority of referrals came from the Henderson Mental Health Center's Family Resource Center intake specialist. The goal of the Family Resource Center Team was to assist Broward Sheriff's Office with linking at-risk Broward County families with services that would meet their behavioral health needs and thereby promote the preservation of the family. In an average month, approximately 1,000 child abuse referrals were received by the Broward Sheriff's Office Child Protective Investigators, and about 120–200 families per month were deemed to have low to moderate risk of child removal from the home. These cases were referred to the Family Resource Team. Some families were being reported the first or second time for potential abuse, and the goal of the program was to prevent future incidents of abuse. Of these incidents, about 40 percent were related to domestic violence. The intake specialist reported referring nearly all of these cases to Broward County Safe Start, unless the perpetrator was still in the home. In those cases, she assigned them to a case coordinator at Henderson, who offered up to three months of wraparound services but sometimes was able to refer the family to Safe Start later on, once the family was deemed to be relatively safe.

In many cases, the child most in need of the intervention, or the "target" of the intervention, was clear upon referral into the program, and, in these cases, the primary caregiver and that

**Figure B.2**
**Model of Broward County Safe Start**

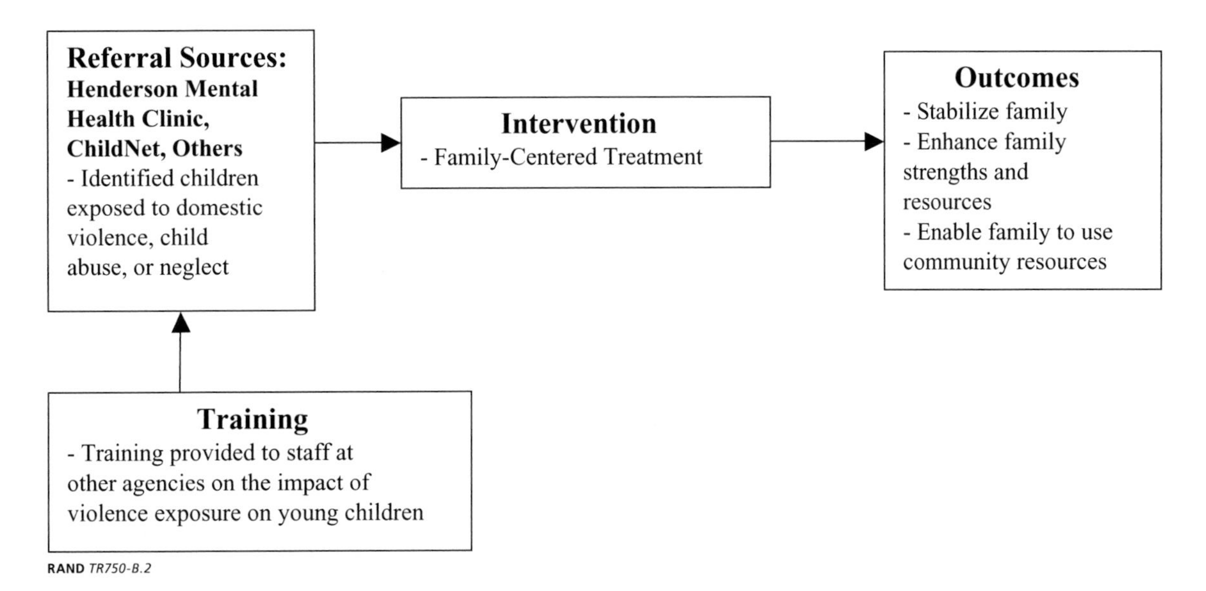


RAND *TR750-B.2*

child were recruited to participate in the research project, although the entire family participated in the intervention. In other cases, more than one child in the 0–8 age range had been exposed to violence, and all were the focus of intervention within the FCT model.

In the beginning of the project, community partner agencies had difficulty referring families because of the control group. Henderson Mental Health Center was required to ensure services for every family, so referring to an agency that would only provide services to a random half of families immediately was not thought to be workable. With a change in staffing at Broward County Safe Start in early 2007, IFCS changed its control group procedures to include a detailed protocol for providing referrals after the baseline assessment, checking in with families monthly, mailing information on referral possibilities if families could not be reached by telephone, and details about when to remove a family from the wait list and offer immediate services (a credible threat by the perpetrator, failure to follow safety plan or protect child, etc). This enhanced usual care protocol allowed Henderson Mental Health Center to fulfill its obligations to the family and made it possible to refer families, knowing some services would be provided.

However, other agencies were still reluctant to refer into the program. Particularly, domestic violence agencies had concerns about IFCS's practice of sometimes including the perpetrator in FCT. In about 25–30 percent of cases, Broward County Safe Start staff reported inclusion of the perpetrator at some point in the treatment. They worked with the Safe Start Center to arrange training from the Family Violence Prevention Fund for their staff to ensure that they were employing best practices in ensuring safety and empowering women and children with whom they were working, as will be described in the training section. Although the two agencies connected directly to work jointly with many families, at the agency level they were unable to overcome this obstacle. Thus, domestic violence agencies made only one referral during the life of the project.

### Services

Table B.2 summarizes service delivery for those who received services through the Broward County Safe Start program. Broward County had started with two therapists at the beginning of Year 1 and quickly expanded to five therapists. Throughout Year 2, they had 5–6 therapists, which was ramped up to 7–8 therapists in Year 3 (through March 2009).

Social workers were master's-level therapists who went through an extensive training in FCT before they were certified to treat cases. FCT was documented via a detailed "Wheels of Change" treatment manual (Painter and Smith, 2004), augmented by weekly didactic seminars and monthly trainings to augment the intervention techniques, as well as live training and supervision.

The Broward County Safe Start Program prided itself on being able to "join" with the family and to help the family meet its own goals. Program staff told us that if they could "get in the door" for the first appointment, they were almost always able to continue with the family. The site went through the OJJDP-sponsored engagement training by Mary McKay for the Safe Start sites and said staff were happy to see that they already did most of the things suggested. The family specialists also worked closely with the other agencies, and thus they were able to explain to the family how they were able to contact it and that they were there to help support the family and keep it together (to distinguish themselves from an agency that might remove the child from the home).

**Table B.2**
**Service Delivery for Enrollees in the Broward County Safe Start Intervention**

| | Year 1 | Year 2 | Year 3 (9 months) |
|---|---|---|---|
| Average quarterly caseload per therapist | 2.9 | 5.1 | 7 |
| Total number of individual therapy sessions | 75 | 491 | 268 |
| Total number of family therapy sessions | 301 | 970 | 606 |
| Total number of case management contacts | 32 | 251 | 284 |

FCT was reported to be implemented as planned, with one major exception. The plan to include three levels of services, depending on family need, proved to be infeasible, largely because the families referred to were judged to need the highest level of service. The staff members' perception was that the partnering agencies were referring the families with the most severe problems, since many of the agencies already offered the type of stabilization services offered in lower levels of intensity. In addition, the IFCS originally began its work in Broward County by asking a mental health agency to give them their "hardest" case and provided services pro bono to prove themselves to staff at this agency by helping this family. Thus, the staff reported feeling as if they had built a reputation for helping families in great need prior to beginning their Safe Start project. Further, their home-based services were seen as advantageous, because families had transportation issues and could not attend regular sessions at a mental health clinic or other community agency.

In addition, the gendergram that was proposed was not ultimately used because the supervisors believed that that the therapists needed to focus on the basic concepts within the FCT model, and saw the focus on gender to be more complicated and not necessary for every family. Supervisors reported that this method would be particularly useful when working with perpetrators of violence, but that they felt the Family Centered Evaluation included in the basic FCT model was adequate for the families they worked with in this project.

IFCS fit the Safe Start Program into its ongoing services: Each therapist had a few Safe Start cases along with a mix of other families in their caseload. New families to the program were assigned to a therapist based on their primary language and therapist availability, and that therapist worked with the family for the assessment phase as well as the intervention phase.

The Safe Start program was able to enroll families effectively, but often had difficulty tracking and locating families over time as well as difficulty offering the intervention following the family's time on the waiting list. Program staff noted that Broward County had many families coming from the north for the winter and many people coming from other countries. Thus, many families left the county, sometimes even leaving the United States, and thus were difficult to track.

There were other components of the Broward County Safe Start program that helped shape the implementation. These are described in the box titled "Broward County Safe Start Additional Program Components."

### Broward County Safe Start Additional Program Components

**Quality Assurance.** New staff were trained first via the model manual to learn core concepts and through video examples of the intervention in action, followed by shadowing a senior therapist, followed by demonstration of adherence to 14 core skills with a family (as observed by the trainer for the region). Thus, all staff were certified prior to delivering services on their own. Cases were reviewed by staff in weekly group sessions for peer feedback and biweekly for individual supervision. There were also bimonthly supervision meetings by the project director for training and case presentations.

**Training.** Over the first two years, Broward County Safe Start participated in and/or conducted 24 trainings. Most of these trainings were focused on clinical issues (33.3%) or training on other interventions (33.3%). There were fewer trainings on engaging families or issues related to child welfare. Various staff participated in the clinical training on topics such as women in distress and working with resistance in family-based care. During 2007 and 2008, there were also multiday trainings delivered by the Family Violence Prevention Fund to augment clinicians' skills in working with the families experiencing domestic violence, sometimes including the perpetrator.

**Policies and Protocols.** The Broward County Safe Start program developed or changed policies related to improving the enrollment process and provision of services. Criteria were developed to assign children/families in the treatment group to the most appropriate of the three levels of treatment; however, these criteria were later abandoned when the tiers of services were eliminated. The enrollment procedure was also modified to meet evaluation requirements. Broward also changed a policy to improve the method used to track case management services provided to Safe Start families and to increase access to the information from just IFCS to the Family Centered Specialists and Regional Directors. Final adjustments to policy were increased engagement with the control group, requiring at least one phone call per month, to increase the safety of those families during their waiting period and to avoid high attrition rates after a six-month wait period.

**Program Outreach.** The large majority of Broward's program advocacy efforts consisted of presentations to various community groups to educate them about the program and gain support and referrals. In addition to the presentations, relationships were made with a few key judges at domestic violence court–sponsored events.

**Resources and Costs.** Broward County Safe Start did not provide information about program resources or costs for the purposes of our cost analysis.

## Summary

Family-Centered Treatment®, delivered through the Broward County Safe Start program, offered a different type of treatment than was available in Broward County for children exposed to violence and their families. Whereas many agencies offered concrete support and crisis intervention, the Safe Start program's in-home, intensive services augmented these other services, and many families were referred to the program, particularly by the Henderson Mental Health Clinic.

The Safe Start program built a local reputation for working with "difficult" families, and thus appeared to be a resource to some of the agencies working with families who had experienced domestic violence. This resulted in them implementing their full model with most families, offering the full four to six month program that combined stabilization, psychoeducation, and skill building, as well as their intensive services that attempt to improve family functioning. However, their approach, which includes the abuse perpetrator in the therapy at some points, was controversial with some agency partners and made some agencies wary about referring families into the program.

Successes of the program included steady referrals into the project and a positive reputation in the community overall. Challenges related to tracking these highly mobile families and establishing trust with community partners who were concerned about their work with perpetrators. As a program that has promise, the successful implementation of the program in this environment would allow the outcomes to be evaluated, to show whether this approach can be successful, and to what degree.

**Data collection for this program summary included:**

- Key informant interviews with key program staff and community partners
  - Program Director
  - Social workers
  - Supervisors and regional directors
  - Research Coordinator
  - Family that had been through the treatment program
  - Intake specialist at referral agency
  - IFCS Vice President
- Case review of randomly selected treatment and control group cases
- Review of online training program
- Quality assurance checklist completed by the clinical supervisor
- Quarterly activity reports on services, training, policies and advocacy
- Grant application
- Green Light notes
- *Safe Start: Promising Approaches Communities Working Together to Help Children Exposed to Violence* (Safe Start Center, 2008).

## 3. Chelsea Program Description

### Chelsea Safe Start

- **Intervention type:** Group therapy, home visits, and care coordination
- **Intervention length:** 3 months
- **Intervention setting:** Clinic and in-home
- **Target population:** Children who have been exposed to violence
- **Age range:** 0–17
- **Primary referral sources:** Mental health and pediatric units of the Chelsea Health Care Center, the Chelsea Police Department's Police Action Counseling Teams, the Harbor Area Department of Social Services, and public schools
- **Types of violence exposure:** Domestic violence, community violence.

### Program and Community Setting

The Chelsea Safe Start program is located in the city of Chelsea, Massachusetts, approximately two miles north of Boston. According to the 2000 Census, the city of Chelsea had a population of 35,000. Children younger than age 5 represented 8 percent of the total population. Fifty-eight percent of the population was white; 7 percent, black; 48 percent, Hispanic; slightly less than 5 percent, Asian; and less than 1 percent, Native American. Approximately 23 percent of the population indicated "Other" as their race on the 2000 Census. In 1999, the per capita income was $17,127,[5] and a little more than 23 percent of the population was living below the federal poverty line.[6]

Chelsea residents experience high poverty levels (more than twice the statewide average), low education levels, high rates of unemployment, and high crime. Violence-related injuries in Chelsea are six times the statewide rate at 160 per 100,000 (Massachusetts Department of Public Health, Bureau of Health Statistics Research and Evaluation, 2000). One study found that between 8 and 20 percent of high school students reported carrying a weapon on school grounds during the past month (Massachusetts General Hospital, 2004). In addition, child maltreatment rates in Chelsea appeared to be increasing at the time of the proposal.

The Chelsea Safe Start project was housed within the Massachusetts General Hospital Chelsea (MGH) Health Care Center. Intake data from MGH's domestic violence program found that 93 percent of all program clients had children; 30 percent of those had children younger than 6 years old, and 15 percent were pregnant at intake (Massachusetts General Hospital, 2004).

Prior to the Safe Start project, there were programs and organizations in Chelsea to help children and families stabilize after exposure to violence. The MGH Chelsea Health Care Center provided basic mental health services, such as individual counseling and family group counseling. Although the health care center occasionally offered group therapy, it was not a consistently one of the treatment options and did not follow a specific curriculum. There

[5] This is the 1999 per capita income reported in 2005 dollars; the 1999 per capita income as reported in the census is $14,628.

[6] Information is taken from the 2000 Census and can be found at the Census website (U.S. Census Bureau, no date).

were also existing partnerships between the Chelsea Police Department and the Harbor Area Department of Social Services to develop and implement programs, including

- Police Action Counseling Team (PACT) program—a team consisting of mental health clinicians and police officers who provide on scene responses to 911 calls involving domestic violence incidents in which children were exposed to violence
- Chelsea Children's Advocacy Team (CHAT) program—a mental health intervention aimed at meeting the clinical needs of children exposed to domestic violence through comprehensive mental health assessments, ongoing clinical services, and case management.

Despite these efforts, there were perceived gaps in services such as outreach, follow-up, and coordination of care for high-risk families. To address these needs, Chelsea designed its Safe Start program to provide a continuum of care that sought to identify, respond to, and refer children exposed to violence. With this approach, the program aimed to provide services that would lessen the impact of exposure to violence and promote healthy growth and development in children exposed to violence. The exposure was mainly to domestic violence, but exposure to community violence was also included in some cases.

### Chelsea Safe Start Partner Agencies

**MGH Chelsea Health Care Center.** The Chelsea Health Care Center is part of the Massachusetts General Hospital. Established in 1971, the center provides comprehensive primary, specialty, and urgent adult and pediatric health care, mental health services, and other social services, such as a food bank. To meet the needs of the large immigrant population, the center staff are fluent in 20 different languages. The center was the lead agency of the Safe Start project, and the center staff provided all Safe Start intervention services.

**Chelsea Police Department.** The Chelsea Police Department was established in 1857. The department works collaboratively with community-based programs in Chelsea to address youth and family issues. For example, the PACT program was established in 1998. PACT is a crisis-intervention team that responds with the police when there is domestic violence or child abuse and neglect. A school resource officer was assigned from the police department to the Safe Start program. The officer participated in Safe Start team meetings and made referrals to the program.

**Harbor Area Department of Social Services.** The Department of Social Services (DSS) is the state agency responsible for the safety and protection of child victims of abuse and neglect. The Harbor Area DSS office participated in the Safe Start multidisciplinary team meetings and referred clients to the Safe Start program.

The Safe Start program originally developed by Chelsea targeted children from birth to age 6 who had been exposed to violence. Chelsea's plan for outreach and care coordination had three main components: group therapy, home visits, and case coordination. Although these components were previously available at the Chelsea Health Center, Safe Start would strengthen and coordinate these services for children exposed to violence. The Chelsea Safe Start proposal to OJJDP outlined how the program would identify and assess children and families exposed to violence, develop comprehensive treatment plans, and provide individual, group, and family treatment. Chelsea designed the program to receive referrals internally from the obstetrics, pediatrics, mental health, and primary care units of the health care center as well as from a long list of external referral sources, including the police department, the DSS, and schools.

The Chelsea program was selected by OJJDP as one of 15 Safe Start sites across the country. After receiving the grant, Chelsea went through OJJDP's Green Light process to prepare for program implementation and evaluation. At the time, the Chelsea Safe Start program staff felt that there was a mismatch between what they applied for in their proposal and what emerged during the Green Light process, particularly around the relative intensity of the research component and the relationship between the research design and the treatment to be delivered under Safe Start. During the Green Light process, it proved challenging to educate clinical staff about the research-driven approach and relieve some anxieties about how the research component might affect clinical care. The clinicians were particularly concerned that the project might force decisions about provision of clinical care (i.e., sending clients to set of treatment options defined as the Safe Start intervention), rather than leaving that up to the clinician. The Safe Start program staff fostered buy-in by bringing the staff together for meetings and trainings. By involving their partners in the Green Light process, Chelsea was able to explain the research component and allow their partners to help design the programmatic details. For example, based on feedback from the clinicians about feeling uncomfortable excluding older children from treatment, Chelsea expanded the age range to include children up through age 17.

## Intervention

The Chelsea Safe Start intervention model included three main components: group therapy, home visits, and case coordination. The intervention period lasted approximately 12 weeks for the group therapy and up to one year for the case coordination. Home visits were used to conduct a onetime assessment of the family's situation. These visits were optional, occurring for families that requested them. The services were primarily provided at the clinic, except for the home visits, which were conducted at the family's home. To be eligible for Safe Start services, the child had to have been exposed to domestic or community violence. In addition, the child and parent/caregiver had to understand either English or Spanish and receive medical services from medical staff at MGH Chelsea.

### Therapy

The therapy component primarily involved group therapy models designed for different age groups, including Rainbow Dance for children from birth to age 3, Kids' Club for ages 4 to 6, Cool Youth for ages 8 to 12, and the Teen Group for ages 12 and up. Each of the group therapy programs focused on attachment, regulation, and competency, using trauma-informed interventions, techniques, and methods.

***Rainbow Dance.*** For children from birth to age 3, Chelsea used Macy's curriculum to work on parent-child development as well as mind-body connections (Macy, 2007; Macy et al., 2003). The model is based on the notion that there are body-based manifestations of trauma, so the curriculum focused on attachment and affect regulation. The model used music, movement, and storytelling for relaxation, attunement, and attachment. Because the participants usually entered the process stressed, the program started with movement and then worked on behavior expectations for children. The sessions were held weekly and there was no maximum or minimum numbers of sessions.

***Kids' Club.*** For children ages 4 to 6, Chelsea used a group curriculum developed for the Massachusetts DSS using best practices gathered from the literature (Cohen et al., 2005). The 12-session curriculum focused on feelings, safety, personal space, family structure, use of kind words, and problem-solving.

***Cool Youth.*** This group therapy for 8-to-11-year-olds used a 12-week interactive group therapy curriculum developed for the Massachusetts DSS (Northnode, 2007). The children and parents met at the same time but in separate groups. The curriculum for the children focused on violence exposure, with sessions on feelings, abuse, safety planning, family changes, substance abuse, solving conflicts, sexual abuse, and children's rights. The curriculum for the parent group focused on helping parents understand the children's experiences and symptoms. The curriculum was flexible to allow the parents to express what was currently occurring with the family.

***Teen Group.*** This group therapy for adolescents 12 to 17 years old was loosely based on the attachment, self-regulation, and competency (ARC) framework (Kinniburgh et al., 2005). With this model, the group worked toward improving affect and regulation. The therapists focused on helping the teens identify the things that drive their feelings and then understand their choices for handling them. There was also a concurrent parent group that was relatively unstructured. During the parent group, the therapist stressed talking with the teens about what happened and helping make them feel safer.

***Other therapy.*** Clinicians from the Mental Health Unit also provided individual, dyadic, and family therapy as needed. Based on the child's needs or strengths, the clinician chose an appropriate therapeutic approach based on a menu of options (e.g., psycho-education, ARC, relationship strengthening, social skills, and parent education). For the dyadic therapy, the clinicians used a blend of play therapy, cognitive behavioral techniques, elements of the ARC framework, and parent education, depending on the child and parent.

### Home Visits

For Safe Start families with children ages 0–7, the in-home assessment was conducted once for all families who wanted one by a Safe Start team member and additional staff from the clinical team as appropriate. The home visitor used a checklist adapted with permission from the Kaiser Family Foundation and the Harvard Center for Mental Health and Media. The checklist included sections on child supervision; environment/safety; and media, computer, and video games. The purpose of the assessment was to observe these areas and then to provide supports, such as advocacy, education, resources, and case management.

### Case Coordination

Case coordination was conducted by a multidisciplinary team that met weekly to discuss and review each family's progress. These meetings were attended by six social workers, a pediatrician from the health care center, a representative of a domestic violence advocacy group, and the psychologist who is the unit chief for the mental health unit. The multidisciplinary team developed a treatment plan based on the home visit, medical assessment, and evaluation assessment. The treatment plan specified which model of care each family and child would receive.

The case coordination involved helping families gain independence and self-sufficiency to take actions necessary for safety through communication, education, service facilitation and coordination, advocacy, and identification of and referrals to appropriate resources. The case coordination also involved monitoring service provision in terms of appropriateness, utility, and cost-effectiveness as well as coordinating among resource providers in areas such as mental and physical health, education, food and clothing, transportation, job training, safety, and law and criminal justice. Case coordination continued throughout the families' involvement in treatment up until the last assessment.

The intervention was conducted in the context of a rigorous outcome evaluation as required by OJJDP (see the box titled "Chelsea Safe Start Evaluation" for a description).

### Chelsea Safe Start Evaluation

**Design.** This uses a comparison group design.

**Treatment versus comparison group services.** In addition to receiving any services or supports from the referring agency, those who were assigned to the treatment group received group therapy, home visits, and care coordination. Those in the comparison group received only the services and supports they were already receiving from the health care center.

**Data collection.** Data were collected through longitudinal assessments of child-level outcomes.

**Enrollment.** The site originally planned to enroll 600 families over the four-year period (300 in each group). Funding ended prematurely for the National Evaluation. By the time it ended, enrollment had taken place over two years and seven months and resulted in 71 in the treatment group and 11 in the comparison group.

## Implementation

Figure B.3 provides a diagram to show Chelsea's implementation of their intervention. The following description of the program implementation is the result of data collected for the national evaluation. See Appendix A for a full discussion of the data collection methodology employed at each of the Safe Start sites.

### Referrals

When Safe Start began in 2006, Chelsea envisioned that the program would receive referrals from a long list of agencies and community organizations in addition to internal referrals from obstetrics, pediatrics, the mental health unit, primary care, and the community health team. In practice, most of the referrals were from the mental health and pediatric units of the health care center, with the bulk of them from pediatricians. Safe Start program staff indicated that the families were more comfortable talking to their pediatrician, whom they saw more regularly, and were more receptive to a referral related to violence exposure in that setting. Further, the state began to require that all well-child visits include a symptom checklist for mental health and behavioral issues. These checklists allowed providers to detect violence exposure more often and also to understand the impact on child mental health over time. Other internal referrals came from individual clinicians in the mental health unit who were treating mothers with issues related to violence.

**Figure B.3**
**Model of Chelsea Safe Start**

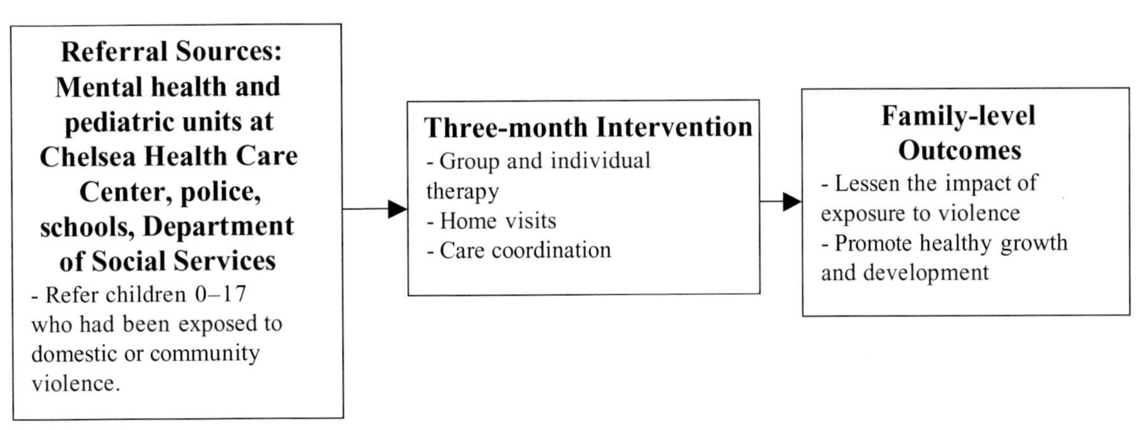


RAND *TR750-B.3*

These internal referrals were further facilitated by the strong relationships that Safe Start program staff had with staff in the other units of the health care center. From the beginning, the program staff also included a pediatrician on the multidisciplinary team that met weekly to discuss families. This helped strengthen the relationship between the pediatric unit and the mental health unit in particular. The participating pediatrician reported that his involvement with Safe Start helped him understand the role of the mental health unit in the health care center, and he shared information about Safe Start and the mental health unit with the rest of his department.

Chelsea did receive some referrals from outside of the health care center, including from the Chelsea Police Department's Police Action Counseling Team, local schools, the DSS, and Harbor Communities Overcoming Violence. Regardless of the external referral source, the child's primary care physician at the health care center had to make a referral as well. The PACT made referrals when it responded to a call involving a child exposed to violence and the family was receptive to being referred. The parents of many of the DSS referrals had already sought care at the health care center. In these cases, the referral specified Safe Start as the Department's recommended service provider.

To encourage referrals from external sources, program staff convened monthly family violence meetings for community agencies. The community partners reported that these meetings helped increase their understanding of each other's roles, helped build trust among the agencies, and helped the agencies gain comfort working with one another. The meetings provided an opportunity for each agency to describe its role and culture and the services it offered for families with children exposed to violence. The monthly family violence meetings also provided an opportunity to discuss specific cases and determine what could be done by the participating agencies.

In the beginning of implementation, the referrals were received by different staff members in the health care center. The Safe Start program staff soon learned that the referrals did not always make it to the program because of the decentralized process. Chelsea consolidated the process so that all of the referrals for violence exposure flowed through the mental health unit intake coordinator. The coordinator screened the cases to confirm their eligibility and then contacted the Safe Start program staff with the referral. The referral was then discussed at the weekly multidisciplinary team meeting and assigned to a clinician to make the first contact with the family.

For this initial contact between the assigned clinician and the parent, the clinicians asked the parent to come in alone to discuss the situation in a one-hour meeting. The clinician then spent time with the child in a separate visit that typically lasted 30 minutes. After these meetings, the clinician decided on an appropriate treatment plan, depending on the unique circumstances with the family.

Normally, the clinician introduced Safe Start to the family after these initial meetings, but this was altered if the family was under stress, including needing safe housing or immediate medical help. Chelsea program staff reported that most of the children were referred for exposure to domestic violence, with very few related to child abuse, neglect, or community violence. It often took a few visits to resolve safety, housing, or other issues and begin to discuss mental health needs and possible participation in Safe Start. Chelsea reported that it was not able to introduce the Safe Start program to some families because families were dealing with safety (from perpetrator) or immediate housing issues. After the initial meetings, the Safe Start program coordinator introduced Safe Start to the family, obtained consent, and completed the baseline assessment.

The clinicians found that, although it was difficult to get the families enrolled, families often wanted to stay in treatment once they started, and it was sometimes difficult for the clinicians to end services. Clinicians shared that families became very attached to them and the services and were reluctant to end a relationship that was considered safe and nurturing.

### Services

Table B.3 summarizes average quarterly caseloads for Safe Start program staff and service delivery for those who received services through the Chelsea Safe Start program. Chelsea had 4–6 clinicians providing therapy during the first year of implementation. During Year 2, the program had 8–13 therapists providing services. In the third year of implementation, 7–10 therapists delivered services (through March 2009).

**Table B.3**
**Service Delivery for Enrollees in the Chelsea Safe Start Intervention**

| | Year 1 | Year 2 | Year 3 (7 mos) |
|---|---|---|---|
| Average quarterly caseload per therapist | 2.5 | 2.7 | 6.4 |
| Total number of home visits | 13 | 34 | 2 |
| Total number of group therapy sessions for parents | 42 | 42 | 26 |
| Total number of group therapy sessions for parents and children (Rainbow Dance, Kid's Club) | 13 | 22 | 20 |
| Total number of group therapy sessions for youth (Cool Youth) | 26 | 30 | 22 |
| Total number of group therapy sessions for adolescents (Teen Group) | 9 | 45 | 11 |
| Total number of individual therapy sessions | 89 | 168 | 54 |
| Total number of joint therapy sessions | 34 | 40 | 8 |
| Total number of family therapy sessions | 0 | 7 | 10 |
| Total number of case management meetings | 25 | 69 | 11 |

### *Therapy*

Families involved with the Chelsea Safe Start program varied in their readiness for treatment. According to the clinicians, if the referral came from a pediatrician who identified violence exposure during a routine medical exam, families were less often ready to engage in treatment. However, if the family was referred to Safe Start during a visit to the mental health unit, then they were more often prepared to begin therapy. The clinicians found that therapy required having a parent who really wanted to start mental health services. If this was not the case, patients tended to come to the health care center for other services and supports but not therapy.

Chelsea's efforts to engage families in treatment capitalized on its presence in the community and long-standing relationships with many of the families. Because most of their referrals came internally, families were already familiar and comfortable with receiving services at the health care center. Chelsea Safe Start provided basic supports to families, including taxi fare and food. Chelsea also worked to maintain families' engagement in the therapy sessions by hosting dinners and open houses. These were generally well attended. According to the program staff, they worked to create a warm atmosphere at these functions, where the parents and children could interact with the clinicians, group leaders, project director, and clinic director.

Despite efforts to engage families, Chelsea found that it was difficult for families to come to the clinic for therapy even when they lived close by. According to program staff, the mobility or transience of the population made retention an issue. The families usually returned to the health care center when they were in need of health services again, but maintaining steady engagement for therapy was challenging. Chelsea also struggled with cultural issues around the stigma of mental health. For example, many of their clients belonged to racial/ethnic minority groups (e.g., Latino) who were concerned about seeking mental health services and thought it was a sign of weakness or brought shame to the family.

Chelsea's approach to the therapy component of the intervention was open-ended. The clinicians reported that the families cycled in and out as needed, depending on what was happening in their lives. Although there was a lot of interest in the group therapy, the schedule sometimes made it difficult for families to attend. In some cases, the children would come and the parents would not.

For the group therapy sessions, children were placed in the different groups, depending on their developmental functioning. Although there were age ranges for each group, the clinician made the determination about which group was most appropriate after assessing the child. The Safe Start clinicians reported that they had usually seen the families who were assigned to their group in the clinic before the first group session. However, if the family was seen by another clinician, then they might not have met before the first group session.

- The Rainbow Dance group (birth to age 3) was scheduled weekly on a continuous basis. When the sequence of songs and movements in the curriculum was completed, they would start up again. If there were more than three families at any one session, then two clinicians led the group. The clinicians found that families typically came in spurts, when it was convenient. With each session, Chelsea responded to the parental needs by providing activities for the parent and child (and siblings) that would encourage bonding and allow the parent to focus attention on the child.

- The Kids' Club group for 4-to-6-year-olds was also dyadic, with parent-child pairs but no siblings participating in the 12-week program. Each one-hour session built on the last and involved snacks, songs, opening and closing routines, and a curriculum that focused on safety and helping children feel good about themselves. The curriculum was followed loosely, but the group was flexible to allow for children to express their concerns.
- For the Cool Kids group, one clinician conducted the group with the children while another clinician met separately with the parents. Chelsea started this group at the beginning of the school year and completed 12 weekly 90-minute sessions. In January of the school year, they formed a second group. In the simultaneous parent group, the clinicians focused on how to talk to the children about the violent event(s) that they experienced and how to make the children feel safer. If parents reported using corporal punishment at home, the clinicians tried to work with them to shift to other methods of discipline.
- Depending on the mix of adolescents, the clinicians would conduct up to four simultaneous groups: (1) teen girls, (2) teen boys, (3) teen boys with behavior issues, and (4) parents. The clinicians chose a theme for each session and then selected from a menu of activities. The curriculum for the teen group was more open, so the clinicians could meet the needs of the group. Sometimes they adjusted the curriculum based on the need and requests of the teens, such as when a teen missed a prior group. Girls' groups focused on self-esteem, partner violence, mind and body, and identity. Boys' groups concentrated on interacting with others and anger management. The optional parent groups were offered only if there was demand for them. When they were offered, parent groups focused on self-care, relaxation, and developmental and trauma awareness.

Clinicians also provided dyadic and individual therapy as needed within the Safe Start program. Staff reported that dyadic therapy was typically used for younger children but was also used with adolescents. For the dyadic therapy, there was not a set curriculum; the therapeutic technique depended on the child. The clinicians reported that the dyadic work took a family-systems approach that focused on problem-solving for concrete situations such as physical health, shelter, and food. Once the basic needs were addressed, the clinician would move on to help the family understand trauma symptoms using ARC principles. The individual therapy also varied, depending on the diagnosis and symptoms. According to the clinicians, about half of the parents received monthly individual therapy. The teens also received individual therapy as needed.

#### *Home Visits*

Chelsea Safe Start program staff conducted home visits for most or all of the families enrolled in Safe Start. Usually, the home visit took place about four to six weeks after the baseline assessment. Home visits were used for assessment rather than treatment. The home visits involved the Safe Start project director and a clinician as appropriate. The home visit entailed an assessment of the child's home life, including safety issues (e.g., guns in the home), environment (e.g., household cleanliness), media exposure (e.g., television content with violence), and child supervision (who is responsible for monitoring and when).

#### *Case Coordination*

Case coordination began with case management. The mental health unit had two case managers (one for adults and one for children). The Chelsea Safe Start program also had a case manager, but this position was not filled consistently throughout implementation. Clinicians also did a lot of case management as needed, including services coordination with schools, in-home services, the DSS social worker, and the pediatrician.

The multidisciplinary team, which included social workers, a pediatrician, a psychologist, and a representative of a domestic violence advocacy group, met weekly to discuss the families. They started by reviewing new referrals to Safe Start and determining who would work with the family, taking into consideration which clinician knew the family or worked with a parent or sibling. According to the clinicians, assigning families during the weekly meeting meant reduced wait time for services for the Safe Start families because the clinicians could determine their docket of cases and how families would fit in the priority queue. This approach avoided the potential delays associated with obtaining data through other administrative methods. After assigning the referrals, the team reviewed ongoing cases. The number of cases reviewed each week varied, depending on the current needs of the families. The Chelsea Safe Start program staff considered the meetings to be very important, since meetings allowed them to collectively discuss the families that were facing the most difficult issues. For each family, the multidisciplinary team would start by determining what service mix was necessary to stabilize the family. The clinician assigned to the family then developed a treatment plan that included all of the services needed. The treatment plan was usually prepared for the parent and target child, although siblings were sometimes included. The clinician updated the treatment plan every 90 days.

According to Chelsea's Safe Start program staff, the involvement of the pediatrician on the multidisciplinary team was unique. Before Safe Start, there was no mechanism for coordinating mental health referrals with a primary care pediatrician. With Safe Start, there was intensive communication about what was happening with the child through the weekly multidisciplinary team meetings. The pediatrician would provide medical consultation during the meeting but also assessed the training needs among pediatric staff at the health center, organized the appropriate trainings, communicated key issues about Safe Start children to pediatric colleagues, and acted as liaison between Safe Start and MGH/Chelsea. In this way, the pediatrician was part of the Safe Start team and interacted with the mental health unit to create a strong linkage between the two parts of the health care center.

Families that needed services after two years were able to access services. For Chelsea program staff, the long-term relationship meant they were able to see the families mature and develop a set of coping skills.

There were other components of the Chelsea Safe Start program that helped shape the implementation (see the box titled "Chelsea Safe Start Additional Program Components").

### Chelsea Safe Start Additional Program Components

**Quality Assurance.** Chelsea Safe Start therapists had prior training and experience in group and individual interventions with children from birth to age 17 and their families. The site's ongoing training efforts included annual teaching on ARC principles using case examples. New therapists were trained on the group therapy models prior to conducting any groups. The therapists also had access to any relevant manuals or materials related to the group therapy options and ARC. Clinical supervision was provided through weekly Children Exposed to Violence team meetings, peer supervision meetings, and team consultation meetings. Adherence to the program models was monitored via quarterly treatment plans, with measurable outcomes for each case.

### Chelsea Safe Start Additional Program Components (continued)

**Training.** In the first two years of the program, Chelsea Safe Start conducted and/or participated in 36 trainings. These trainings mostly focused on the provision of clinical care (50%), child welfare issues (14%), and referral processes (11%). Session topics included the ARC framework, family violence, and issues around immigrant mental health and human trafficking.

**Policies and Protocols.** The Chelsea Safe Start program developed or revised policies to improve their overall efficiency and delivery of services. Specifically, Chelsea created an email distribution list for Safe Start clinical team members and the Department of Social Services staff and supervisors; changed protocols so that when a Massachusetts Department of Social Services Child Abuse/Neglect Report was filed, MGH/Chelsea Security was notified if there were any concerns that the situation might warrant their involvement; established a service delivery process for the HAVEN program, which consisted of on-call MGH domestic violence advocates; and developed a new procedure for when a medical evaluation was needed immediately for a child removed from their home.

**Program Outreach.** The Chelsea Safe Start program gave a number of presentations to various community groups to discuss the Safe Start program, gain support, and initiate collaboration or a partnership.

**Resources and Costs.** Chelsea Safe Start did not provide information about program resources or costs for the purposes of our cost analysis.

## Summary

Although the Chelsea Health Care Center treated children exposed to violence prior to Safe Start, there was limited coordination and structure to the services. With Safe Start, it appears that Chelsea was able to improve communication both internally and with community agency partners to provide more coordinated care for children exposed to violence. With their weekly multidisciplinary team meetings focused on children exposed to violence, Chelsea strengthened relationships between the mental health and pediatric units of the health care center. The meetings provided an opportunity to share information, discuss treatment strategies, and plan next steps for specific families. Further, families who were referred to the program from outside the health care center had faster entry into care at the Chelsea health care center. Since the team would discuss these families and develop a treatment plan, the families did not have to go on waiting lists for services.

Safe Start program staff also reported that Safe Start allowed them to expand and formalize their group therapy options in response to the needs of the families. Prior to Safe Start, it was more difficult to provide group therapy because of a lack of staff and resources. With Safe Start, Chelsea developed a team of clinicians trained and available to provide group therapy. The group therapy curriculum is also more standardized now.

The Chelsea Safe Start program experienced some challenges engaging and retaining families with children exposed to violence. Despite offering food and other basic supports, the families referred to Safe Start often did not fully engage in the program. The stress of their lives, including issues of economic and housing stability, made it difficult for them to consistently engage in the Safe Start program. They cycled in and out services, which made it difficult to provide the complete intervention model.

**Data collection for this program summary included:**

- Key informant interviews with key program staff and community partners:
  - Safe Start project director
  - Safe Start program manager
  - Safe Start therapists
  - Chelsea Health Care Center pediatrician
  - Massachusetts General Hospital Community Benefits Office staff
  - Chelsea Police Department staff
- Tour of the Chelsea community and Chelsea Health Care Center
- Observation of two group therapy sessions and a recruitment open house
- Case review of randomly selected treatment group cases
- Quality assurance checklist completed by the project director
- Quarterly activity reports on services, training, policies, and advocacy
- Grant application
- Green Light notes
- *Safe Start: Promising Approaches Communities Working Together to Help Children Exposed to Violence* (Safe Start Center, 2008)
- Home visit protocol, treatment plan template, group therapy curriculum materials.

# 4. Dallas Program Description

## Dallas Safe Start

- **Intervention type:** Project SUPPORT intervention, including therapy, case management, and child mentorship
- **Intervention length:** 6 months
- **Intervention setting:** In-home
- **Target population:** Children exposed to domestic violence exiting domestic violence shelters with their mothers
- **Age range:** 3–9
- **Primary referral source:** Three domestic violence shelters

## Program and Community Setting

The Dallas Safe Start program was located in Dallas County, Texas, and functioned within Dallas County. As of the 2000 Census, the population in the county was approximately 2.2 million; 58 percent of which was white; 20 percent, black; 30 percent, Hispanic; with the remainder consisting of other racial and ethnic groups. Of the total population, 8.2 percent were younger than 5. The 2000 U.S. Census also reported that Dallas County per capita income was $26,465,[7] with about 13.5 percent of the population living below the poverty line.

In 2004, the year the Dallas Safe Start program was proposed, there were 182,087 incidents of family violence in Texas. During that same period, 11,983 adults and 17,619 children were housed in domestic violence shelters. Nonresidential services were provided to 36,858 adults and 16,203 children in the state (Texas Council on Family Violence, 2006). In Dallas County, approximately 1,500 adults and 1,200 children were provided residential domestic violence shelter in 2003 (Southern Methodist University, 2004).

Although Dallas-area domestic violence shelters provided counseling and case management services, these services were often brief in duration (e.g., the average stay at The Family Place shelter was 22 days) and delivered during a difficult period of transition, often characterized by considerable confusion and uncertainty for both mother and children (Southern Methodist University, 2004). Dallas-area shelters also offered continuing counseling and support services following shelter exits, but mothers with children faced multiple barriers to accessing these and other community-based services. Barriers such as a lack of transportation (particularly transportation manageable with several young children), work schedule conflicts, and lack of child care were among those cited as typical in the Dallas area. Indeed, these barriers to services were typical of those faced by mothers across the state seeking to obtain mental health and support services for their children after their shelter exit (Jouriles et al., 2001).

The Dallas Safe Start project was initiated with the goal of helping to fill a gap in mental health services for children exposed to domestic violence. For two key reasons, the project partners focused on providing these services specifically to children exiting shelters with their mothers. First, this is a population most at risk for mental health problems related to domestic violence (Jouriles et al., 2001). Second, existing mental health services were limited and difficult to access for families exiting domestic violence shelters in the Dallas area.

---

[7] $26,465 is the 1999 per capita income in 2005 dollars. The 1999 per capita income was $22,603.

In this context, the development of the Dallas Safe Start program built on an existing research partnership between Southern Methodist University (SMU) researchers and The Family Place domestic violence shelter. Their prior research collaboration studied aggression among children exposed to domestic violence who had resided in The Family Place shelter. The OJJDP solicitation for the Safe Start program offered the opportunity for the partners to expand their activities to include testing the effectiveness of an intervention for these children. The partners recruited the Genesis Women's Shelter to join the effort prior to the award of the Safe Start grant. A summary of the Dallas Safe Start partners is provided in the box titled "Dallas Safe Start Partner Agencies."

Like the other Safe Start programs, the Dallas Safe Start partners received notice of their selection by OJJDP in August 2005 and commenced preparations for implementation by following the steps of the initiative's Green Light process. In this process, in collaboration with OJJDP and RAND, the program expanded its eligibility criteria, at the request of OJJDP, to include mothers who after exiting the shelter return to live in a home with a domestic violence perpetrator. Previously, eligibility required mothers to reside separately from a violent partner, primarily because of safety concerns. Safety protocols were reviewed and enhanced as a result of this change.

### Dallas Safe Start Partner Agencies

**Department of Psychology, Southern Methodist University.** Southern Methodist University (SMU) is a private university in Dallas, Texas. Its Department of Psychology houses the developers of Project SUPPORT, the intervention implemented in the Dallas Safe Start program. Department of Psychology faculty engage in both teaching and research activities in the Dallas community. Doctoral students in SMU's Department of Psychology provide mental health services to clients in a variety of settings under the clinical supervision of its teaching and research faculty. This is the lead agency in the Safe Start program.

**The Family Place.** The Family Place is the largest domestic violence service provider agency serving the Dallas area. It is a nonprofit organization providing emergency shelter, crisis counseling, transitional housing, supervised visitation services, victim advocacy, and case management services to adult female victims of domestic violence and their children.

**Genesis Women's Shelter.** Genesis Women's Shelter is a nonprofit domestic violence service provider organization offering both residential and nonresidential services in the Dallas area. Residential and transitional housing services are available for women and children seeking shelter due to domestic violence. Nonresidential services include crisis and group counseling, community referrals, parenting classes, and child and adolescent therapy.

**Salvation Army Family Violence Program.** This program within the Salvation Army nonprofit charitable organization provides residential shelter services, including counseling and referral, to adult women domestic violence victims and their children in the Dallas area.

## Intervention

The invention provided by the Dallas Safe Start program was entitled Project SUPPORT. It was originally developed and evaluated by the SMU partners in the Safe Start program. Project

SUPPORT was designed for use with children who exhibit clinical levels of conduct problems upon exit from domestic violence shelters with their mothers. The intervention was developed to address children's mental health problems related to domestic violence exposure, particularly conduct problems and symptoms of depression and trauma. Indications from early evaluations of the model showed promise for improving symptoms among children ages 4 to 9 exiting domestic violence shelters in the Houston, Texas, area (Jouriles et al., 2001; McDonald et al., 2006).

Project Support was a home-based intervention involving a two-person team: a therapist and a child mentor. The intervention was intended to begin as soon as feasible after the shelter stay and to consist of 24 weekly one-hour sessions provided over a maximum of six months. The home-based delivery of the intervention was intended to remove transportation as a barrier to services, the hardship of which is particularly significant for mothers of several young children who rely on public transportation. Moreover, clients were expected to feel more comfortable in a home-based setting and to be afforded the opportunity to practice skills in their real-life setting, all of which the program expected would increase the effectiveness of the intervention.

### Therapy

The therapeutic intervention sessions delivered by the therapist combined case management (referred to in the model as "social and instrumental support") and parent training for mothers in nurturing and child behavior management skills. Both of these components were provided by a single therapist within the context of weekly treatment sessions of 60–90 minutes in length. The therapists were doctoral-level graduate students in the SMU Department of Psychology, working under the supervision of the Safe Start project leader.

The nurturing and child behavior management skill components of the intervention sessions employed a behavior training model that involved assessing mothers' current knowledge and skills and providing education and training to enhance a specific skill set. As cited in the program's "Child Behavior and Management Skills" training manual, the following 11 skills were taught to the parents:

1. Listening
2. Comforting
3. Praise and Positive Attention
4. Directives
5. Rewards and Privileges
6. Reprimands and Redirecting
7. Ignoring
8. Rule Setting
9. Time Out
10. Withdrawing Rewards and Privileges
11. Marking Time Out.

The skill training involved therapist and parent role-play and therapist coaching of parents during observed parent-child interaction. Targeted skills were introduced progressively, and work on each skill continued until parents demonstrated its mastery.

Project SUPPORT also directed its therapists to devote some share of each session to case management–type activities. Thus, therapists were trained to work with clients to ensure that the family's basic needs were being met. This may have involved assisting with obtaining such needs as food, clothing, legal assistance and advocacy, rental assistance, child care, transportation, employment assistance, health care, and utilities assistance. Therapists were trained to both make referrals and assist clients with accessing these services to whatever extent needed by the client. Project SUPPORT builds case management in as a central component based on the evidence that families are less likely to benefit from therapy if their basic needs go unmet (McDonald et al., 2006).

#### Child Mentors

Project SUPPORT also included "child mentors." These were staff who went with therapists to each home-based session, for the purpose of entertaining and working with any children present in the home while their mother was engaged in a session. In advance of the home visit, the child mentors were expected to plan and prepare interesting and age-appropriate activities that they would engage in with the children while the mother was working individually with the therapist. Also, mentors were charged with establishing positive, supportive relationships with the children by using praise and providing positive attention and generally entertaining them while their mother was engaged with the therapist. This served the function of reducing the sources of parental distraction that can be problematic within a home-based setting. The child mentor component was not expected to produce its own outcomes (such as reduce child conduct problems). Instead, it was intended to help constructively entertain children so that mothers could fully engage in the therapy sessions.

The intervention was conducted in the context of a rigorous outcome evaluation as required by OJJDP (see the box titled "Dallas Safe Start Evaluation" for a description).

### Dallas Safe Start Evaluation

**Design.** The study design was randomized controlled effectiveness.

**Treatment versus control group services.** Families randomly assigned to the treatment group received home-based case management and skill-based family therapy provided by a therapist, accompanied by a child mentor. Those in the control group received monthly contacts from Safe Start program staff providing referrals to community resources and assistance with accessing these services.

**Data collection.** Data were collected through longitudinal assessments of child-level outcomes.

**Enrollment.** The site originally planned to enroll 160 families over the study period (80 per group). Funding ended prematurely for the National Evaluation. By the time it ended, enrollment had taken place over two years and eight months and resulted in 31 families in the treatment group and 37 in the control group.

## Implementation

Figure B.4 diagrams the implementation of the Dallas Safe Start intervention. The Dallas Safe Start program received Green Light approval from OJJDP to begin implementation in June 2006, and services began for treatment group clients in October 2006. The following description of the program implementation is the result of data collected for the national evaluation. See Appendix A for a full discussion of the data collection methodology employed at each of the Safe Start sites.

**Figure B.4**
**Model of Dallas Safe Start**

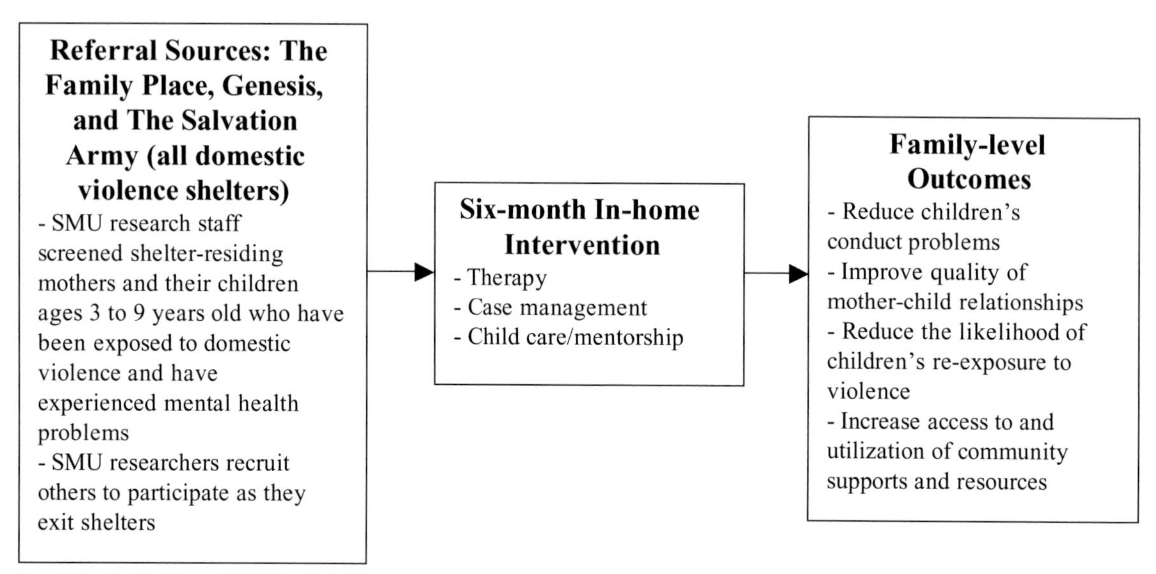


RAND *TR750-B.4*

## Referrals

Referrals to the Safe Start project came exclusively from within the three participating domestic violence shelters. The Safe Start program initially began with the involvement of two referring domestic violence shelters. About six months after services began, as part of an effort to increase enrollment, the Salvation Army Family Violence Program became the third domestic violence shelter recruited to join the Safe Start partnership.

Staff at all shelters provided access for SMU research staff to identify and attempt to recruit potentially eligible families, but staff were not actively involved in making referrals. At the time of its initial implementation, the eligibility criteria for the Dallas Safe Start program specified mothers who

- had sought shelter because of physical relationship violence and had reported at least one incident of physical violence directed toward them by an intimate partner during the previous six months
- had at least one child living with them between 3 and 6 years of age and moved no further than 25 miles from the participating shelter upon shelter exit
- had at least one child in the target age range who had been exposed to domestic violence and was determined to be experiencing elevated levels of mental health problems
- were not actively psychotic or experiencing severe drug or alcohol problems, and the target child was not identified as having a pervasive developmental disorder or mental retardation
- spoke and understood English well enough to participate in therapy sessions and research interviews conducted in English.

The process of identifying eligible families began with SMU researchers regularly reviewing lists of shelter admissions, looking for children in the target age. When such families were identified, SMU research staff would locate the mother within the shelter to introduce her to the opportunity to have her child screened for participation in the Safe Start program. Children of consenting mothers were then assessed for psychological adjustment using the Child Behavior Checklist (CBCL; Achenbach, 1991). Those children who showed elevated levels of internalizing or externalizing adjustment problems (defined as a CBCL score of 60 or higher) were deemed appropriate for Project SUPPORT services and therefore were eligible for the study. SMU researchers also confirmed eligibility on the remaining criteria and remained in regular contact with eligible families until the time of their shelter departure.

After families departed from the shelter, SMU researchers contacted them to arrange for the first research assessment, reconfirm eligibility criteria, and undertake the process of officially enrolling the family in the study. At the completion of this baseline assessment, eligible families were then randomly assigned to the treatment group (receiving the Project Support intervention) or to the control group.

The control group received monthly contacts from SMU research staff offering case management services. These consisted of offering to assist families to locate and connect with providers offering services to meet basic needs, such as food, clothing, housing, and legal assistance. For control group families facing particular difficulty, SMU research staff made collateral contacts with service provider agencies and provided transportation to critical services, such as food bank distribution centers.

Despite the SMU researchers' prior experience with implementing Project SUPPORT in a research-based context, the pace of recruitment of families into the Dallas Safe Start project was much slower than expected. To help address this challenge, three months after implementation, the Dallas Safe Start project obtained permission from OJJDP to expand its target age range from ages 3–6 to ages 3–9. Following this change, recruitment continued to lag behind projections. Thus, about 17 months after implementation, the program obtained permission from OJJDP to expand recruitment beyond those receiving shelter services to include families utilizing the nonresidential services (such as support groups and legal assistance services) of The Family Place domestic violence organization. All other eligibility criteria remained the same. Also, as previously discussed, a third shelter was added to the recruitment pool in an effort to increase enrollment.

During our process evaluation, we gathered information about the reasons for the slower-than-anticipated pace of recruitment. One reason cited by program staff was that the life circumstances of the families in the program's target population were characterized by high levels of stress and extreme hardship, such as poverty, housing instability, lack of transportation, unemployment, health care needs, inconsistent access to food, and a host of other difficulties. These severe life difficulties were not eliminated when mothers with young children took refuge from domestic violence during a temporary shelter stay. Thus, program staff reported the overwhelming nature of the difficulties faced by this population and how these problems discouraged the mothers from consenting to participate in an intervention program, even when that intervention promised to help improve the families' life circumstances. The research context of the intervention added an additional layer of challenge to recruitment, in that eligible families could not be told in advance exactly what type of intervention they would receive. Program staff thought that the uncertainty of group assignment may have been a factor in discouraging participation for some families.

Safe Start program staff also indicated that the process of screening for eligibility using the CBCL was time consuming (approximately 30–45 minutes) and thus discouraged participation among some mothers. Our interviewees also reported that, on occasion, one shelter resident's negative view of participation would discourage other shelter residents from agreeing to participate. This problem was viewed as relatively short lived, however, due to the relatively high turnover among shelter residents.

### Services

Table B.4 summarizes service delivery for those who received services through the Dallas Safe Start program. Dallas had from one to five doctoral-level graduate students serving as therapists at any one time during the project. Each therapist typically had one case. Together, the therapists conducted a total of 75 family therapy sessions in Year 1, 58 in Year 2, and 15 in Year 3 (through March 2009). Because the intervention was designed to provide both mental health and case management services within these sessions, the program further documented the amount of time in each session spent on each component. Specifically, in Year 1, the therapists delivered 20 sessions (or 27% of the 75 total sessions) in which more than half of the time was spent focused on case management-type activities. In Year 2, 14 (24%) of the 58 total sessions were focused mostly on case management. During the third year of implementation, six (40%) of the 15 total sessions focused primarily on case management. Sessions in which time was divided equally between mental health and case management activities numbered 30 (40%) in Year 1, 9 (15%) in Year 2, and 0 in Year 3. Sessions in which more than half of the time was spent focusing on mental health issues numbered 25 (33%) in Year 1, 35 (60%) in Year 2, and 9 (60%) in Year 3. The differences between the implementation years in session time allocation are discussed in a subsequent section.

In coordination with the therapy sessions, the Safe Start program staff provided a total of 74 mentorship/child care sessions in Year 1, 47 in Year 2, and 13 in year 3.

### Therapy

According to the Safe Start project leadership, it appeared that the therapy sessions were delivered generally as the model was intended. However, modifications were made to the program to address challenges that emerged in implementation. Key among these changes was an alteration to formalize the amount of time spent by therapists in each therapy session on the case management and skills training components. The model was initially designed with a great degree of flexibility in each session, allowing therapists to first attend to case management needs, which for clients were often seen as the most pressing needs. It became clear that the high level of basic needs for many clients meant that many of the initial sessions were spent mostly or entirely on case management, leaving little time to move on to the mental health

**Table B.4**
**Service Delivery for Enrollees in the Dallas Safe Start Intervention**

| | Year 1 | Year 2 | Year 3 (8 mos) |
|---|---|---|---|
| Average active quarterly caseload per therapist | 1.1 | 1.0 | 1 |
| Total number of family therapy sessions | 75 | 58 | 15 |
| • Number of these sessions consisting mostly of case management | 20 (27%) | 14 (24%) | 6 (40%) |
| • Number of these sessions consisting equally of mental health therapy and case management | 30 (40%) | 9 (15%) | 0 |
| • Number of these sessions consisting mostly of mental health therapy | 25 (33%) | 35 (60%) | 9 (60%) |
| Total number of mentorship/child care sessions | 74 | 47 | 13 |
| Total number of motivational interviewing sessions | 6 | — | — |

component. Some of the therapists reported that, at the end of the six-month intervention, some clients simply "ran out of time" to work on mastering the list of targeted skills because so many sessions had been consumed by case management activities. In addition, the therapists found that some clients had difficulties making the transition to working with their therapists on issues of parent-child interaction in later sessions after having spent numerous early sessions working with their therapists to obtain food stamps, housing assistance, affordable child care access, legal assistance with child custody issues, and the like.

To address these challenges, in the first year of implementation, the decision was made to allocate the session time between the two major activities more evenly. Specifically, starting with the first session, no more than half of every session should be allocated to case management activities. As Table B.4 shows, in the data reported by the program, the distribution of time devoted to each activity did appear to shift toward sessions spent mostly focused on mental health (33% in Year 1 versus 60% in Years 2 and 3). The therapists indicated that this was a positive modification to the program. They viewed it as a good way to balance the importance of helping clients meet their basic needs for stability and safety, while making it actually possible to complete the skills training component of Project SUPPORT within the six-month intervention window.

The change in session time allocation to allow for more focus on mental health issues, however, did not lessen the intervention's intention to help ensure that their client's basic needs were being met. Because of the extreme difficulty of the families' daily circumstances (lack of affordable housing, access to food and clothing, access to health care, etc.), program staff reported that involvement in the work was extremely emotionally and time intensive. Thus, program supervisors needed to be very attentive to the issue of staff burnout. Supervisors within the program reported a need to constantly monitor staff for morale and signs of compassion fatigue.

One reported challenge was the difficulty in determining the most appropriate and effective method of engaging fathers in the intervention, when they were present. The program therapists reported that this occurred only in two cases (at the time of our interviews) but had raised issues in terms of safety concerns and issues of determining "who the client is" when conflicts arose between parents. The model had not initially been designed to include potentially abusive fathers, and thus the program was in the process of gaining experience on which to base future protocols. In the two cases handled to date, the therapists reported working very closely with their supervisors and Project SUPPORT model developer, Renee McDonald, to address their unique issues on a case-by-case basis.

Another challenge raised by the program therapists was that of racial and cultural differences between the therapists (all or mostly white) and the clients (mostly non-white) that sometimes presented challenges. Therapists reported that they sometimes had to devote extra attention to overcoming the distrust of clients who may have experienced race-based mistreatment in the past. The therapists said that the difficulty was sometimes compounded when the broader family or social circle of the client were also distrusting of a white therapist, which sometimes led to their lack of support for the client's participation in the program. Thus, therapists reported needing to be aware of the potential for race- and culture-based dynamics in intervention sessions and to work to overcome these barriers by building rapport and trust overtime.

Finally, during the initial Green Light process, the Dallas Safe Start program elected to add a motivational interviewing component to the intervention, as an effort to maximize the research-based information that might be gleaned from the program. Motivational interviewing refers to a brief method of counseling that attempts to increase client motivation and engagement in therapy (Gance-Cleveland, 2007). The intent was to conduct a substudy of the efficacy of motivational interviewing in this population by randomly assigning half of the treatment group to receive motivational interviewing as part of the first session of the planned intervention. The remaining half of the treatment group would receive the planned intervention without this component. In practice, the motivational interviewing technique was used in only six cases before the program discontinued its use. The program staff reported that it proved to be unnecessary in each of the six cases where it had been used. This, combined with the lower-than-expected enrollment in the study overall, led the program leadership to anticipate little benefit for continuing the use of motivational interviewing in this context.

#### *Child Mentoring*

According to the Safe Start project team leadership, the child mentors served the important function of entertaining children during the home-based therapy sessions. The child mentors reportedly served well in their role of making it possible for mothers to focus more fully on the sessions, rather than trying to simultaneously participate in the session and supervise young children. The project leadership also reported that the child mentors also contributed to the safety of therapists delivering the home-based services. Safety was raised as an issue, because some of the participants lived in high-crime areas and in volatile situations involving a domestic violence perpetrator. Some therapists did not report concern for their safety, but the project leadership felt that two-person teams were an important safety precaution for delivering the home-based intervention for domestic violence victims.

The greatest challenge to implementing the child-mentoring component was maintaining a consistently available pool of mentors to go out to scheduled sessions. The mentors were students drawn from SMU's Department of Psychology and trained by its research staff working on the Safe Start program. Thus, the academic calendar the students worked on did not always match the calendar of service provision. At times when a trained child mentor was not available to go with a therapist for a home-based session, program staff reported that one of the Safe Start data collection team from the Department of Psychology would go with the therapist to entertain the children. This staff substitution reportedly worked adequately to allow mothers to focus their attention on the therapy session, the key goal of the child mentorship component.

There were other components of the Dallas Safe Start program that helped shape the implementation (see the box titled "Dallas Safe Start Additional Program Components").

### Dallas Safe Start Additional Program Components

**Quality Assurance.** At the onset of the project, therapist competence was formally assessed through participation in six videotaped role-play situations that the therapist was likely to encounter. The model developers and community partners also provided training on delivery of the model, family violence, and safety issues to all therapists who provided services to families. For clinical supervision and assurance of model fidelity, each family therapy session was videotaped and coded, and the model developer observed selected sessions and assessed therapist competence using a systematic review protocol. The therapists had access to program and implementation materials. Case review, discussion, and ongoing training and updates also took place in weekly group meetings. Peer-to-peer training occurred with newer therapists working in a team with more experienced therapists as part of the training process, under the supervision of the model developer.

**Dallas Safe Start Additional Program Components (continued)**

**Training.** In the first two years of the Dallas Safe Start program, the program conducted and/or participated in 17 trainings. The majority of these trainings were focused on Safe Start processes (53%), domestic violence (24%), and the clinical intervention (12%). Topics for training were mostly related to implementation of Project SUPPORT.

**Policies and Protocols.** Dallas Safe Start did not provide information about new or revised policies or protocols on their quarterly activity reports.

**Program Advocacy.** Dallas Safe Start did not provide information about program resources or costs for the purposes of our cost analysis.

**Resources and Costs.** In the first two years of SSPA, Dallas Safe Start used most of its resources for its staff, including project director, recruitment and retention specialist, and data collection specialist. Remaining funds were used for general office supplies and travel to support home visits.

## Summary

Based on our observations, the Dallas Safe Start program implemented its planned intervention, Project SUPPORT, largely as intended. Overall, the Safe Start therapists reported a feeling of confidence in the success of the intervention. In their view, this was due to the program's orientation toward "meeting mothers where they are" and focusing on building on a mother's existing nurturing and child management skills. Although the model was clearly structured and delivered in a series of specific steps that parents must follow to demonstrate mastery of each individual skill, the therapists were afforded flexibility to modify how they worked with each client in proceeding through the steps, depending on the client's level of need. The program staff indicated that intensive training, practice, and supervision were important for therapists to adequately prepare them for successfully employing this more subtle and customized method of model delivery. They reported that much of the clinical supervision within the Dallas Safe Start program focused on working with the therapists to develop and enhance their own skills in delivering this structured, yet flexible model.

One important innovation for ensuring full model delivery was the program's shift toward striking a balance in each treatment session between case management and therapy. This modification reportedly made delivery of the model more feasible in the midst of the often troubled circumstances of the program's target population. One respondent explained the program's philosophy as "you still have to parent, even in a crisis." The Dallas Safe Start program appeared to have identified a promising method of model delivery that made space for both parenting and crisis circumstances, within the context of a single combined session. These observations relate specifically to the delivery of the model, however, and not to the response of families to this more rigid session-time allocation. Collection of data on the latter was beyond the scope of this report.

One goal of the program was to provide whatever services were necessary to help alleviate hardships, and the life circumstances of many of the Safe Start clients were characterized by ongoing hardships in the extreme. This made program service delivery a very intensive commitment on the part of staff. Thus, a close level of supervision of staff well-being appeared to be an important feature of this program model, helping to ensure that therapists have adequate emotional reserves and personal boundaries to constructively deliver the intended services over time.

It is possible that the barriers to program model delivery would be lessened by seeking to include therapists whose racial and cultural characteristics were more closely matched to those of the client population. The Dallas Safe Start program staff reported that it had success in overcoming such challenges with individual clients over time, but increasing the diversity of the therapist pool could at least reduce some initial challenges.

**Data collection for this program summary included:**

- Key informant interviews with key program staff and shelter staff:
  - Project director and model developer
  - Therapists
  - Child mentors
  - Shelter staff
  - Participant recruiter staff
  - Assessment staff
- Case review of randomly selected treatment and control group cases
- Quality assurance checklist completed by the clinical supervisor
- Quarterly activity reports on services, training, policies, and advocacy
- OJJDP grant application
- Green Light notes
- *Safe Start: Promising Approaches Communities Working Together to Help Children Exposed to Violence* (Safe Start Center, 2008).

## 5. Dayton Program Description

### Dayton Safe Start

- **Intervention type:** Child-Parent Psychotherapy (CPP) and case management
- **Intervention length:** 6–12 months CPP; up to the end of the evaluation (case management)
- **Intervention Setting:** In-home
- **Target population:** Children exposed to domestic violence
- **Age range:** 0–5
- **Primary referral source:** Nurse home-visiting program

## Program and Community Setting

The Dayton Safe Start program was located in Dayton, Ohio. In 2003, the population of Dayton was approximately 162,000 residents, with slightly more than 7 percent of them children younger than age 5. Dayton was 53 percent white and 43 percent black, with very small Asian and American Indian populations. The per capita income was $15,547, with 23 percent of the population living below the poverty line.[8]

Dayton, Ohio, is located in Montgomery County, the fourth-largest county in Ohio. At the time of the project, Montgomery County had significantly higher violent crime rates; poorer social, health, and economic indicators; and disproportionately higher rates of child abuse than the rest of the state. Based on information from the Montgomery County Court of Common Pleas data, between 2000 and 2002 there were 788 domestic violence cases with charges filed against a defendant (Artemis Center for Domestic Violence Alternatives, 2004).

Prior to Safe Start, there were limited resources in the Dayton community for young children exposed to violence. To address this need, the Dayton Safe Start project came together as a collaborative endeavor of the Artemis Center for Alternatives to Domestic Violence, Brighter Futures (a home-based nurse visitation program), and the Young Children's Assessment and Treatment Services (YCATS) program of Samaritan Behavioral Health, Inc., with Artemis as the lead agent (see the box titled "Dayton Safe Start Partner Agencies" for a brief description of each partner agency).

In 2004, these agencies began to work together on the issue of infant mental health. Shortly before the grant opportunity, Artemis contracted with Samaritan Behavioral Health to learn more about infant mental health and to enable them to serve children under age 5. Artemis had been referring these young children to the YCATS program but wanted to increase its capacity to serve the mother and child at the same location. In response, YCATS staff began to teach the Artemis child therapists about infant mental health and working with parent-child dyads using the Lieberman model of CPP. At the same time, the Brighter Futures nurse home-visiting program had also contracted with Samaritan Behavioral Health for more generalized training on infant mental health.

With these initial steps into infant mental health, the partners came together to develop the capacity to serve the mental health needs of very young children exposed to violence. In preparing the proposal, Artemis's executive director first approached Artemis's clinical director and

[8] Information taken from the 2000 Census and can be found at the Census website (U.S. Census Bureau, no date).

the child therapy program to determine their level of interest. She then invited Brighter Futures and Samaritan Behavioral Health to join the collaboration and convened the collaborators to clarify details and write the grant. Together, the partners wanted to increase the community's capacity to provide mental health services to infants and very young children who had been exposed to violence and to offer those services in conjunction with services for the mothers.

The program that was originally developed by the collaborating partners targeted children 0–2 years of age who had been exposed to violence. *Exposure to violence* was defined as the mother having experienced physical or emotional abuse from her partner and the child having been within range to see, hear, or otherwise experience it. The partners designed a program for Artemis to offer CPP and case management in the client's home with referrals from the Brighter Futures nurses. YCATS would provide training, clinical supervision, and data collection.

## Dayton Safe Start Partner Agencies

**Artemis Center for Alternatives to Domestic Violence.** Artemis was founded in 1985 as an alternative to shelter-based care for victims of domestic violence. Artemis assists in providing a domestic violence hotline, which received about 90 calls per week during peak hours at the time of the proposal. The hotline is staffed by an advocate or supervisor who talks through the woman's circumstances, sometimes during a series of calls, and then connects her with Artemis's services. Artemis's advocacy and outreach services include advocates in the criminal court, at the job center, and at the Children's Services Bureau to help clients navigate the systems. Artemis also runs support groups, including a group for women who resort to violence in response to their own victimization, education groups, and open support groups. Artemis started its child therapy program in 1987 in response to the fact that children were being exposed to violence and that the cycle of violence would continue without intervention with the child. The child therapy program provides individual therapy, family therapy, and parent education, depending on needs. With funding from grants and private donations, Artemis is able to provide its services free to clients.

**Young Children's Assessment and Treatment Services.** Since 1970, YCATS has provided mental health diagnostic, intervention and prevention services, and developmental services to children ages 0–5. YCATS works with community agencies, such as Head Start, Help Me Grow, and public and private preschools and day care centers, to deliver mental health training and consultation as well as diagnostic and intervention services. YCATS therapists assess the children and then treat the majority of them in the home with child therapy, play therapy, or other appropriate therapies.

**Brighter Futures.** Established in 1996, Brighter Futures is a nurse home-visiting program based on the Olds model. The program targets mothers ages 24 and younger who have a child younger than age 3. The program is designed to improve birth outcomes, physical and emotional health and development of the child, and parental economic self-sufficiency. All Brighter Futures clients receive in-home nurse visits, referrals for therapy, and advocacy services.

The Dayton program was selected by OJJDP as one of 15 sites across the country. After receiving the grant, Dayton went through the Green Light process to prepare for program implementation and evaluation. Dayton also used this period to educate people both internally and externally about the goals and overall purpose of the initiative. Whereas the collaborators were eager to get started, the staff found it very helpful to lay the groundwork for the project before launching treatment. Throughout the project, the executive director worked to establish and maintain community relationships.

## Intervention

The Dayton Safe Start program involved two main components: intensive, long-term CPP and case management through an advocate. The intervention period lasted approximately one year. All of the services were provided in the client's home.

### Child-Parent Psychotherapy

The therapy component involved parent-child dyadic therapy using the Lieberman model. CPP is a relationship-based intervention designed for use with children ages 6 and younger. It can be used with any child whose relationship to his or her parent or other primary caregiver is impacted by negative circumstances, including family violence. CPP integrates psychodynamic, attachment, trauma, cognitive-behavioral, and social learning theories (NCTSN, 2008). There are two components in CPP: assessment and treatment, with information gained during the assessment used to inform the treatment component. In the intervention component, child-parent interactions are the focus of six intervention modalities aimed at restoring a sense of mastery, security, and growth and promoting congruence between bodily sensations, feelings, and thinking on the part of both child and parent and in their relationship with one another (NCTSN, 2008).

The Dayton site delivered weekly, one-hour CPP sessions in the home. The therapist conducted an initial home visit in conjunction with the advocate if possible. The therapy was then delivered during weekly sessions in the client's home. In implementing CPP, the Safe Start therapist worked on identifying and talking about the abuse using techniques in the *Don't Hit My Mommy* book (Lieberman and Van Horn, 2005) to help the parent understand the child's behavior and symptoms. During the Green Light process, Dayton specified that the therapy would continue until 75 percent of the treatment goals were met, usually by about 24 weeks. If 75 percent of the treatment goals were not met, there was a possibility of up to 24 more sessions as long as adequate progress had been made and there had been regular participation in the sessions.

### Case Management and Coordination

The case management component was made available for each family throughout its therapy and beyond that for up to four years through the life of the project. The case management was provided by an advocate who accompanied the therapist on the first home visit. The advocacy involved such case management activities as assistance with housing, employment, and transportation issues. The advocate also incorporated domestic violence education into the case management.

The intervention was conducted in the context of a rigorous evaluation as required by OJJDP (see the box titled "Dayton Safe Start Evaluation" for a description).

### Dayton Safe Start Evaluation

**Design.** This randomized control effectiveness trial was focused on child outcomes.

**Treatment versus control group services.** In addition to receiving any services or supports from the referring agency, those who were assigned to the treatment group received CPP and case management from Artemis staff. Those who were assigned to the control group received only the services and supports they were already receiving from the referring agency.

**Dayton Safe Start Evaluation (continued)**

**Data collection.** Data were collected through longitudinal assessments of child-level outcomes.

**Enrollment.** The site originally planned to enroll 160 families over the four-year period (80 in each group). Funding for the National Evaluation ended prematurely. By the time it ended, enrollment had taken place over two years and nine months and resulted in 25 families in the treatment group and 24 in the control group.

## Implementation

Figure B.5 diagrams Dayton's implementation of its intervention. The following description of the program implementation is the result of data collected for the national evaluation. See Appendix A for a full discussion of the data collection methodology employed at each of the Safe Start sites.

### Referrals

From the program's inception in the spring of 2006 until early 2008, Dayton Safe Start relied solely on the Brighter Futures nurse home-visiting program for referrals. The Brighter Futures protocol included a questionnaire on the mother's relationships and domestic violence that was completed at intake, at 3–6 months, and at 12 months into the Brighter Futures program. When the Brighter Futures nurses administered the questionnaire and detected violence, they were supposed to refer the case to Safe Start. Once a referral was received, the project director assigned the case to an YCATS data collector so that the baseline assessment could be scheduled and completed in the client's home. After the assessment, the project director implemented the random assignment procedures and informed the referring party about the results. Within two days of completion of the assessment, the family was contacted by the therapist (for intervention families) or the advocate (for control families).

**Figure B.5**
**Model of Dayton Safe Start**

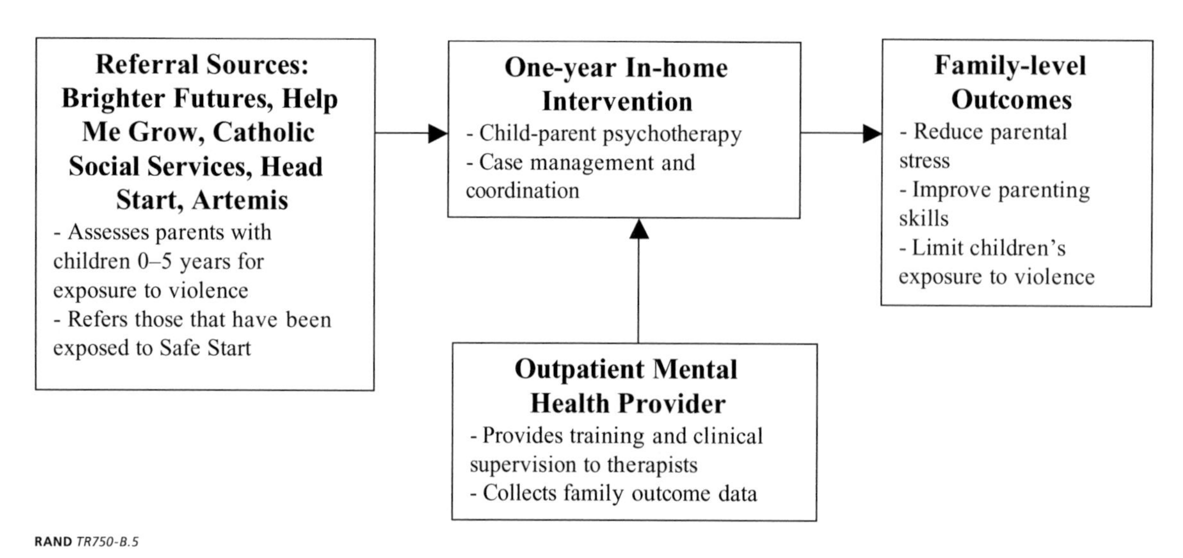


RAND *TR750-B.5*

After absorbing a backlog of cases that were identified during the Green Light process, Artemis received very few new referrals from the Brighter Futures nurses. There were several reasons identified by Artemis and Brighter Futures staff for the slower than expected rate of referrals.

- Client readiness. The nurse supervisors reported that it took time to build the relationship with the client to the point where it was safe and the client was receptive to a discussion of domestic violence.
- Nurse training. According to the supervisors, when Brighter Futures had staff turnover, the new nurses needed to learn how to identify and assess domestic violence in addition to all of their Brighter Futures activities. The nurses had varying experience and comfort levels with assessing clients for domestic violence, which made referring clients challenging.
- Research design. The research design posed challenges to maintaining a steady flow of referrals from the Brighter Futures nurse home-visiting program. The nurses reported that the close relationships they developed with their clients made them reluctant to refer because they did not want them to be assigned to the control group and not get the services.

In an attempt to remedy these problems, the Safe Start therapist and advocate met regularly with the nurses to build rapport and alleviate any concerns that Safe Start would interfere with the nurse's work with the client. Nonetheless, the slow pace of referrals continued, and the program began to explore options for expanding its referral sources.

In the spring of 2008, Dayton Safe Start added Help Me Grow, a local Head Start program, the Catholic Social Services Parent Link program, and Artemis as referral sources. Because some of these additional referring agencies or programs provide services to children up to the age of 5, the program also simultaneously increased its eligible age range from 0–2 to 0–5.

Help Me Grow is Ohio's statewide early intervention program for children ages 0–3. With a combination of federal, state, and local funding, each county in Ohio implements Help Me Grow. Like Brighter Futures, Help Me Grow is an in-home intervention in which service providers offer early childhood education and health screenings in addition to family-centered services for children at risk for developmental delays.

The Dayton Head Start program provides preschool children of low-income families with a comprehensive program to meet their emotional, social, health, nutritional, and psychology needs.

The Catholic Social Services' Teen Link program offers education and support to pregnant and parenting young people to help them gain confidence and understanding about their parenting role. Their services include home-based parenting education for expecting teen parents or teen parents with a child less than three years of age.

### Services

Table B.5 summarizes the average quarterly caseload and service delivery for those who received services through the Dayton Safe Start program during the first three years of implementation (through March 2009). Dayton had one therapist who was a licensed professional counselor devoted full time throughout the life of the project. The case management was provided by a full-time advocate who had experience with the population and who had held other positions at Artemis.

**Table B.5**
**Service Delivery for Enrollees in the Dayton Safe Start Intervention**

| | Year 1 | Year 2 | Year 3 (9 months) |
|---|---|---|---|
| Average quarterly caseload per therapist | 5.4 | 8.5 | 4.8 |
| Average quarterly caseload per advocate | 4.5 | 6.5 | 6.8 |
| Total number of CPP sessions | 120 | 117 | 102 |
| Total number of case management contacts | 338 | 282 | 422 |
| Total number of case coordination meetings | 194 | 150 | 246 |

### *Child-Parent Psychotherapy*

During the initial contact with intervention families, the therapist evaluated the family for crisis and lethality and completed safety planning. The next step was an initial home visit, which the therapist and advocate conducted together whenever possible. For these visits, the Safe Start staff reported that the families were typically in some degree of chaos at the time of the referral. Although the referral might have been related to a crisis that prompted the nurse to refer, the program staff saw the difficult living situations as chronic. The Safe Start staff observed that the women referred typically lived in pronounced poverty, had long histories of violence, had experienced multiple traumas, and had family histories of violence.

Overall, Safe Start staff found during the initial home visits that the women were often not ready to talk about domestic violence or participate in therapy when they first became engaged with Safe Start. As a result, the program staff concentrated on educating mothers about domestic violence, building independence, and developing rapport with their clients during the early sessions. Although this took time and resources, the Safe Start program staff found it necessary to address safety and basic needs before starting therapy in order to provide the women with the stability they needed to engage in mental health treatment.

Once therapy started, the therapist reported that the women consistently did not understand how therapy might help the relationship with their children. According to the therapist, domestic violence and mental health were not a priority for these women, who had a lot of issues to confront that took precedence over bonding with the child. The Safe Start program staff also noted some challenges to providing the therapy in the home. The program staff reported that the homes were often chaotic, which made it time consuming for the therapist to learn the client's story and understand the family and the circumstances. Once they were able to earn the client's trust, the program staff found that they were able to take big steps forward in terms of their ability to start working on the parent-child relationship.

### *Case Management and Coordination*

The advocate provided most of the advocacy services, although the therapist also did some advocacy and case management while actively engaged with the families. The advocate and therapist worked very closely together. The advocate assisted with stabilization of the life situation for both mother and child by providing case management and resources, with a focus on the achievement and maintenance of safety. This involved the advocate helping the mother secure a range of services, such as legal assistance, housing, health care, and accessing the criminal justice system, as well as regularly reviewing and monitoring the safety plan. The advocate found that the client stayed engaged with Safe Start as long as the program staff followed through on what they told the client they would do, clarified their roles with the client, and allowed the client to tell them when the pace or intensity of the services and supports needed to be adjusted.

There was some coordination with other service providers for families referred from Brighter Futures. Brighter Futures had done some training with Safe Start staff about how to work with the population and how to work in the home. Brighter Futures had a history with the families, and sharing some of that history informally at the staff meetings that the Safe Start program staff attended helped Safe Start work with the families. The Safe Start therapist attended some monthly Brighter Futures meetings, which allowed for informal communication, but there was no formal, structured process for coordinating. With its focus on domestic violence, Safe Start freed the Brighter Futures nurses to work on issues related to healthy development. Nonetheless, there were some issues around roles, particularly around the advocacy component and who was taking care of which needs of the client.

There were other components of the Dayton Safe Start program that helped shape the implementation. These are described in the box titled "Dayton Safe Start Additional Program Components."

### Dayton Safe Start Additional Program Components

**Quality Assurance.** The site's CPP training efforts included initial clinician training for both the child therapist and advocate that involved discussion of the books by one of the model developers and related articles. The therapist had access to these materials as well as an infant mental health handbook. The clinical supervisor served as both a supervisor and mentor, meeting weekly with the therapist to review the session protocols and analyze how the sessions went; discuss progress, next steps, and termination planning; assess how well the therapist could reframe the client's status and adapt his or her style to meet the client's circumstances; and utilize the intervention techniques and provide updates related to the intervention.

**Training.** In the first two years of Dayton Safe Start, the program conducted and/or participated in 29 trainings. The majority of these trainings were focused on domestic violence (31%), mental health interventions (24%), and the clinical intervention used for Safe Start (14%). Topics for training ranged from dating violence to the effects of trauma on children.

**Policies and Protocols.** Dayton worked closely with its primary referral source on policies and protocols related to making and responding to referrals. These efforts involved streamlining the referral process, improving communication between Safe Start and the referring agency, and facilitating information-sharing among those involved with the families. Dayton Safe Start also helped the county-level criminal justice subcommittee on domestic violence add a section on children exposed to domestic violence that includes suggestions to police officers on interacting with children as well as information about symptoms that children may exhibit after exposure to an existing criminal justice protocol on domestic violence.

**Program Outreach.** The site's outreach efforts included advocating with the state job program regarding the practice of sanctioning mothers who choose not to cooperate with child support even when the reason involves threats from the battered fathers. Locally, Dayton Safe Start met with the Children's Advocacy Center to enhance collaboration regarding children exposed to violence.

**Resources and Costs.** In the first two years of SSPA, Dayton Safe Start used most of their resources for several staff members needed to implement the program, including the child therapist and advocate. Office supplies, costs for advertising, and assistance for clients comprised most of the remaining OJJDP funds.

## Summary

By selecting an established therapeutic intervention, the partners in Dayton increased the local capacity to treat very young children who witness domestic violence. The community had already been trying to move toward providing infant mental health for children exposed to violence prior to receiving the grant. Safe Start enabled Artemis to expand and strengthen this focus and to work with a different clientele in a different setting.

In the course of implementing its intervention, Dayton learned some valuable lessons about treating this population. Because of the complexity of the families' problems, staff found it imperative that the client have an advocate to address the layers of issues that must be resolved before the client was ready to work on the parent-child relationship. Dayton also found that the Safe Start therapist could not do her work without the case management/advocacy component. Further, the process of building rapport and trust took time, so the overall length of the intervention stretched to encompass this initial phase of relationship-building. Rather than moving forward with the therapy regardless of the situation, the Safe Start program staff allowed the client to set the agenda until there was readiness to address the domestic violence and work on the parent-child relationship.

The setting also provided challenges and opportunities. From the outset, the partners decided to provide the therapy in the home. The therapist found that the homes were often very chaotic, with many distractions. It was difficult to find the time and space to focus on and deliver the treatment. Yet, by bringing the treatment to the home, the therapist thought that she was able to demonstrate her commitment to the family and the importance of child and family functioning. According to the prior experiences of Artemis staff, the population served by Safe Start would not have come to a clinic or office for treatment, so bringing the intervention to the home was the only way to reach them. Once trust had been established, the therapist was able to delve into improving the parent-child relationship.

Dayton struggled with enrollment throughout the project. The Brighter Futures nurses were not able to provide a steady flow of referrals to Safe Start. Although they worked closely with the target population, the nurses reported that they were still building relationships with clients and this made introducing domestic violence issues difficult. In order to refer more consistently, Safe Start program staff felt that the nurses needed to learn how to identify and assess for domestic violence. Some were more willing and comfortable with domestic violence issues than others.

**Data collection for this program summary included:**

- Key informant interviews with key program staff and community partners:
  - Artemis agency director
  - Artemis clinical supervisor
  - Safe Start therapist
  - Safe Start advocate
  - YCATS director
  - Brighter Futures director, coordinator, supervisors and nurses
  - Artemis therapist for the KIDS program
  - Artemis financial director
- Case review of randomly selected treatment and control group cases

**Data collection for this program summary included (continued)**

- Quality assurance checklist completed by the clinical supervisor
- Quarterly activity reports on services, training, policies, and advocacy
- Grant application
- Green Light notes
- *Safe Start: Promising Approaches Communities Working Together to Help Children Exposed to Violence* (Safe Start Center, 2008).

## 6. Erie Program Description

### Erie Safe Start

- **Intervention type.** Individualized therapy, case management, and parent education groups
- **Intervention length:** 6 months
- **Intervention setting:** In-home, clinic, school, or day care depending on client's preference
- **Target population:** Children who had been physically or sexually abused, witnessed domestic violence, victim of any violent crime, or witnessed violent crime
- **Age range:** 0–8
- **Primary referral sources:** Children's Advocacy Center, Office of Children and Youth

### Program and Community Setting

The Erie Safe Start program is located in Erie, Pennsylvania. In Erie County, there were approximately 101,400 residents, with slightly more than 7 percent of them children younger than age 5. In 2005, approximately 80 percent of the population was white, 15 percent was black, and 5 percent was Asian or American Indian. The per capita income was $14,972, with about 19 percent of the population living below the poverty line.[9]

In 2005, Erie County's Office of Children and Youth (OCY) received about 625 reports of child abuse and neglect. About 20 percent of these were substantiated after the investigation (Children's Advocacy Center of Erie County, 2004). The usual response in the community is for OCY caseworkers to help make arrangements for counseling, medical care, and physical resources needed by the family. Law enforcement responds to calls involving children exposed to violence and conducts criminal investigations. The District Attorney's Office determines whether there is enough evidence to prosecute the perpetrator. For cases involved with both the OCY and law enforcement, the Children's Advocacy Center (CAC) provides forensic interviewing and case coordination for approximately 350 cases per year.

Prior to the Safe Start project, the CAC maintained close relationships with the agencies and organizations that work with children exposed to violence. CAC did this mainly through its Board of Directors, which included community and business representatives. For the most part, the directors and the agency and organization staffs had worked together and known each other either personally or by reputation for a number of years. The relationships appeared to be based on a combination of personal knowledge of the agency or staff member as well as the services that are provided, informal communication, and mutual trust among the agencies and organizations.

Despite these relationships and focus, the resources in the community for children exposed to violence prior to Safe Start were limited and fragmented. To address this need, the CAC decided to respond to the Safe Start request for applications and led a community effort to increase the capacity to serve these children (see the box titled "Erie Safe Start Partner Agencies" for descriptions).

The Safe Start program originally developed by the CAC targeted children ages 0–12 who had been exposed to violence (defined as being physically or sexually abused, witnessing

[9] Information taken from the 2000 Census and can be found at the Census website (U.S. Census Bureau, no date).

domestic violence, being a victim of any violent crime, or witnessing violent crime). Erie's intervention involved an integrated treatment team approach with three main components: therapy, case management, and parent education groups. The case management and parent education components of this integrated treatment program were unique because they were not previously available for this population. The Erie Safe Start proposal outlined how the program would bring existing therapy options to families earlier and coordinate that treatment across different community agencies. Erie designed the program to receive referrals from the CAC, the OCY, the District Attorney's Office, and the Crime Victim Center (CVC).

After receiving the OJJDP grant, Erie went through the Green Light process to prepare for program implementation and evaluation. The Erie Safe Start program staff reported that they had not anticipated the lengthy and involved Green Light process, but they did appreciate the opportunity to clarify their plans and revise their projected enrollment totals. During the early part of implementation, they expanded their age range and revised their eligibility criteria to remove a requirement related to the recency of the violence exposure. Both of these changes were made to increase the pool of possible participants.

### Erie Safe Start Partner Agencies

**Children's Advocacy Center.** The Children's Advocacy Center of Erie County, Inc. (CAC) is a nonprofit organization created in 2001 as the result of a two-year community planning process. The CAC was designed to reduce additional trauma that abused children might face as they navigate the criminal justice and child protection systems. The CAC also works to improve coordination, investigation, and communication involving cases of child maltreatment. To achieve these objectives, the CAC conducts forensic interviews (i.e., neutral, fact-finding assessment) of children utilizing trained personnel with expertise in working with children of all ages. The CAC also facilitates reviews of all child abuse cases by a multidisciplinary team, as well as a work group that designed and implemented the countywide Child Abuse protocol. The organization also provides training to area professionals and brings in national speakers. The CAC relies on grants, donations, and fundraising efforts to fund their services.

**Crime Victim Center.** The Crime Victim Center (CVC) provides free confidential crisis and supportive counseling services, education, and advocacy to any crime victim. Established in 1973 as a rape crisis center, the CVC expanded in 1986 to include victims of other violent crimes. The CVC helps prepare children for the criminal justice process and provides advocates to accompany victims, children, and families to court. The CVC relies on government support, donations, and fundraising.

**The Achievement Center.** The Achievement Center is an early intervention service provider serving children ages 0–3 in Erie County since 1923. The Achievement Center focuses on providing treatment for children with physical disabilities, developmental delays, emotional/behavioral problems, and autism spectrum disorders. The Achievement Center also offers play therapy for children suffering from trauma.

## Intervention

All families referred to Safe Start received a developmental screening to assess child and family functioning. The Erie Safe Start intervention model included three main components: individualized therapy, case management, and parenting education groups. The intervention period lasted approximately six months. Most of the services were provided at the CAC, although the program staff did develop the capacity to provide mobile therapy if the client preferred, based on a need that developed as they began to work with the families.

#### Individualized Therapy

The therapy component of Erie's integrated treatment program was relatively unstructured and largely driven by the needs of the parent and child. The assigned therapist conducted an initial home visit, guided by a written protocol designed to gather information about the child's developmental history, the family situation, and the home environment through questions and observations by the therapist. The therapist then used all the information gathered from the developmental screening and home visit to develop a treatment plan for the family, with flexibility in how the treatment was delivered and the amount of effort spent in any area. The types of therapy might include dyadic therapy, play therapy, or family therapy. The plan listed each problem area with short-term outcomes, methods for addressing the problem, frequency, person responsible, and target date. This treatment plan was reviewed by the integrated treatment team and signed by the parent, therapist, and treatment team.

During the six-month intervention period, the treatment plan was regularly reviewed, again using a standard protocol. Depending on the family's needs, the treatment plan might have involved individual therapy for the child or parent, or joint therapy for the parent and child or family.

#### Case Management

The case management involved contacting the family members regularly to connect them with services, notifying them about the research assessments, and helping with any obstacles. The case management continued after the six-month intervention period for 1.5 years until the last assessment.

Erie Safe Start also convened the integrated treatment team each week to discuss and review each family's progress. The Safe Start case manager and therapists as well as someone from the OCY and the CVC attended these treatment team meetings.

#### Parent Education Groups

The parenting group component was developed and modified by the original project director with the goals of expanding parent knowledge, improving parent-child bonding, and providing child management and child protection skills. There was a standard curriculum for the 12 weekly 90-minute sessions, with materials and a participant workbook for each session; eight sessions were conducted with parents only and four were conducted with parents and children together. The first four sessions focused on psycho-education; the next four, with both the parents and children, focused on parent-child attachment and bonding; and the final four focused on the parent's role as leader of the family. For each session, there were two facilitators. One facilitator worked with the parents and the other worked with the children. For the joint parent-child sessions, the program had one facilitator for each participating family.

The intervention was conducted in the context of a rigorous evaluation as required by OJJDP (see the box titled "Erie Safe Start Evaluation" for a description).

## Erie Safe Start Evaluation

**Design.** This randomized control effectiveness trial was focused on child outcomes.

**Treatment versus control group services.** In addition to receiving any services or supports from the referring agency, those who were assigned to the treatment group received individualized therapy, case management, and parent education. Those who were assigned to the control group received only the services and supports they were already receiving from the referring agency. Both groups received a developmental screening that is not part of usual care.

**Data collection.** Data were collected through longitudinal assessments of child-level outcomes.

**Enrollment.** The site originally planned to serve 360 families over the four-year period (180 in each group). Funding for the National Evaluation ended prematurely. By the time it ended, enrollment had taken place over three years and resulted in 85 families in the treatment group and 87 in the control group.

## Implementation

Figure B.6 diagrams Erie's implementation of its intervention. The following description of the program implementation is the result of data collected for the national evaluation. See Appendix A for a full discussion of the data collection methodology employed at each of the Safe Start sites.

### Referrals

When the program started in 2006, Erie Safe Start had thought it would receive referrals from the CAC, the OCY, the District Attorney's Office, and the CVC. However, these referral

**Figure B.6**
**Model of Erie Safe Start**

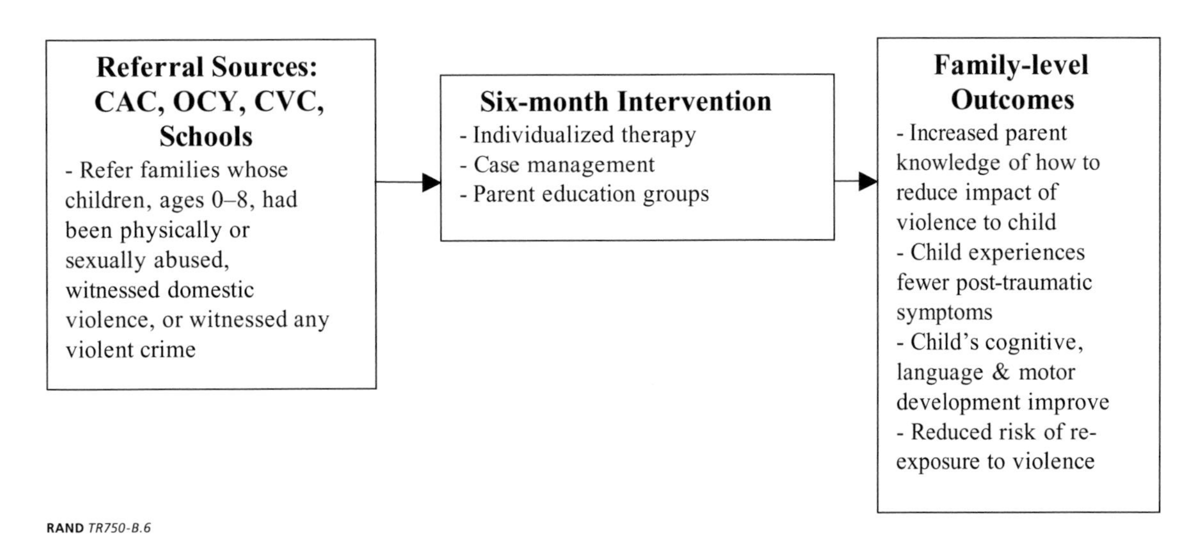


RAND *TR750-B.6*

sources were either not referring clients or not referring enough clients to meet the needed enrollment numbers. As the referral issues deepened, Erie Safe Start experienced some staff turnover. Part way through 2007, a new CAC executive director and Safe Start project director started. Both brought renewed energy and commitment to the project. Together, they developed a multipronged approach to increasing referrals that included

- outreach to some of the places that were not referring at all, such as the Achievement Center, the court system, and the District Attorney's office
- education for the agencies that were referring, such as the OCY, the CVC, and schools
- promotion of Safe Start internally within the CAC.

In their outreach to some of the community agencies that were not referring families, the Safe Start program staff indicated that agencies lacked information about the program and its value. For example, detectives from the police department who were co-located at the CAC did not know about Safe Start. The project director developed a new database to track their outreach efforts and coordinate their communication with new and existing partners. In the process of educating community partners and clearing up any confusion, the staff felt like they generated a lot of enthusiasm and support for the project.

Among those who were referring families, but not at the expected pace, there were similar issues. At the OCY, referrals were slow at the beginning because the agency was the focus of an investigation that led to a significant reorganization and several staffing changes. Once the situation eased, the Safe Start program staff reintroduced the project and developed processes for intake and ongoing workers to make referrals. Within the CAC, the Safe Start program staff worked closely with those coordinating the CAC's intake process to ensure that all families who met the criteria were being referred.

The program's internal and external outreach efforts with new and existing referral sources dramatically increased referrals in the middle of 2007.

### Services

Table B.6 summarizes average quarterly caseloads for Safe Start program staff and service delivery for those who received services through the Erie Safe Start program during the first three years of implementation (through March 2009). Erie had a mixture of full- and part-time dedicated Safe Start therapists and part-time contracted mobile therapists. The case management was provided by two CAC case managers. The parenting education groups were conducted by the project director. At the beginning of the project, the project director's clinical responsibilities were limited to the parenting groups. During 2007, Erie restructured the budget to have the project director spend 50 percent time in program development and administrative duties and 50 percent in clinical services providing therapy at the CAC and conducting the parent education groups. The therapy session totals and case management contacts in Table B.6 reflect how Erie refocused their service delivery to provide more therapy and less case management from Year 1 to Year 2.

**Table B.6**
**Service Delivery for Enrollees in the Erie Safe Start Intervention**

| | Year 1 | Year 2 | Year 3 |
|---|---|---|---|
| Average quarterly caseload per therapist | 3.3 | 3.5 | 4.6 |
| Average quarterly caseload per case manager | 13 | 25 | 32 |
| Total number of caregiver individual therapy sessions | 28 | 55 | 142 |
| Total number of child individual therapy sessions | 26 | 62 | 345 |
| Total number of caregiver group sessions | 32 | 11 | 64 |
| Total number of joint therapy sessions | 5 | 37 | 203 |
| Total number of caregiver and child group therapy sessions | 16 | — | 22 |
| Total number of case management contacts | 408 | 284 | 760 |

### *Developmental Screening*

Once they received a referral, the Safe Start program staff immediately called and attempted to set up an appointment for a developmental screening conducted at the CAC. At the appointment, the Safe Start program staff completed a developmental clinic intake form and administered the Battelle Developmental Inventory for children up to age 8, which is a widely recognized instrument to assess the development of young children. For children ages 8–12, program staff used the Vineland Adaptive Behavior Scales. The developmental screening tools were followed by the baseline research assessments. For both treatment and control families, the project director summarized the results of the developmental screening in a written summary that was sent to the family.

According to the Safe Start program staff, the families referred often had multiple stressors but did not necessarily recognize the need for help in the form of mental health treatment. They felt that the developmental screening gave them a structured tool to help identify needs and engage the families in recognizing and responding to the needs.

### *Therapy*

For those families randomized into the treatment group, staff asked the parent a few additional questions about the current concerns related to the child. They then determined whether the therapy would be delivered in-home by a mobile therapist or at the CAC based on what was convenient for the family. Over time, they found that many of the families preferred in-home services as opposed to clinic-based treatment, especially in families with multiple children. After the developmental screening, the family was assigned to a therapist who conducted a home visit and developed the treatment plan.

The therapy component was driven by the needs of the parent and child and could have involved individual child therapy, joint parent-child therapy, caregiver group therapy, caregiver individual therapy, or family therapy. When working individually with the child, the therapists reported that they often used some form of play therapy or directive therapy about the trauma. The therapists had access to different workbooks on traumatic stress and indicated that they used these to find activities appropriate to the situation. When working individually with the parent, the therapists reported that they focused on psycho-educational skills, parenting, attachment, and interaction. When working with the parent and child or the family, the therapists said that they incorporated more directive structured family therapy. They also observed play and modeled the interaction between the parent and child.

### *Case Management*

For the case management component, a case manager provided most of the support, although the therapists also reported doing case management while they were actively engaged with the families. The case management involved contacting the family to follow through with referrals to services identified through the developmental screenings. Safe Start continued to offer case management after the six-month intervention period. If the family was no longer involved with therapy, the case manager reported that she or he attempted to reach each family at least monthly to connect with services, notify them about upcoming assessments, help with such obstacles as food and transportation, and make collateral calls to Head Start or early intervention.

### *Parent Education Groups*

During the implementation period, the 12-week parent group component was delivered four times. At certain points during the implementation, the Safe Start program staff sometimes had to wait for enough parents to be referred to begin a new set of sessions. For those parents who were unable or unwilling to attend the group sessions, the therapist delivered the materials during regular therapy sessions.

The Safe Start program staff indicated that the group sessions were very well received. Safe Start provided child care and transportation assistance in the form of gas cards or bus tokens to encourage participation. According to program staff, participating families became connected to one another and expressed a desire to have additional sessions. In response to this demand, the program staff began offering a monthly support group for those who had finished the parent group curriculum and wanted to remain connected with each other and Safe Start.

The Safe Start program staff reported that the families who participated in the parenting groups had experienced a great deal of violence. They felt that the group setting allowed the families to share their experiences with others in similar situations and to allow the caregivers to practice ways to interact with their children. In many cases, the program staff reported that the parents had been victims of abuse themselves as children. In these cases, the Safe Start program staff connected the parents with the CVC so they could receive services to help them process these childhood experiences.

There were other components of the Erie Safe Start program that helped shape the implementation. These are described in the box titled "Erie Safe Start Additional Program Components."

## Erie Safe Start Additional Program Components

**Quality Assurance.** Staff who delivered intervention services were training in the intervention model and the implementation process. In addition, staff participated in weekly treatment team meetings and individual clinical supervision. During these meetings, the team reviewed assessment and intervention techniques, discussed strategies for engaging clients, and outlined specific treatment goals. Individual clinical supervision sessions were used to address potential difficulties, suggest appropriate approaches, and assess therapist competence. In addition, the CAC developed a process of reviewing and modifying model-driven, family treatment plans with clinical staff to ensure fidelity to the model.

### Erie Safe Start Additional Program Components (continued)

**Training.** In the first two years of Erie Safe Start, the program conducted and/or participated in 21 training sessions. The majority of these sessions were focused on child welfare issues (57%) and Safe Start processes (19%). Other topics focused on engaging families, domestic violence, and the clinical intervention. Topics were focused primarily on child abuse, with a few sessions on the Safe Start program and recruiting and retaining families.

**Policies and Protocols.** The policies and protocols that the Erie site developed focused primarily on internal procedures for receiving referrals, determining eligibility, and making home visits.

**Program Outreach.** In terms of the site's outreach and advocacy efforts, the project director met with a statewide group to discuss improving responses for maltreated children. Locally, Erie Safe Start engaged various public and private agencies to discuss the project, the services available, and the referral process.

**Resources and Costs.** In the first two years of SSPA, Erie Safe Start used most of its resources for its staff, including their project director, case manager, and crime victim director. Remaining funds were used for office supplies, therapeutic play equipment, testing supplies, and incentives.

## Summary

Prior to Safe Start, there was a perceived gap in services for children in Erie County suffering from trauma. With Safe Start, the CAC was able to expand the range of options available to these families to include therapy, parent education, and case management. According to program staff, because they were offering more services to these families, the CAC also stayed involved with these families for a much longer period of time. This more lengthy involvement helped provide more continuity and coordination among the agencies involved with these families.

By expanding the referral options in the community, Erie learned of the real need for trauma-focused treatment for children exposed to violence. According to their staff and directors, the referring agencies appreciated having a way to bring more services to families. Further, Safe Start program staff found that the families referred were relatively easy to engage. According to them, the developmental screenings and treatment plans allowed Safe Start to offer families a range of services in different settings. By offering tailored and flexible services to families, the CAC appears to have helped engage families in addressing the trauma issues.

Erie's tailored approach to services also brought with it some challenges. For the therapy component, the program did not have a standard protocol to follow for each family. Staff assessed each family's need at the developmental screening and then selected the appropriate therapy option. Although this allowed the program staff to be very responsive to client needs, it made monitoring the cases more challenging. Because the parent education group was not required, Erie sometimes had to wait long periods for enough families to express interest before starting a new session. Although the content of the parent education was offered individually, some families were left without a key component of the intervention for much of their treatment period or were not exposed to potential benefits of the group setting.

**Data collection for this program summary included:**

- Key informant interviews with key program staff and community partners:
  - CAC agency director
  - CAC project director
  - Safe Start therapist
  - Safe Start case manager and data collector
  - OCY intake supervisor
  - CVC director
  - Achievement Center therapist
- Case review of randomly selected treatment and control group cases
- Quality assurance checklist completed by the project director
- Quarterly activity reports on services, training, policies, and advocacy
- Grant application
- Green Light notes
- *Safe Start: Promising Approaches Communities Working Together to Help Children Exposed to Violence* (Safe Start Center, 2008).

## 7. Kalamazoo Program Description

### Kalamazoo Safe Start

- **Intervention type:** Head Start School Intervention Project (a classroom intervention), teacher training, and parent training program
- **Intervention length:** 26 weeks
- **Intervention setting:** Head Start classrooms
- **Target population:** Children exposed to violence
- **Age range:** 3–5
- **Primary referral source:** Head Start

### Program and Community Setting

The Kalamazoo Safe Start program is located in Kalamazoo County, Michigan. As of the 2000 Census, about 238,600 people were living in the county, 6.5 percent of whom were younger than age 5. The population in Kalamazoo was about 85 percent white, 10 percent black, 3 percent Hispanic, 2 percent Asian, and less than 1 percent Native American or Pacific Islander. The 1999 income per capita was $25,454,[10] and 12 percent of the population was living below the poverty line at that time.[11]

According to Kalamazoo's original proposal for the Safe Start initiative, 2,029 child maltreatment complaints were investigated by the child protective services agency serving Kalamazoo County in 2003, with more than 30 percent of them substantiated for abuse/neglect. The Kalamazoo Family Court received 278 child abuse/neglect petitions, and more than 200 children were removed from their homes, resulting in a total of 695 children living in some type of out-of-home care during 2003 (Western Michigan University, 2004). Domestic violence reports to police totaled 2,430 in 2003, with 1,288 of these resulting in criminal charges filed by the Prosecuting Attorney's Office (Kalamazoo Assault Intervention Program, 2004).

Collaborative work in Kalamazoo began in 2000, when the Southwest Michigan Children's Trauma Assessment Center (CTAC), the lead agency for the Safe Start program, was established at Western Michigan University. This center was established to develop expertise for the comprehensive assessment of maltreated children. The CTAC received a grant from the Substance Abuse and Mental Health Services Administration to participate in the National Child Traumatic Stress Network in 2003, for a four-year project to develop a school-based curriculum to train professionals across Michigan in child trauma, among other goals.

Thus, prior to Safe Start, the CTAC had worked with Kalamazoo Public Schools to develop the School Intervention Program for 4th- through 7th-grade children. This program

---

[10] This is the 1999 income per capita reported in 2005 dollars. The 1999 income as reported in the 2000 census is $21,739.

[11] This information is taken from the 2000 Census unless otherwise stated. The data can be found on the census website (U.S. Census Bureau, no date).

was designed to address the needs of children impacted by prenatal and/or postnatal trauma and to foster their ability to feel safe in the learning environment. However, Kalamazoo's Safe Start proposal to OJJDP noted that the major gap in existing services was that no referral for assessment or treatment took place prior to the emergence of developmental, emotional, or behavioral problems. Many of these issues might not be recognized until the children entered school, even though the problems might exist earlier. According to the Safe Start partner agencies, the existing system of care presumed that children younger than age 5 were more resilient than older children, and thus less likely to be referred for the impact of exposure to violence (Western Michigan University, 2004). Moreover, younger children who were referred for services received interventions that did not approach the targeted behavior as a possible by-product of exposure to violence. This led directly to the Kalamazoo Safe Start proposal to develop an intervention for younger children enrolled in the Head Start program that would explicitly link behavior problems with violence exposure (Western Michigan University, 2004).

As originally proposed, the Kalamazoo Safe Start program targeted children 3 to 5 years of age who were enrolled in Kalamazoo County Head Start, spoke English or Spanish, and whose parent had endorsed at least one indicator of CEV. These indicators included whether the child had seen another child harmed or threatened by an adult, seen two or more adults fighting, seen somebody arrested, heard gunshots in the neighborhood, heard an adult threaten to harm another adults, or feared being beaten up or shot. All children in the classroom could participate in the activities, not only the ones that had been exposed to violence. The Head Start School Intervention Project (HSSIP) was planned to include training of teachers and staff, a curriculum for Head Start classrooms, and optional parent training meetings. After developing the intervention materials and pilot-testing the program in the first year of the project, the Safe Start team planned to implement the curriculum themselves, by training social workers (referred to as "school interventionists") in the second year of the program and having the teachers observe the implementation. In the third year, school interventionists would co-lead the curriculum with teachers, and then teachers would lead the curriculum in the fourth year. "Parent interventionists" would lead parent group meetings, to run concurrently with the HSSIP curriculum.

As a secondary goal, the Safe Start project would establish a "core team" of staff from several agencies to collaborate in evaluating current practices and developing policies that improve and sustain the systematic response to young children exposed to violence in the county (see the box titled "Kalamazoo Safe Start Partner Agencies" for more details).

The Kalamazoo program was selected by OJJDP as one of 15 Safe Start sites across the country. After receiving the grant, Kalamazoo went through OJJDP's Green Light process to prepare for program implementation and evaluation. Unlike the other Safe Start sites, Kalamazoo's had planned a pilot test of the program during the 2005–2006 school year and requested OJJDP's permission to proceed with the pilot test as planned during the Green Light process. This allowed them to make use of the 2005–2006 school year, instead of waiting to implement until the following school year. Thus, the Green Light process focused on the specifics of their evaluation plan to randomize classrooms to Safe Start and control classrooms for the remaining three years (2006–2009). The Safe Start program staff reported that the Green Light process was new and different for them, as staff had prior research experience and were used to running programs on their own, but that they felt supported and that communication was good overall.

## Kalamazoo Safe Start Partner Agencies

**Southwestern Michigan Children's Trauma Assessment Center, Western Michigan University.** Created in 2000 in recognition of the fact that exposure to traumatic events can affect child functioning within the cognitive, affective, behavioral, and physiological domains, the CTAC assesses the impact of trauma on children ages 3 months to 14 years, with a focus on children entering the foster care system due to experiencing child abuse and/or neglect. The CTAC was housed within the Trauma Center of Western Michigan University and was the lead agency for the Kalamazoo Safe Start project, providing the Safe Start staff and coordinating all aspects of the project.

**Kalamazoo County Head Start.** This Head Start program provides early learning experiences for economically disadvantaged children and their families, encouraging intellectual, social, and emotional growth to enhance prereadiness skills prior to kindergarten. The program uses a standardized Head Start curriculum that emphasizes early literacy. Family services are also provided, including social services, education/employment, adult literacy, and health services. In 2009, Head Start included 24 classrooms at 12 different sites and served the entire county. In the Kalamazoo Safe Start project, the Head Start program was engaged as a partner, participating in training and consultation, helping to recruit families, and helping to deliver the intervention in the HSSIP classrooms.

**Project REVOC.** This was a multiagency public and private partnership developed specifically for the Safe Start project, whose activities focused on young children exposed to violence in Kalamazoo County. Called the Kalamazoo Collaborative Initiative for Reducing the Effects of Violence on Children, or Project REVOC, this group consisted of Southwestern Michigan's Child Trauma Assessment Center, Kalamazoo County Head Start, Community Mental Health and Substance Agency, Family Court, and the Early Intervention Program.

## Intervention

The Kalamazoo Safe Start program involved a 26-week HSSIP curriculum, along with teacher and staff training and an optional parent curriculum.

### Head Start School Intervention Project Curriculum

The HSSIP school curriculum was adapted from the school-aged School Intervention Project. The curriculum consisted of six core elements. Within the general framework provided by the six core elements, there were specific "units" that set out for teachers the concrete activities that they were to engage in with the students in the classroom.

The six core elements of the curriculum were as follows:

1. **Feeling safe.** Students who do not feel safe usually have great difficulty regulating stress and their emotions. The curriculum was designed to build a level of safety and calm that is necessary for learning to occur.
2. **Making and keeping friends.** This component focuses on relational difficulties that are pervasive for children exposed to violence. Children learn different ways to communicate what they are feeling. The goal is for children to solve or avoid problems through good communication and to be nurtured within relationships.

3. **Calming mind and body.** In this aspect of the curriculum, students are instructed on how to deal with regulating their emotions, such as hyperalertness and sensitivity to changes within the environment. This part of the curriculum emphasizes calming strategies for both students and teachers.
4. **Feeling good about learning.** Students who feel safe, are able to regulate their own emotions, and have the support of school staff when they are struggling are more likely to have positive academic outcomes.
5. **Making meaning of experiences.** The curriculum helps children to understand that the environment is not always dangerous and that some adults can be trusted.
6. **Literacy.** Strategies to promote literacy were woven into the curriculum covering the first five components.

The five units within the curriculum were (1) Learning About School, (2) Learning About Self, (3) Learning About Community, (4) Learning About Friendship, and (5) Saying Goodbye. Within each unit, there were structured activities that build both social/emotional skills and literacy. Also included in the curriculum were professional development worksheets that allowed staff members to develop their own intervention plan for the classroom that tied into the structured activity, laid out according to the "plan-do-study-act model," which encourages staff to create an intervention plan, detail action steps, outline what action steps could be taken, and identify possible outcomes of the action.

The manual for the HSSIP was developed during the Safe Start pilot testing period and contained goals, activity length, materials needed, instructional procedures, key points, and tips to ease implementation. For example, one lesson in the "Learning about School" unit was "Time Capsule." The goals of this activity were to help the student experience how things change over time, because children exposed to violence "often have a poor sense of future or time" (Kiracofe et al., 2005). For this activity, students decorated name tags with pictures of themselves and placed them in a safe place, to be opened at the end of the school year. The manual pointed out key points relevant to anxiety that might come up during the activity (that the child may become frustrated while decorating the image or may not want to place the image in the capsule) and how to work around those issues. It also described tips on how to weave in literacy goals, such as how to introduce a calendar, how to emphasize the starting sound of each child's name, and how to read the names of the months aloud. The manual provided between one and five activities each week over the 26-week curriculum.

#### Teacher and Staff Training

The professional training for Head Start teachers and staff was a series of training slides and handouts, designed to help Head Start staff understand the link between CEV and changes in behavior, emotions, physiology, and learning. The curriculum is described in more detail in Appendix C of this report. In addition to a two-day training at the beginning of the school year delivered by Safe Start staff, ongoing consultation with school interventionists was planned to occur weekly or biweekly, in teams of teachers and aides who worked in each classroom. During these meetings, Head Start staff members could describe concerns or challenges related to specific students. Safe Start school interventionist staff members were prepared to put those issues in the context of violence exposure (as appropriate) and suggest strategies for response that would be consistent with the curriculum. For instance, a Safe Start staff member might explain that a child's aversive behaviors at the beginning of the school day might be in part a reaction to not feeling safe in the classroom, and that the teacher and aide could help by reassuring the student about safety, rather than punishing him or her. Central to this approach was the goal of improving the management of the child and the understanding that Head Start staff members have of their students—in essence, as stated by Safe Start staff, to go from seeing their difficult behavior as "being willfully disobedient" to seeing it as "striving for survival needs."

#### Parent Curriculum

The parent groups were designed to meet bimonthly for twelve 90-minute meetings, drawing on evidence-based approaches, such as Parent Child Interaction Therapy (PCIT; Chaffin et al., 2004; Hood and Eyberg, 2003), The Incredible Years (Webster-Stratton, 1994; Webster-Stratton, 1998), the Sanctuary Model (Bloom, 2005), START (Systematic Training to Assist in the Recovery from Trauma; Benamati, 2002), and TARGET (Trauma Adaptive Recovery Group Education; Ford and Russo, 2006). They aimed to provide specific and age-appropriate information about psychological, emotional, behavioral, social, and academic problems associated with CEV and to help foster the development of the child in three domains: trust, autonomy, and initiative. These parent groups were co-facilitated by two parent interventionists and organized in collaboration with Kalamazoo Head Start staff.

For example, one group's agenda began with a check-in procedure (ratings of parent's stress levels and control levels); taught some specific coping skills (linking thoughts and feelings), which included an arts activity that parents could also do with their children afterward (e.g., making play dough) that was done for the purpose of teaching them a pleasant, child-focused activity they could do with their child; and then closed with a centering activity (balancing a peacock feather on the palm of your hand) that was done for the purpose of teaching them how to calm themselves and focus on an external object rather than their own thoughts and worries.

Transportation and dinner were provided for the parents who attended, and their children were also provided dinner and games and supervision in an auditorium in the building. Attendance was planned as optional, with parents of all children participating in the intervention invited. Parents were also given an incentive for attendance—a $10 gift card per family per session attended. The parent training was not manualized but rather consisted of a series of agendas and parent materials.

The intervention was conducted in the context of a rigorous evaluation as required by OJJDP (see the box titled "Kalamazoo Safe Start Evaluation" for a description).

### Kalamazoo Safe Start Evaluation

**Design.** This randomized controlled effectiveness trial focused on child outcomes, with classrooms randomized.

**Treatment versus control group services.** In addition to the regular Head Start curriculum and services, children assigned to intervention classrooms received the HSSIP curriculum, and their teachers and staff members (bus drivers and aides) received training about CEV. Their parents were invited to participate in the optional parent curriculum. Children assigned to the control classrooms received the usual Head Start curriculum and services only.

**Kalamazoo Safe Start Evaluation (continued)**

**Data collection.** Longitudinal assessments were performed on child-level outcomes.

**Enrollment.** The site originally planned to enroll 162 families over the four-year period (81 in each group). The site modified plans to include a pilot test of the program in the first year, and then to include 356 families across three years. Funding for the National Evaluation ended prematurely, but Kalamazoo had completed its proposed collection by the time it ended, and expanded data collection as feasible within the constraints of funding. Over the three years, the site enrolled 231 children in the treatment group and 201 in the control group.

## Implementation

Figure B.7 diagrams Kalamazoo's implementation of the intervention. The following description of the program implementation is the result of data collected for the national evaluation. See Appendix A for a full discussion of the data collection methodology employed at each of the Safe Start sites.

### Project REVOC

The Project REVOC committee met regularly for the first year to 18 months of the project, focusing on the needs for additional evidence-based treatments for children exposed to trauma, and identified PCIT (Hembree-Kigin and McNeil, 1995) as a practice that would be beneficial in Kalamazoo. The group worked with the Safe Start Center to arrange training in PCIT for community-based therapists that would be available in the Kalamazoo catchment area but

**Figure B.7**
**Model of Kalamazoo Safe Start**

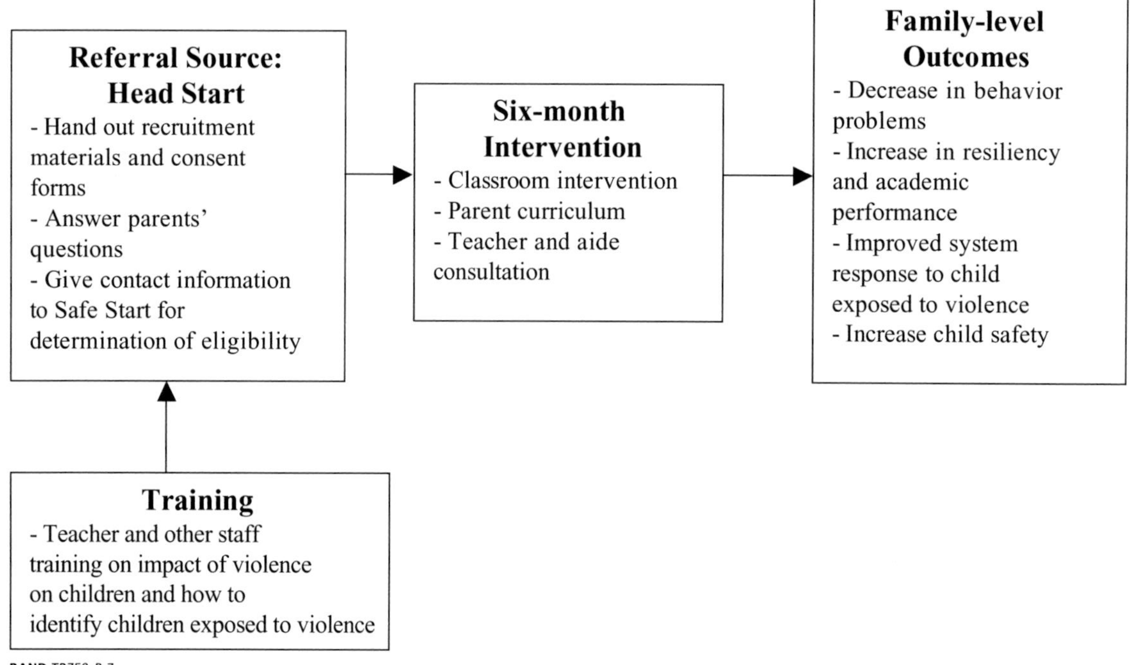


RAND *TR750-B.7*

unrelated to the Head Start Safe Start activities. After the completion of this task, attendance and commitment to the committee gradually dwindled down to the point that only the CTAC and Head Start staff were attending regularly, so the committee meetings were discontinued. Safe Start staff reported that the more focused agenda of bolstering evidence-based care for children exposed to violence worked better to engage community agencies than the broad focus on children exposed to violence. They also reported some difficulty in fully engaging local domestic violence agencies in the project, at least in part due to the focus on children, which was outside of their immediate missions.

### Recruitment

Kalamazoo Safe Start was able to implement the program generally as planned within the county Head Start classrooms, and they credit this to the buy-in that they had with key staff in the Head Start administration. The director and deputy director of Head Start collaborated with Kalamazoo Safe Start to select classrooms, assign children to classrooms, and arrange transportation in order to meet the needs of the project. The deputy director also participated in the trainings, observed intervention activities, and did much of the planning for the parent group meetings, which took place at the Head Start administration building.

Recruitment for the project began with Head Start teachers, who handed out the consent forms with an introductory letter to parents at the beginning of the school year, collected back signed forms, and gave them to the Safe Start staff members (for separate recruitment into the outcome evaluation research, discussed in detail in a separate report). All 12 children in each intervention classroom were exposed to the intervention, regardless of whether they took part in the research project.

### Services

Table B.7 summarizes service delivery for those who received services through the Kalamazoo Safe Start program. Throughout the first three years of implementation (through March 2009), Kalamazoo had one or two school interventionists (social workers) who delivered the intervention, along with the teachers and staff assigned to the specific intervention classrooms, as well as conducting the consultation sessions with teachers and aides. Two other staff members designed and delivered the parent group sessions. There were also research assistants, parent coordinators, and social workers who provided support throughout implementation.

#### *School Intervention Program (HSSIP) Curriculum*

The pilot test of the curriculum and development of the manual in the first year resulted in a detailed manual to be used in the rest of the project. Once the actual project began, the implementation proceeded about as expected. Safe Start activities were fit into the school day between required school elements, such as meals, outdoor time, and teeth brushing. The activities were

**Table B.7**
**Service Delivery for Enrollees in the Kalamazoo Safe Start Intervention**

| | Year 1 | Year 2 | Year 3 |
|---|---|---|---|
| Total number of classroom curriculum sessions | 425 | 374 | 455 |
| Total number of parent group therapy sessions | 59 | 11 | 17 |
| Total number of consultation meetings | 84 | 78 | 28 |
| Total number of classroom observations | 531 | 130 | 0 |

presented to the children as optional, offered as one possible activity that students could choose to participate in or not. Thus, not all students in the intervention classrooms took part in all Safe Start activities.

However, Head Start teachers and aides were not always able to carry out the activities as originally planned. At the beginning, the teachers and aides often used the opportunity of having an additional "hand" (the school interventionist) in the classroom to take care of some other task in the classroom or elsewhere in the building, and thus were not able to observe the activities as expected. In the following year, they were expected to begin participating in delivering the activities as co-leaders, but often were not able to do so because of the same types of competing demands. However, by the third implementation year, at least some teachers and aides were participating more fully, and some were leading the activities as intended.

#### *Teacher and Staff Training and Consultation*

The professional training was conducted at the beginning of each school year, once the intervention classrooms had been identified. In the first year, the presentation was largely didactic, and trainers received feedback from the trainees that it was overly so. In the second and third years, they modified the training to address this by presenting more vignettes and scenarios to engage the staff more.

Each Head Start classroom was staffed with a team consisting of a teacher, and aide, and/or a bus driver, such that there was a two- or three-person Head Start team for each set of 12 children. Bus drivers were included on these teams because they are the only direct contact with parents in some cases (picking up and dropping off children at the home) and spend a good deal of time with the children while en route. (However, there were not enough bus drivers to have one in each classroom.) Some teams served two classrooms per day (morning and afternoon), depending on the Head Start site. The plan to bring all these Head Start teams together weekly for consultation proved infeasible, as the staff members were unable to leave the classroom at the same time without engaging help, and the bus drivers were often off-site. Instead, the meetings included whoever was available and sometimes had to be canceled entirely.

Safe Start staff observed that the training and consultation meetings required a careful tone, so that the Head Start teams did not feel like they lacked skills or knowledge that the "experts" had. The Safe Start staff reported that they took great care to listen more to the Head Start teams than to offer advice, to understand the team's perspective, and to try to support them as much as possible. At the same time as the Safe Start staff were trying to change some of the fundamental ways that the Head Start teams might approach some children, they had to find a way not to blame the teacher, aide, or bus driver, but rather to focus on the needs of the child.

For example, Safe Start staff noticed early on that the teachers were trying to enforce a "rule" that all the children sit with crossed legs during portions of the classroom instruction. The Safe Start staff were tempted to question this policy, in recognition that many children would have trouble sitting still in a particular position, but instead waited for it to come up in consultation. When it did, Safe Start staff were able to support the teacher by acknowledging how hard it must be to enforce this, when children, particularly those exposed to violence, have trouble resting their bodies. This discussion occurred when the Head Start supervisor happened to be sitting in and was able to say that it was not actually a rule and that the teacher did not need to try to enforce it.

In general, Safe Start staff found the integration of the information they were offering to the Head Start team to be slower than expected. They thought this was partly because of competing demands for the teacher's attention and partly because of the difficulty in changing a culture in the classroom that values order and discipline over understanding the children's emotional needs. However, in the second and third year of the program, the Safe Start program staff reported some improvements in both the participation level of teachers and aides, with some teachers taking over the activities, and ways that teachers and aides were working with the children.

Safe Start program staff also noted during the first year of implementation some possible tensions related to race/ethnicity, with most of the teachers being white and many of the aides and students being African-American. They had wanted to include some discussion of differences in discipline and behavioral expectations in their training and consultation, and Head Start agreed that they could begin to broach this topic of cultural differences in the second year of the project.

#### *Parent Group Meetings*

Attendance at the biweekly parent groups was optional during the six-month implementation period, and only small numbers of parents took part. Safe Start staff found the groups to be challenging at first, with some parents wanting to use the groups for disclosure of their own violence exposure or hardships, rather than on learning parenting skills and information about the children. Safe Start staff reported that parents said the most important part of the groups was being together and providing support for one another, rather than the specific activities. There was also a sense that this group activity provided a "break" for many, since they could have dinner there for themselves and for their children, and they knew their children were safely being looked after. Thus, the groups may have served as respite and support, in addition to providing information and skills building as originally conceived.

There were other components of the Kalamazoo Safe Start program that helped shape the implementation. These are described in the box titled "Kalamazoo Safe Start Additional Program Components."

### Kalamazoo Safe Start Additional Program Components

**Quality Assurance.** Each of the intervention components was delivered in this project by the developers of the component, assisted by other staff. Thus, they were able to monitor fidelity to the model as it was implemented. HSSIP was documented in a detailed manual, and the developers were assisted by interns. They also used session adherence logs and attendance records to record each staff person's activities. Supervision occurred live, following activities, and on a weekly basis. Parent Group meetings were documented by handouts given to parents, log of attendance and incentives, and agendas for each meeting. Teacher training and consultation were documented by the slides used in the training.

**Training.** During the course of the first two years, Kalamazoo Safe Start conducted and/or participated in 111 training sessions. Most of these training sessions were focused on child welfare (26%) and clinical intervention (21%) issues. Topics of these sessions included training on complex trauma, parent support groups, and how to use assessment tools with Head Start students. As described earlier in this section, Kalamazoo Safe Start created a School Intervention Project curriculum that they used with teachers and other staff throughout the course of the year. This curriculum focused on issues affecting children exposed to violence, including safety, interpersonal relationships, and self-regulation to deal with stress.

### Kalamazoo Safe Start Additional Program Components (continued)

**Policies and Protocols.** The Kalamazoo Safe Start site implemented one major new policy. Early during program implementation, a network of home-based, outpatient, public, and private therapists were trained in Parent-Child Interactive Therapy (PCIT), an evidence-based intervention for children exposed to violence between ages 2 and 7 and their caregivers. There was an identified gap in services for children exposed to violence with regard to treatment resources for young children. PCIT-trained therapists were identified by the Project REVOC meetings as a needed resource. The network of therapists, 16 in total, committed to the provision of PCIT for children exposed to community violence in Kalamazoo and surrounding communities. The training eventually developed into regular, weekly conference calls with feedback, plus feedback and discussions on written reports from supervisors. In addition, the Safe Start Center developed an evaluation protocol for the training.

**Program Outreach.** The site held monthly Project REVOC meetings to report on Safe Start activities and community needs related to young children exposed to violence. These meetings continued throughout the duration of the program. Kalamazoo met with various representatives of a university-based foundation to discuss different funding sources for the April 2008 Safe Start Conference that the site planned. The site also sent letters and made phone calls in April 2008 to solicit donations to support the conference as well as raise awareness of the CTAC's involvement in the Safe Start program.

**Resources and Costs.** In the first two years of SSPA, Kalamazoo Safe Start used most of their resources for their staff, including their project director, school interventionist, parent coordinator, and clinical supervisor. Remaining funds were used for consultants (primarily Head Start) and general office supplies.

## Summary

The Kalamazoo Safe Start project combined a Head Start classroom-level curriculum for children ages 3 to 5 who had been exposed to violence, with training and consultation for the Head Start teachers and aides as well as an optional parent group that ran biweekly through the six-month intervention period. The classroom-level curriculum was offered to all children in the intervention classrooms and consisted of a series of lessons delivered through the week. Thus, the intervention was partly direct, with group activities within the classroom, and partly indirect, with training and consultation to improve knowledge and empathy among teachers, aides, bus drivers, and parents who attended the parent groups.

Project REVOC, a committee convened to guide the Safe Start project and, more broadly, interventions focused on children exposed to violence, helped to start off the project and culminated in training of community therapists in a parent-child therapeutic technique. After this, it was discontinued.

Kalamazoo Safe Start benefited from a close partnership with Kalamazoo County Head Start, enabling the program to recruit families readily for the project from within Safe Start classrooms, schedule training and consultation with teachers and aides, and make arrangements for the delivery of the parent groups. Kalamazoo Head Start also was fully engaged in the research component of the project. Thus, the complex logistics of delivering an intervention in this setting were minimized via an outstanding partnership that was evidenced through joint planning and investment of resources from Head Start.

Kalamazoo Head Start staff note that the intervention involved more than engaging in the actual intervention activities because it focused on changing the culture of the classrooms from one in which behavior is seen as "good" or "bad" and in need of teacher control to one in which the unique behavior of each child is seen in the context of a search for safety and healing from violence exposure. This cultural shift was challenging and demanded more time than originally expected by the Safe Start leadership. Ultimately, the Safe Start staff saw that teachers were implementing the activities and taking ownership of the curriculum by the end of the project.

Training of Head Start staff shifted over time from a more didactic, expert approach to a more interactive approach, and the teacher consultations took on a supportive approach as well, as evidenced by teacher comments that the teacher consultation sessions provided an outlet for the stress they experienced in the classroom. Parent groups, which had been planned to cover specific topics in parallel to the classroom curriculum, took on a more supportive function for parents than expected.

**Data collection for this program summary included:**

- Key informant interviews with key program staff and community partners:
  - Kalamazoo Safe Start director and project director
  - Classroom school interventionist and interns
  - Parent interventionists
  - Data collectors
  - Head Start administrator
  - Head Start teachers and aides and bus drivers
  - Safe Start budget administrator director
  - Parent participants in parent group meetings
- Observation of HSSIP curriculum implementation
- Observation of parent curriculum meeting
- Observation of consultation meetings
- Case review of randomly selected treatment group cases
- Quality assurance checklist completed by project director
- Quarterly activity reports on services, training, policies, and advocacy
- Grant application
- Green Light notes
- *Safe Start: Promising Approaches Communities Working Together to Help Children Exposed to Violence* (Safe Start Center, 2008).

# 8. Miami Program Description

## Miami Safe Start

- **Intervention type.** Infant mental health (IMH); dyadic CPP and Heroes group sessions
- **Intervention length:** 6 months (IMH), 10 weeks (Heroes)
- **Intervention Setting:** Domestic violence shelters and transitional housing, homeless shelters, and child and family clinics
- **Target population:** Children residing in specific shelters who have been exposed to domestic violence, community violence, and/or experienced abuse or neglect; or court-referred children with verified maltreatment allegations for clinic-based treatment
- **Age range:** Birth to age 12
- **Primary referral sources:** Shelter staff, juvenile court

## Program and Community Setting

The Miami Safe Start program is located in the county of Miami-Dade in Florida. According to the 2000 Census, Miami-Dade County had a population slightly less than 2.3 million, 6.5 percent of which was younger than age 5. In 2000, about 70 percent of the population was white, 20 percent black, about 1.4 percent Asian, less than 1 percent Native American, and about 57 percent Hispanic. In 1999, the per capita income was $21,658,[12] and approximately 18 percent of the population was living below the poverty line.[13] Rates of child maltreatment and domestic violence included more than 17,155 cases of child abuse reported between 2000 and 2003 in Miami-Dade County (Consortium for Children in Crisis, 2004).

The Miami Safe Start program built on earlier collaborative work within Miami-Dade County through three separate projects. First was a project called Prevention and Evaluation of Early Neglect and Trauma (PREVENT) in the Miami-Dade Juvenile Court, which developed treatment and assessment protocols for young children in the court system. This work led to recognition of developmental delays and impaired parenting in this group and the realization that very few services were offered for the younger children. As a result, the work expanded to a second state-funded project, the "Infant and Young Children's Mental Health Pilot Site," which identified three intervention sites: Miami, Sarasota, and Pinellas Counties. In Miami, the project implemented CPP for court-referred babies and toddlers. This project was followed by the OJJDP-funded Miami Safe Start Initiative (Phase I), a collaboration—involving a Juvenile Court (dependency division), the University of Miami, and Early Head Start—for children who were maltreated or who witnessed violence at home. Court-referred children in Early Head Start and their primary caregivers participated in the CPP intervention. Based on three program evaluations, the CPP intervention showed gains in parental sensitivity, child-parent interaction, and behavioral and emotional parental and child responsiveness and affect

[12] This is the 1999 income per capita converted to 2005 dollars; the 1999 per capita income as reported in 1999 dollars is $18,497.

[13] All of the above information was taken from the 2000 Census and can be found on the Census website at (U.S. Census Bureau, no date).

(Adams et al., 2003). Reunification rates for children and their parents were high, and no re-entry was seen into the child welfare system for the participating children in the six months after treatment (Osofsky et al., 2007). These three projects together used the term "Infant Mental Health" to describe the use of assessment and intervention (CPP) for very young children within Miami-Dade County.

Despite the success of this work, the collaborative still saw unmet needs for children outside the court system. For the Safe Start Promising Approaches proposal, the collaborative decided to expand to include the Miami-Dade County Department of Human Services system of child care providers and domestic violence divisions, which worked to support families experiencing domestic violence and outside of dependency court supervision, as well as the University of Miami's Department of Social Work. The prior collaborative, along with the Department of Human Services, called itself the Consortium for Children in Crisis and applied for the Safe Start Promising Approaches funding to expand services for children ages 0–18 by delivering services on-site in domestic violence shelters. The Miami Safe Start program had the following goals:

1. Expand clinical training in infant mental health.
2. Provide clinical services to underserved populations ages 0–6.
3. Deliver effective dyadic therapy in shelters for the first time.
4. Expand implementation of the group Heroes program for children ages 5–18.
5. Establish a more seamless community response system among providers within Miami-Dade County for children exposed to violence.

Miami's Safe Start proposal described how its program would address these five goals. In terms of training, the program planned to train more professionals in the Infant Mental Health (IMH) CPP model, including training others to be trainers in this model, thereby increasing the capacity to deliver this intervention in the community. Coupled with the CPP treatment would be an extensive assessment of the child and parent-child relationship. Also proposed were trainings for Miami-Dade County's Child Development Services staff (subsidized child care providers) in CEV and child maltreatment with the goal of improving child care practices when working with these children.

In terms of clinical services, the program proposed to increase the age range for use of Infant Mental Health (IMH) and to use a detailed assessment of parent-child interaction and development as well as dyadic parent-child psychotherapy for children 0–6. Also in the proposal was the Heroes program, developed at the University of Miami School of Social Work, for children ages 5–18. Expansion of this program to domestic violence shelters for implementation of both interventions was also planned. Finally, service would be extended to children of different ages (specifically, the underserved 4–5 year olds) and new intervention delivery sites, and to conducting outreach and training efforts across the counties.

In working through the OJJDP Green Light process to prepare for the national evaluation, some specific plans were formalized and altered. First, the age range for both IMH and the Heroes programs was changed. For the Heroes program, the upper age limit was reduced from 18 to 11, in recognition that the domestic violence shelters allowed women to bring young children, but not teenage boys, into the shelters. Second, the lower age limit for IMH was increased for infants to six months to bring it in line with the intervention model. Finally, the inclusion criteria for the two programs were changed so that there would be no age overlap, because the site did not have specific ideas about how to choose between IMH and Heroes for the 5-year-old children. Thus, children up to 60 months would receive IMH, and those 60 months or older would receive Heroes.

The domestic violence shelters chosen to provide referrals to Miami Safe Start project were two Department of Human Services transitional housing shelters (Inn Transition North, Inn Transition South) and the Lodge, a short-term emergency shelter operated by a private nonprofit group called Victim Response, Inc. Miami Safe Start proposed to deliver IMH and Heroes intervention services in both Inn Transition South and the Lodge, and Inn Transition North would serve as the source of the comparison group participants. This latter group would receive enhanced case management services consisting of a thorough assessment and feedback to caseworkers at the facility to improve case management and match family needs to possible community referrals.

The planned sites' recruitment of families for intervention changed during the course of the intervention—with elimination of one domestic violence shelter, expansion to two homeless shelters, and addition of a court-referred program for IMH. This point is explained in more detail below, and the ultimate partnering agencies are presented in the box titled "Miami Safe Start Partner Agencies."

## Miami Safe Start Partner Agencies

**Linda Ray Center.** The Linda Ray Center is a program within the University of Miami Department of Psychology and was founded in 1991. The center develops and delivers programs to improve the outcomes for Miami's at-risk children and families. The program's goal is to lay a foundation for school readiness, to build parenting skills, and to help families create safe environments. Evidence is collected on program effectiveness to share with the community and other partners. Services are funded by the Miami-Dade County Public Schools, the Florida Diagnostic and Learning Resources System of the Florida Department of Education, and research and demonstration funds from federal agencies. This agency was the lead for the Miami Consortium for Children in Crisis Safe Start site.

**Miami-Dade County Homeless Trust/Community Partnership for Homeless, Inc.** The Homeless Trust was established in 1993 and oversees the implementation of the Community Homeless Plan and administration of a 1 percent food and beverage tax. Its mission is to end homelessness in Miami-Dade County. The Homeless Trust partnered with Community Partnership for Homeless, Inc., a local private nonprofit agency that provides the direct services, with three levels of care: emergency housing, transitional housing, and permanent assisted housing. The Safe Start program operated in the emergency housing level, in both of the two Homeless Assistance Centers (HACs) in the county (opened in 1995 and 1998). These HACs operate as intake centers into the homeless assistance system of care, providing shelter, showers, food, clothing, mail, and telephones, along with counseling and development of a case plan for each individual. This agency collaborated to provide referrals and access to families within the shelters, space for interventions, and coordination of case management.

**Miami-Dade County Human Services Violence Intervention and Prevention Services.** This agency operates a number of services related to violence, including hotlines, victim assistance centers, emergency shelters, and two transitional housing shelters: Inn Transition North and Inn Transition South. These shelters receive referrals from any of the Homeless Trust agencies and involve the Junior League of Miami to help support their programs. This agency collaborated to provide referrals and access to families within the shelters, space for interventions, and coordination of case management.

**Miami Safe Start Partner Agencies (continued)**

**11th Judicial Circuit of Florida, Administrative Office of the Courts.** The court contains a Juvenile Division that handles delinquency and dependency cases, including child abuse and neglect, failure to protect (domestic violence), and other forms of child maltreatment. The administrative judge in the Juvenile Division helped to create the original Safe Start Dependency Court Intervention Project and participated by referring cases to Safe Start for IMH treatment at the Linda Ray Center.

## Intervention

The planned interventions included the PREVENT assessment, CPP for children ages 6 months to 60 months, and the Heroes groups for children ages 60 months to 12 years. The original plan called for mothers and their children who were residing in the three domestic violence shelters to be referred by shelter staff, assessed for eligibility by Safe Start staff, and enrolled in the age-appropriate program. Later, these services were expanded to two homeless shelters, and a court-referred IMH program was implemented at the Linda Ray Center, as will be discussed below.

### Infant Mental Health: PREVENT Assessment and Child-Parent Psychotherapy

The PREVENT assessment was conducted for all families with children in the 6-to-60-months age range, including those in the enhanced case management group. The assessment included several paper and pencil forms (depression inventory, parenting stress inventory) as well as a developmental assessment, gathering of background and pediatric health information, and a structured, videotaped parent-child interaction observation. This assessment was used for determining need for the intervention and to establish baseline functioning for the CPP intervention model. The assessment was administered twice: before treatment and at the end of treatment. The videotaped structured assessment of parent-child interaction was reviewed by the therapist and parent together, with the therapist pointing out strengths and areas needing attention. The parent-child assessment (Osofsky et al., 2007) included an unstructured playtime (with specific toys), a clean-up period, three tasks of various sorts, child separation from parent, and reunion. Eligibility for the IMH program required that the assessment reveal particular problems in the parent-child relationship in terms of affect/mood (e.g., blunted or angry affect), intrusiveness (e.g., overly directive, repeated commands), behavioral responsiveness (e.g., teasing, indifference), emotional responsiveness (e.g., unable to read child's cues), or discipline (e.g., overly harsh or derogatory comments).

CPP had been developed by Alicia Lieberman and Patricia Van Horn and then refined by Joy Osofsky for collaboration with the courts via the earlier Safe Start and IMH state pilot projects. It is highly similar to the CPP model implemented by other Safe Start sites. CPP is a relationship-based intervention designed for use with children up to age 6. It can be used with any child whose relationship to his or her parent or other primary caregiver is impacted by negative circumstances, including family violence. CPP integrates psychodynamic, attachment, trauma, cognitive-behavioral, and social learning theories (NCTSN, 2008). There are two components in CPP: assessment and treatment, with information gained during the assessment used to inform the treatment component. In the intervention component, child-parent interactions are the focus of six intervention modalities aimed at restoring a sense of mastery, security, and growth and promoting congruence between bodily sensations, feelings, and thinking on the part of both child and parent and in their relationship with one another (NCTSN, 2008). The intervention was expected to last approximately 25 sessions.

### Heroes

The Heroes program is an arts-based group approach to explore underlying distress related to exposure to violence for school-aged children. The program was developed at the University of Miami and used by its School of Social Work in the community before the development of Safe Start, but the program had not previously been published or evaluated. Each of the 10 group sessions began with a clip from a child-focused animated film, to help engage the children. Then various processing questions were asked of the group, followed by an expressive art activity (music, drawing, role plays, etc.) and a closure activity. At the proposal stage of the project, the manual for this intervention existed only in outline form, but the Safe Start Heroes intervention team developed it into a comprehensive manual during the course of the funded Safe Start project (Calvo et al., 2008). Children were to be included in Heroes groups if they were between the ages of 60 months and 12 years and had experienced or witnessed violence.

The intervention was conducted in the context of a rigorous evaluation as required by OJJDP (see the box titled "Miami Safe Start Evaluation" for a description).

### Miami Safe Start Evaluation

**Design.** The quasi-experimental effectiveness trial focused on child outcomes at two intervention shelters and one comparison shelter. A randomized controlled effectiveness trial (wait-list control group) was used for court-referred children.

**Treatment versus control group services.** In addition to extensive services available in the shelters (health care, child care, job training, etc.), families assigned to the treatment group received IMH or Heroes from therapists at shelters, or IMH at the clinic. Families assigned to the control group received enhanced case management: Some assessment results were given to the case manager at the shelters staff, and a resource book with specialized service information was given to staff and families. Court-referred families on the waiting list received support and referrals for six months until they were eligible to enroll in the IMH intervention.

**Data collection.** Data were collected through longitudinal assessments of child-level outcomes.

**Enrollment.** The site originally planned to enroll 175 families over the four-year period (30 in each group for Heroes, and 58 in each group for IMH). Funding for the National Evaluation ended prematurely. By the time it ended, enrollment had taken place over two years and six months and resulted in 84 families in the treatment group and 59 in the control group.

## Implementation

Figure B.8 shows Miami's implementation of its intervention. Miami's plan changed over time: Work was discontinued in one of the shelters and expanded to two additional homeless shelters using the same protocols. However, as noted in Figure B.8, Miami also expanded work to include IMH treatment at the Linda Ray Center for court-referred families whose children

**Figure B.8**
**Model of Miami Safe Start**

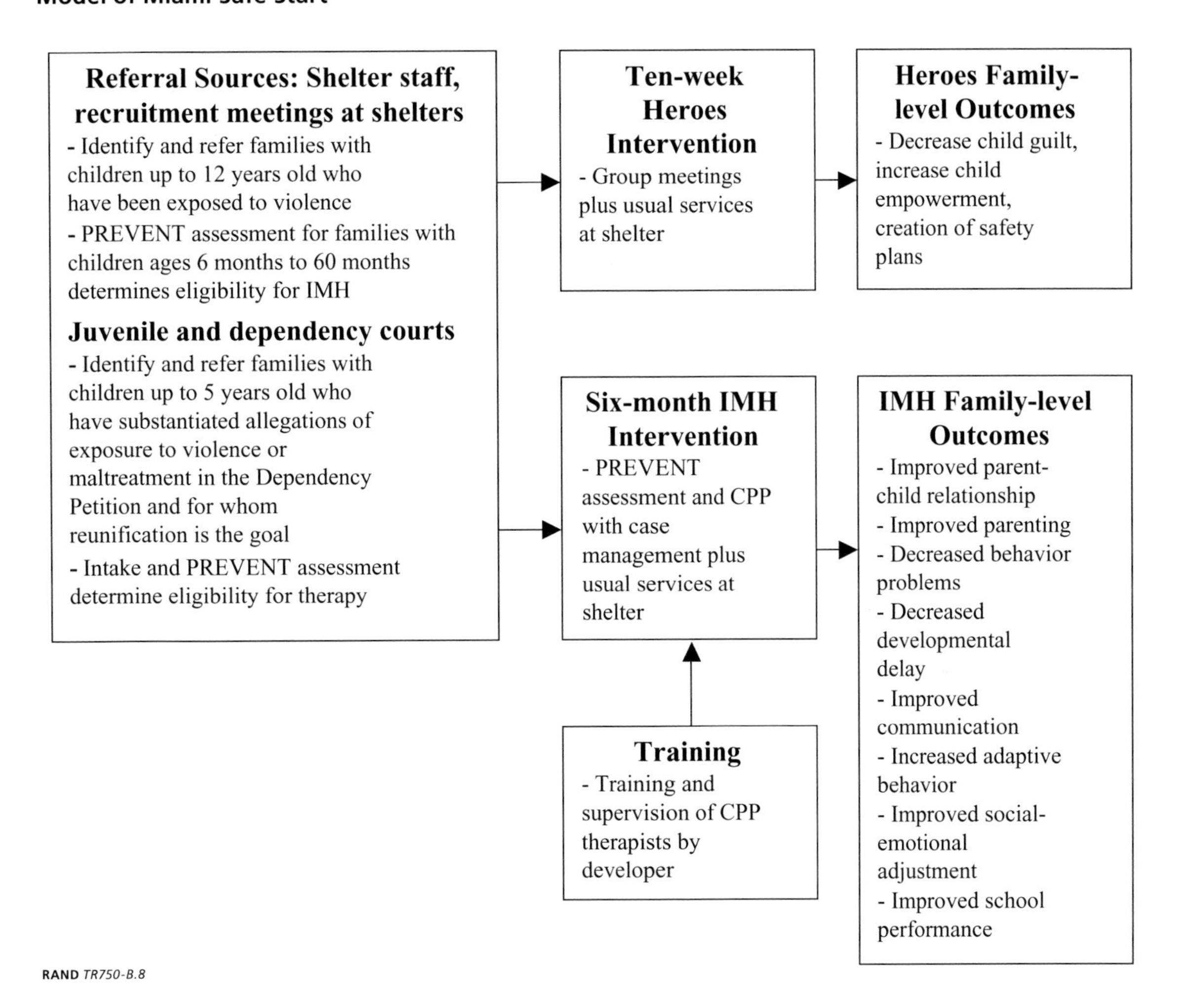


RAND *TR750-B.8*

had verified maltreatment. This intervention was similar to that developed in their earlier Phase 1 Safe Start work, including interaction and reporting to the court during the course of treatment. These changes will be explained in the section below.

The following description of the program implementation is the result of data collected for the national evaluation. See Appendix A for a full discussion of the data collection methodology employed at each of the Safe Start sites.

## Referrals

The referral plan for Miami's Safe Start program specified that shelter staff would refer interested families to the project, and the Safe Start staff would assess for eligibility and interest in the program. Inn Transition North housed 20 families at a time, who typically stayed six months to one year, whereas Inn Transition South housed 55 families, with stays of 1 to 2 years. In both cases, exceptions could be made for families to stay longer. Thus, turnover in families was low and only a portion of the families residing in these apartments were eligible for the project based on the age of their children. The referral plans appeared to work well at the two Inn Transition shelters, but were also augmented by having one of the Safe Start staff members attend the shelters' weekly group meetings to introduce the program, meet new families, and arrange appointments for the assessment with those who were interested. Thus, recruitment of families was successful and allowed the program to serve as many families as intended.

At the third shelter, referrals were more difficult. The Lodge was designed as a short-term emergency shelter, serving women and their children who had just fled violent situations and were therefore experiencing a great deal of stress. Their lengths of stay were short, and the shelter was usually filled to capacity, with virtually no space for assessments or intervention to occur on site. The Safe Start staff members were not allowed in the living areas and were required to stay in the public areas, making it difficult to connect with families directly without the help of the shelter staff. In addition, shelter staff appeared to have some concerns about the project and did not encourage families to participate in it. Specifically, according to Safe Start program staff, there were concerns about the focus on child abuse and maltreatment and the potential for reporting child abuse to authorities. A final problem noted by Safe Start staff is that the families were highly mobile upon leaving the shelter, and thus it was very difficult to complete treatment. After about six months of Safe Start implementation and repeated attempts to address these issues with the Lodge staff and administration, it was decided to stop work at this shelter.

Because the other two remaining shelters had limited capacity and high turnover, the Miami Safe Start program began discussions with the Homeless Trust organization to explore working in its regular homeless shelters, recruiting those exposed to violence. These meetings identified a mutual interest in working together, and eventually a plan for adding the two HACs operating in Miami-Dade County—the North/Central HAC and HAC-South. Work in these shelters began in the fall of 2007, about a year after the original project began. HAC-South would serve as the enhanced case management site, and North/Central HAC would serve as the IMH/Heroes site. Recruitment at these sites operated in much the same way as at the domestic violence shelters, with a combination of staff referral and direct recruitment at group meetings.

Finally, in the spring of 2008, Miami Safe Start sought approval from OJJDP to add an additional component to the study, to increase the number of families receiving IMH services. Families would be referred into the program from the Juvenile Court and receive services at the Linda Ray Center, extending their earlier Phase 1 Safe Start model. In order to evaluate this component, Miami Safe Start developed a randomized wait-list control group design, with some families waiting six months for IMH to begin.

### Services

In working with shelter-based families, questions arose over how to pick the service modality and identify the target child. When more than one child in a family was potentially eligible for the program by virtue of exposure to violence, identification of the "target child" for the program was sometimes difficult. Early on in the project, rules for the research project required that only one child per family participate in the evaluation portion of the project. Program staff, trained in IMH, often thought that the young child and parent-child dyad might be the best focus of treatment, but mothers often focused on the needs for their older child, who was more noticeably disruptive and upset. Concerned that this focus on the older child might not best meet the family's needs, the rule was adjusted so that a child could be included in each intervention (IMH and Heroes), thus serving the needs of the younger child and helping the mother with parenting, and at the same time meeting the needs of the older child via the Heroes groups. Additional siblings were also allowed to take part in Heroes as space permitted.

**Table B.8**
**Service Delivery for Enrollees in the Miami Safe Start Intervention**

| | Year 1 | Year 2 | Year 3 (6 mos) |
|---|---|---|---|
| Average quarterly caseload per therapist | 2.3 | 2.1 | 4.3 |
| Average quarterly caseload per case manager | 11.7 | 28 | 102 |
| Total number of child group therapy sessions | 29 | 33 | 21 |
| Total number of joint therapy sessions | 83 | 54 | 352 |
| Total number of case management meetings/contacts | 441 | 673 | 1322 |

Table B.8 summarizes service delivery for those who received services through the Miami Safe Start program. Miami had three to six therapists (2–4 IMH and 1–2 Heroes therapists, respectively) in Year 1, six therapists in Year 2 (4 IMH and 2 Heroes therapists), and five to six therapists in Year 3. Miami also had one to two case managers throughout the first three years of implementation.

#### *Infant Mental Health*

Implementation of the IMH intervention reportedly went according to plan at the two transitional housing shelters, where families stayed long enough to take part in the entire program and space was available for sessions and storage of play materials and video equipment used in the treatment sessions. However, as noted, challenges with these issues led Miami Safe Start to stop offering Safe Start at the Lodge emergency shelter.

To make up for the loss of the Lodge, the intervention services were expanded to the Central/North HAC in Miami as well as to dependency court-referred children at the nearby Linda Ray Center. Because space was limited at the HAC, those families took a shuttle bus or were transported by the Linda Ray Center van to the center to take part in the IMH services. Despite only a distance of a few blocks, this proved to be an obstacle. There were difficulties in making appointments and for families keeping appointments when the services were delivered outside of the shelter.

Therapists reported that the families in shelters had even more immediate needs due to housing issues than those in the dependency court systems, with whom they had a great deal of experience prior to this project. Thus, a good deal of time within IMH was spent on case management to help families resolve those needs, particularly with the few families at the Lodge. However, therapists also reported being able to engage parents in the dyadic therapy itself and in focusing on parenting and understanding the impact of the violence on their children.

#### *Heroes*

Like IMH, Heroes was also extended to the Central/North HAC. Forming and starting groups for Heroes occurred periodically at each of the two intervention shelters, and these worked well in terms of attendance and logistics. The therapists walked around the campus of the shelter to gather up the children and bring them to a community room, so that mothers were not burdened with bringing children to the session. Therapists reported that mothers were eager for the hour-long break from the children, and that the children liked the groups and were eager to attend them. Observation of one of the Heroes groups confirmed that the children were engaged in the group. The use of children's movies to initiate the discussion, provision of a snack, and experiential arts activities were all popular aspects of the groups, and the children appeared to be attached to the therapists.

#### *Enhanced Case Management*

At the Inn Transition North domestic violence shelter and the HAC-South homeless shelter, enhanced case management was offered as the comparison group for the Heroes and CPP interventions. The PREVENT assessment was summarized for the shelter case manager, and the case manager used this information for the tailored case management that was part of usual services at each shelter. Interviews with case managers revealed that they found the information from these assessments valuable, because there had typically been little focus on young children. Thus, the information about the mental health needs of the child could be integrated into the case plan for parents. In addition, case managers reported that parents were often worried about the impact of violence exposure on their child, and thus were eager to take part and get feedback on how their child was faring.

There were other components of the Miami Safe Start program that helped shape the implementation (see the box titled "Miami Safe Start Additional Program Components").

### Miami Safe Start Additional Program Components

**Quality Assurance.** Training for IMH was conducted by the model developer using detailed training slides, videotapes of parent-child interaction, and reading material on the model. Therapists met weekly with supervisors and in monthly collaborative discussions with the developer and had access to her for ad hoc consultation. PREVENT assessments were videotaped and sent to the developer's team for quality ratings. IMH therapy sessions were also videotaped for use in therapy sessions but not reviewed in supervision. The clinicians for the Heroes groups provided peer-to-peer support and training and met regularly with the original developer for model consultation and a licensed clinician for supervision. During the course of the project, all of the program therapists developed a treatment manual that describes the program in detail.

**Training.** Over the course of the first two years of the Safe Start program, Miami Safe Start conducted and/or participated in 23 trainings. Most of these trainings were focused on infant mental health. Approximately 27 percent of the trainings were focused on child welfare issues, 22 percent of the trainings were clinical, 18 percent were focused on interventions such as Heroes, and 13 percent focused on Safe Start programming in general and systems of care. Topics of sessions included the effects of violence on maltreated young children, infant-parent relationships, and relationship-based assessments. As planned, Miami Safe Start conducted three trainings designed for Child Development Services child care workers.

**Policies and Protocols.** As the Miami Safe Start program was implemented, staff made several changes in sites for recruitment and service delivery, as noted in this section. In addition, Miami Safe Start developed and implemented an evidence-based group model parenting program for parents of children ages 0–3 in the dependency system with identified maltreatment (Project Hand-N-Hand) and also implemented the PREVENT assessment and at least one standardized measure of parenting attitudes before and after intervention for court-referred families. They also designed a template for use when making court reports on family/child progress. Additionally, the site worked on developing new legislation pursuant to requiring that maltreated children ages 0–3 be in quality child care, and they worked with Child Welfare's lead agency to begin planning what the quality assurance section will look like in terms of monitoring agencies and examining fidelity to the parenting curricula.

**Miami Safe Start Additional Program Components (continued)**

**Program Outreach.** Miami's advocacy efforts included presentations to graduate-level clinicians to increase community support and identify additional clinicians interested in the project. They also conducted presentations to external visitors to explain the project and clinical model of assessment and treatment for children ages 0–3 who have been exposed to trauma and violence. Miami Safe Start also held meetings to discuss expanding the program to other populations and prepared law enforcement training on the effects of violence and maltreatment on children younger than age 5 and the services available for children/families in that target group.

**Resources and Costs.** In the first two years of SSPA, Miami Safe Start used most of their resources for its staff, including their project director, research evaluator, and program coordinators. Remaining funds were used for consultants and a partial contribution to rent fees.

## Summary

The Miami Safe Start project provided two different interventions, one for children ages 6 to 60 months, the other for children from 60 months through age 12. Originally slated to work in three domestic violence shelters and to conduct extensive training in the county for child care providers, the program plans changed over time as obstacles were encountered. Eventually the program was implemented in two domestic violence shelters and two homeless shelters, and IMH services were delivered to court-referred families at the Linda Ray Center. This flexibility in adapting to the constraints and barriers at the shelters is noteworthy, given the time and funding constraints for this project.

By the end of the project, consensus among the Safe Start Miami program was that the IMH model was difficult to implement in transitional housing shelters, and that neither intervention was viable in the emergency shelters because of the multiple issues faced by the families, lack of continuity in the shelter, and lack of readiness to focus on child mental health and well-being. Program staff's more familiar and long-standing work with court-referred families stands in contrast. For these families, participation in IMH is required as part of the reunification plan, and thus the court plays a critical role in ensuring participation and completion of treatment. However, therapists reported that, when they were able to engage sheltered families in IMH, they followed the treatment protocol and work on key issues with the dyad, with a slight emphasis on case management. The Heroes groups, on the other hand, were more easily implemented in the transitional housing settings and were well received by staff and families. In the transitional housing shelters, turnover was low because of space constraints and the fact that families that were successfully going through the steps for permanent housing (e.g., job trainings, school) were often granted extensions to stay in the shelters longer.

Also notable were the extensive services offered in usual care at the shelters, augmented by the enhanced case management, which involve an array of services tailored to each particular family. These services are provided to all families in the shelters, although each family may take up different services to different degrees.

**Data collection for this program summary included:**

- Key informant interviews with key program staff:
  - Safe Start program leadership
  - Staff from Inn Transition North and South leadership
  - Staff from HAC-South and Central/North HAC
  - IMH therapists
  - Heroes therapists
- Case review of randomly selected treatment and control group cases
- Observation of IMH therapist training session and interview with trainer
- Observation of Heroes group session
- Quality assurance checklist completed by the project director
- Quarterly activity reports on services, training, policies, and advocacy
- Grant application
- Green Light notes
- *Safe Start: Promising Approaches Communities Working Together to Help Children Exposed to Violence* (Safe Start Center, 2008).

## 9. Multnomah County Program Description

- **Intervention type:** Domestic violence advocacy, CPP, and case coordination and consultation
- **Intervention length:** For all components, flexible depending on meeting goals of case plan
- **Intervention Setting:** In-home and office-based
- **Target population:** Children exposed to domestic violence within a county child welfare population
- **Age range:** 0–6
- **Primary referral source:** Gresham Branch Office of County Child Welfare Services

### Program and Community Setting

The Multnomah County Safe Start program was located in Multnomah County, Oregon, with the intervention services provided in Gresham, Oregon. According to the 2000 Census, Multnomah County's population was almost 661,000, with nearly 6.5 percent being children younger than age 5. County residents were 79 percent white, 6 percent black, almost 6 percent Asian, slightly less than 2 percent Native American or Pacific Islander, and 7.5 percent Hispanic. The 1999 per capita income was $26,486,[14] and about 12.5 percent of the population was living below the poverty line at that time.

Adjacent to the City of Portland, Gresham is located in Multnomah County, the most populous county in Oregon. In the 2000 census, Gresham's population was 90,205 residents, with 8 percent being children age 5 or younger. Gresham's residents were 83 percent white, 3 percent Asian, and 2 percent black, with the remainder representing other races. Nearly 12 percent of residents were Hispanic. The 1999 per capita income of Gresham was somewhat lower than Multnomah County's overall, at $22,935.[15] The share of the population living below the federal poverty line, however, was equal to that of the larger county, at 12.5 percent (Multnomah County, 2004).

At the time of the Multnomah County Safe Start proposal to OJJDP, within the state of Oregon an estimated 33 percent of all domestic violence-related physical assaults and 20 percent of all sexual assaults perpetrated by an intimate partner were witnessed by one or more children (Multnomah County, 2004). Compared with the rest of the state, Multnomah County also reported a higher risk of co-occurring domestic violence exposure among its child abuse cases managed by child welfare services (37% in Multnomah County cases relative to 28% statewide) (Multnomah County, 2004). The proposed Multnomah County Safe Start program was primarily designed to address these kinds of cases, both by providing direct services (discussed below) and enhancing the services available to these families by establishing and enhancing collaboration between child welfare services and domestic violence service providers.

Prior to OJJDP's announcement of the availability of Safe Start funding for SSPA, Multnomah County was interested in implementing a partnership between domestic violence and child welfare service providers and had been holding multiagency discussions about what form such a collaboration might take. This interest stemmed from the fact that although the

---

[14] This is actually the 1999 income per capita in 2005 dollars. The 1999 income per capita as reported in the 2000 Census is $22,606.

[15] This is actually the 1999 income per capita in 2005 dollars. The 1999 income per capita as reported in the 2000 Census is $19,588.

county had well-developed systems of response to domestic violence and child abuse, there was little communication, coordination, or mutual understanding between these two systems. In fact, Multnomah County sought this partnership as a means to help overcome historical tension around the roles and orientation of child welfare workers and domestic violence service providers. Traditionally, child welfare workers have focused on the "best interests of the child," sometimes resulting in negative consequences (such as loss of child custody) for mothers who "fail to protect" children from exposure to domestic violence. At the same time, domestic violence advocates have focused on holding the perpetrator of domestic violence accountable for the exposure, rather than a victimized mother, and historically viewed the child welfare system as blaming and further victimizing abused mothers (Multnomah County, 2004). The county applied for the OJJDP Safe Start award to enable them to pilot-test implementation of a collaborative model that would co-locate domestic violence advocates within a child welfare office (discussed in detail below). The overall goals of the program were as follows:

1. Improve direct services to individual families affected by domestic violence and referred for child welfare involvement.
2. Improve the county's system of care for families by eliminating the tension between the orientation and practices of the domestic violence and child welfare systems (Multnomah County, 2004).

The lead agency in this effort was the county's Domestic Violence Coordinator's Office, which is responsible for fostering interagency relationships to address domestic violence in the county. This office provided the oversight, coordination, and support for the Safe Start program. The services were provided in collaboration with (and to the clients of) the City of Gresham branch of the Oregon Department of Human Services Child Welfare Office. The service providers themselves were employed by partner agencies but relocated for Safe Start to the Gresham Child Welfare Office. Domestic violence advocates were provided by the Volunteers of America Home Free Program and Catholic Charities' El Programa Hispano, whereas a mental health counselor was provided by the Listen to Kids organization (see the box titled "Multnomah County Safe Start Partner Agencies" for descriptions of the partnering agencies). The Safe Start program aimed to "co-locate" these domestic violence service providers within the Child Welfare Office to enhance the domestic violence services provided within the context of child welfare and to help foster integration between these two separate spheres of social service.

The Multnomah County Safe Start program was developed to serve families with children (from birth to age 6) who have been exposed to domestic violence and referred to the Gresham branch Child Welfare Office for protective services assessment due to allegations of child neglect or abuse. As discussed further below, *exposure to domestic violence* was defined as a mother having experienced violence or abuse perpetrated by a present or former romantic partner in the past 60 days. The program did not require that children had witnessed an incident.

As originally developed, the Multnomah County Safe Start program consisted of both direct services to mothers and children and an indirect component, which included advocates providing case consultation and technical assistance to child welfare workers. The latter was intended to enhance and improve the services provided to families who were both impacted by domestic violence and involved with child welfare. The primary component of the direct client services was the provision of domestic violence advocacy to all mothers who had experienced domestic violence. A secondary direct service component was to also offer mothers mental health services (CPP) that focused on addressing the impact of domestic violence on parenting, children, and the parent-child relationship. These services will be discussed in more detail in a subsequent section.

## Multnomah County Safe Start Partner Agencies

**Multnomah County Domestic Violence Coordinator's Office, Department of Human Services.** This office provides leadership and assistance in implementing domestic violence policy adopted by the Multnomah County Board of Commissioners. It staffs the county's Family Violence Coordinating Council, a multiagency partnership focused on community-wide domestic violence prevention and intervention, and provided consultation, support, and technical assistance to organizations and community groups interested in addressing domestic violence. For Safe Start, this office received the grant award and coordinated and oversaw the Safe Start program.

**Gresham Child Welfare Office, Oregon Department of Human Services, Children, Adults and Family Division.** The Oregon Department of Human Services Child Welfare Offices provide voluntary and court-ordered child welfare services through regional branch field offices throughout the state. The offices operate the Multnomah County child abuse and neglect reporting hotline; conduct investigation and assessment of alleged child abuse and neglect; provide case management services; coordinate and oversee foster care, referrals to community services, child advocacy, substance abuse assessment, and counseling; and maintain contracts and partnerships for the provision of a host of other services. The Gresham branch Child Welfare Office served as the location of the Safe Start program, providing the program referrals and housing the Safe Start service providers.

**Volunteers of America Home Free Program.** The Home Free program provides services and support to adult victims of domestic violence and their children. It provides crisis intervention, advocacy, danger assessment and safety planning, housing assistance, support groups for adults and children, and food boxes and other essentials to help meet basic needs. In addition to office-based services, it also provides services through home visits and meeting clients at other community locations. In the Safe Start program, the Home Free program provided one domestic violence advocate to be located at and provide services through the Gresham Child Welfare Office.

**Catholic Charities' El Programa Hispano.** El Programa Hispano is a program housed within the Catholic Charities social service organization. It is a social service program for low-income, Spanish-speaking residents of the Multnomah County metro region, intended to help improve their quality of life and promote cross-cultural understanding. El Programa Hispano has a specific concentration on serving the needs of Latina women victimized by domestic violence and their children. The program provides Spanish-speaking, multicultural advocates to help Latinas navigate the social service and legal systems, provide support and assistance with meeting basic needs, and other advocacy services, such as safety planning. For the Safe Start project, El Programa Hispano provided one Spanish-speaking bicultural domestic violence advocate to be located at and provide services through the Gresham Child Welfare Office.

**Listen to Kids.** Serving the Multnomah County metro region, Listen to Kids (formerly Community Advocates for Safety and Self-Reliance) is a nonprofit organization providing prevention and early intervention programs focusing on child abuse, domestic violence, and sexual assault. Listen to Kids offers a school-based prevention program in elementary and preschool settings. It also offers the Parent Child Involvement Project, which provides groups and home-visiting mental health services for children exposed to domestic violence and their mothers. For the Safe Start project, Listen to Kids provided a masters-level counselor to provide the therapeutic services for Safe Start clients.

The Multnomah County program was selected by OJJDP as one of 15 Safe Start Promising Approaches program sites around the country. After receiving the grant, the Multnomah County participated in OJJDP's Green Light process to prepare for program implementation and evaluation. The program design itself was already well developed, so the Green Light period allowed time for the staff to prepare for implementation. In particular, the Safe Start service providers prepared for physically relocating to the Gresham Child Welfare Office and for spending time "shadowing" child welfare workers as they went about their duties. The staff reported that this period allowed them to become more familiar with the duties and procedures of the Child Welfare staff in anticipation of launching services. The bulk of the time during the Green Light process was focused on developing a feasible evaluation design within the context of a child welfare caseload. Because randomizing clients was not feasible in the child welfare system, Multnomah County proposed a comparison group at another Child Welfare Office.[16]

## Intervention

The Multnomah County Safe Start program involved three main components: domestic violence advocacy, CPP, and case coordination and consultation. For all components, the intervention length was not predetermined and instead was allowed to vary depending on individual need and case plan. The services were voluntary and offered in addition to usual services and procedures of the Gresham Child Welfare Office. Services were provided either in the client's home or in an office or other community setting, wherever was most convenient for the client. Domestic violence advocacy was intended to be the primary service, provided to all clients. Case coordination and consultation among the domestic violence advocates, child welfare workers, and, when applicable, the CPP provider was also expected for all clients. CPP would be offered as an additional service for mothers who expressed an interest in improving their parenting or parent-child relationship impacted by the experience of domestic violence.

### Domestic Violence Advocacy

Domestic violence advocacy services were offered to all mothers with young children referred to child welfare for which a new or recent domestic violence incident (i.e., within the last 60 days) had occurred. These were voluntary services offered to all mothers in addition to the usual Child Welfare services. The domestic violence advocate was physically located in the Gresham Child Welfare Office to facilitate the identification of cases and direct service coordination with child welfare workers.

The initial advocacy services involved conducting a domestic violence–focused assessment of the mother and child's degree of safety and associated needs for protection from an abusive partner. The advocates also assessed whether the family's basic needs were being met for such things as food, clothing, housing, and utilities. The advocate then worked with the mother to develop a safety plan and assisted her as needed to meet the basic needs of

[16] This issue will be discussed more fully, including the criteria for eligibility for the outcome evaluation, in our subsequent report on the topic of the Safe Start outcome evaluation.

herself and her children. This could involve helping mothers access domestic violence–specific resources, navigate the domestic violence–related legal system (police, courts, and restraining orders, etc.), and understand the impact of domestic violence on children and the implications of Child Welfare involvement. The advocates also offered domestic violence victim support groups and provided individual social support, such as accompanying mothers to court hearings. The length of the advocacy services was not predetermined and would continue based on individual need. Ultimately, the model expected that domestic violence–specific advocacy services would improve the mother's life circumstances and functioning, which is necessary for improvement of those of the children.

#### Child-Parent Psychotherapy

The therapy component involved a modification of the Lieberman and Van Horn (2005) model for CPP (discussed further below). CPP is a relationship-based intervention designed for use with children up to age 6. It can be used with any child whose relationship to the parent or other primary caregiver is impacted by negative circumstances, including family violence. CPP integrates psychodynamic, attachment, trauma, cognitive-behavioral, and social learning theories (NCTSN, 2008). There are two components in CPP: assessment and treatment, with information gained during the assessment used to inform the treatment component. In the intervention component, child-parent interactions are the focus of six intervention modalities aimed at restoring a sense of mastery, security, and growth and promoting congruence between bodily sensations, feelings, and thinking on the part of both child and parent and in their relationship with one another (NCTSN, 2008).

In Multnomah County, CPP was delivered in clients' homes by a program staff member with a master's degree in social work, referred to as a "parent-child specialist." The Listen to Kids program internally trained its staff (including the individual it hired to be the Safe Start parent-child specialist) to deliver CPP using the "Don't Hit My Mommy" description of the model (Lieberman and Van Horn, 2005) as the guide. Specifically, the sessions were focused on helping mothers recognize, understand, and respond to the impact of domestic violence on their children and on their own parenting. The intake into the counseling component involved taking information about the family's domestic violence history; reviewing the mother's concerns about her parenting, relationship with her children, and their behaviors; and developing a case plan with the mother setting out goals (tied to the mother's specific concerns) to work toward over the course of the sessions. The home-based sessions were expected to last 60–90 minutes, but the number of sessions or total length was not predetermined. The sessions ended when the goals of case plan were achieved.

#### Case Coordination and Consultation

In addition to the direct services provided to families, the Multnomah County Safe Start program emphasized an indirect component intended to improve services to individual families as well as ultimately result in system-level change for cases that involved both child welfare and domestic violence. Case coordination services included discussions and joint case planning between child welfare workers and domestic violence advocates to coordinate efforts and services to families they are jointly serving. Case coordination involved both formal case review meetings (which could include multiple other service providers, such as the parent-child specialist) and informal conversations as the child welfare workers and advocates interacted with one another around the office or stopped by each other's work spaces to "touch base" about a particular family. The Multnomah County model emphasized the importance of co-location of the advocates within the Child Welfare Office to allow for the informal, spontaneous conversations about needs and progress in individual cases.

The Multnomah County program anticipated that co-location would allow both advocates and child welfare workers to gain a better understanding of each other's approach to working with individual families, including best practices and legal and agency policy requirements. This was seen as a first step in promoting system-level change. The program expected that, as the two sets of service providers interacted more frequently and collaboratively on individual cases, a mutual appreciation would develop and distrust would be reduced. In addition, the program offered cross-training and made advocates available for "technical assistance" consultation to child welfare workers in all of the latter's cases, not just those they were jointly serving. An example would be a case in which the domestic violence had been relatively minor or there was no apparent risk for recurrence. Thus, intensive and ongoing domestic violence advocacy might not be needed, so no advocacy case would be opened. But, as the child welfare worker managed the cases, he or she could seek ad hoc consultation with the advocate if the need did arise.

The Safe Start leadership also convened formal monthly partner meetings wherein all key players in the program and their supervisors discussed progress toward system-level change and worked toward resolving ongoing challenges. These partner meetings were intended to provide a regular forum for identifying and addressing barriers to domestic violence–child welfare collaboration and identifying ways to institutionalize the collaborative practice within the Gresham Child Welfare Office.

The outcome of this formal collaboration was expected to be better, more comprehensive services to families impacted by domestic violence, a reduction in removals of children from their mothers in domestic violence cases, and improved knowledge and practice among child welfare workers in working with families impacted by domestic violence.

The intervention was conducted in the context of a rigorous evaluation as required by OJJDP (see the box titled "Multnomah County Safe Start Evaluation" for a description).

### Multnomah County Safe Start Evaluation

**Design.** The quasi-experimental effectiveness trial focused on child outcomes.

**Treatment versus comparison group services.** The treatment group in the Gresham branch Child Welfare Office received domestic violence advocacy, case coordination, and a modified version of CPP. Study enrollees from the comparison branches of county child welfare offices received child welfare case management services and referrals as usual.

**Data collection.** Data were collected through longitudinal assessments of child-level outcomes.

**Enrollment.** The site originally planned to enroll 160 families over the four-year period (80 in each group). Funding for the National Evaluation ended prematurely. By the time it ended, enrollment had taken place over two years and three months and resulted in 31 families in the treatment group and nine in the comparison group.

## Implementation

Figure B.9 shows the implementation of Multnomah County's Safe Start intervention. The following description of the program implementation is the result of data collected for the national evaluation. See Appendix A for a full discussion of the data collection methodology employed at each of the Safe Start sites.

### Referrals

The referrals for the Multnomah County Safe Start program came exclusively through the Gresham branch of the county's child welfare services office. Eligibility criteria for Safe Start services were as follows:

- Current or recent domestic violence issues were identified as a reason for child welfare referral or as a family issue during the subsequent child welfare investigation.

**Figure B.9**
**Model of Multnomah County Safe Start**

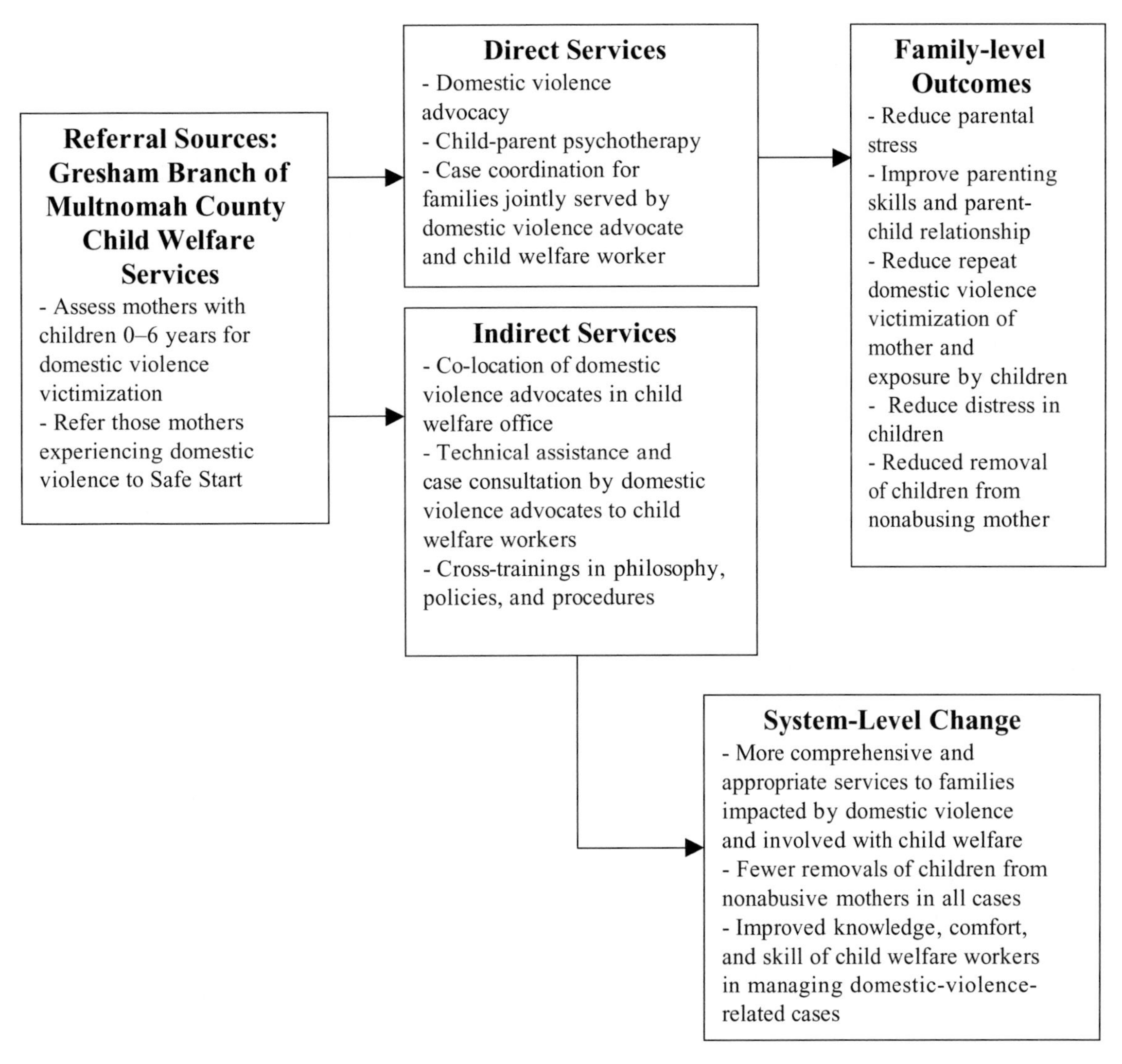


RAND *TR750-B.9*

- Mother (or primary female caregiver) of the children in the case had experienced domestic violence.
- At least one child in the family was age 6 or younger.

Within this group, priority for Safe Start advocacy services was given to families with children at risk of being removed from the custody of a nonabusing mother and families at high risk for repeat domestic violence. Referrals to Safe Start typically were made directly to the domestic violence advocates.

The Safe Start program was designed to receive referrals from the Protective Services organizational unit of the Gresham Child Welfare Office. This unit is responsible for receiving and investigating reports of child abuse and neglect, determining what services are needed, and recommending whether children should be removed from the home. For the Safe Start program, referrals initially came in from a Protective Service supervisor or worker as they reviewed and investigated new cases. Following several months of implementation, the domestic violence advocates also started receiving referrals from child welfare workers in the office's Permanency organizational unit, which is responsible for managing cases that have been open for (typically) more than 60 days. These referrals typically involved new incidents of domestic violence that had occurred within the existing permanency cases.

The Safe Start staff reported that this was both a positive occurrence (indicating that their services were growing in reputation in the office generally) but also a potential sign of some concern. According to Safe Start program staff, the caseworkers working with the Permanency cases operated under a different philosophy of case management, were less familiar with Safe Start, and worked with challenging, often long-standing cases. They indicated a suspicion that some Permanency workers referred mothers to Safe Start expecting that the mother would fail to follow through on the referral or to actively take advantage of voluntary services. This failure then could be used as part of a body of evidence justifying the removal of children from mothers and/or to terminate their parental rights. In short, the staff had mixed feelings about the unsolicited referrals coming from the Permanency side of the Child Welfare Office. RAND's research team did not interview Permanency workers as part of data collection, so we can offer no observations of their perspectives on the program or services.

Upon receipt of a referral, a domestic violence advocate made contact with the mother in the Child Welfare Office when she arrived to meet with a child welfare worker, or the domestic violence advocate traveled with the child welfare worker to meet the mother at her home or other location. The domestic violence advocate presented the Safe Start advocacy services to the mother as a voluntary service, separate from the involvement of and services offered by the child welfare worker. Consenting mothers would then begin working with the domestic violence advocate and would also be offered CPP through the parent-child specialist.

In the first few months of implementation, referrals of mothers to the domestic violence advocates proceeded at a slow pace. According to program staff, the pace picked up dramatically as child welfare workers "warmed up" to the presence of the domestic violence advocates in the office and came to more fully appreciate the type of services that the advocates were able to provide. The increase in referrals was reportedly also related to on-site training from a nationally known expert on domestic violence–child welfare collaborations. This expert, Sue Hubert of the Massachusetts Department of Social Services, delivered a well-received joint training to child welfare staff and the Safe Start service providers that addressed how the roles and functions of both child welfare workers and domestic violence service providers could be seen as complementary and described strategies for improving the collaborative interaction between them.

As a result of the activities, the pace of referrals picked up so much that, within the first year of implementation, the domestic violence advocates reported feeling as if they were serving as many families as possible on their own caseload. They also reported feeling that they could provide ad hoc consultation to child welfare workers on other domestic violence cases, but not actively open an advocacy case themselves. The referral process to the parent-child specialist typically came through the domestic violence advocates; however, after about a year of implementation, the parent-child specialist began to receive some referrals directly from child welfare workers. The pace of referrals to the parent-child specialists, however, did not exceed their caseload capacity during the first two years of implementation.

### Services

Table B.9 summarizes average quarterly caseload per staff and service delivery for those who received services through the Multnomah County Safe Start program. Over the course of implementation, its staff consisted of two advocates and one parent-child specialist. Table B.9 shows services through March 2009, representing just two quarters of implementation in Year 3.

#### *Domestic Violence Advocacy*

The domestic violence advocacy services appear to have been largely implemented as planned. The Safe Start program staff, supervisors, and partners reported an overall positive impression of the services and the integration within the child welfare context. There was reportedly some initial distrust or uncertainty about how the advocate's services could assist the child welfare workers managing their cases, but over time the staff became more familiar with each other and the relationships became more collaborative. That is, understanding and communication between the advocates and the child welfare workers improved, and they began working more closely together on individual cases. As discussed, referrals were initially slow, but then the pace of referrals increased as the partners began to see progress toward promoting communication and understanding between advocates and child welfare workers.

According to Safe Start program staff, despite initial distrust or lack of interest, many child welfare workers came to view the advocates as a useful resource and an important asset to their office. The advocates were able to assist child welfare workers in particular with working with mothers during the often intensive period around the initial referral of the family to child welfare. This was a point at which many families experience considerable turmoil in their lives (such as a lack of safe housing, involvement with the criminal justice system, etc.) and often great fear of the child welfare workers themselves. Although the co-location meant that the advocates at times faced difficulty helping mothers understand the difference between themselves

**Table B.9**
**Service Delivery by the Multnomah County Safe Start Intervention**

| | Year 1 | Year 2 | Year 3 (3 mo) |
|---|---|---|---|
| Average active quarterly caseload per advocate | 18 | 23 | 19.3 |
| Average active quarterly caseload for the parent-child specialist | 10 | 11 | 12 |
| Total number of joint therapy sessions | 199 | 247 | 89 |
| Total number of parent support group meetings | 62 | 82 | 6 |
| Total number of case consultation meetings | 255 | 443 | 257 |

and child welfare workers, they reported feeling generally successful overcoming that difficulty. The advocates and their supervisor reported initial concerns about the confidentiality of their client conversations and records but found after implementation that child welfare workers were understanding and appropriately respectful of advocates' communications with and referrals provided to clients.

By the same token, the increase in the pace of the referrals to the domestic violence advocates after implementation revealed that the partners needed to more clearly define the emphasis of the advocacy services (i.e., the specific family needs on which the advocate needed to focus). That is, because many clients had multiple needs and faced complex issues (such as a lack of access to basic necessities, legal issues, medical problems, extreme poverty, safety concerns, transportation difficulties, extended family structures, mental health issues), there was the potential for advocates to work intensely with a single client for a long time. The size of the advocates' active caseload limited their availability in the office to consult with child welfare workers. This issue raised concerns among the Safe Start partners, because if advocates were unable to take new cases and unavailable in the office for case consultation, then the system-level change the program sought was jeopardized.

In response, during the first year of implementation, the Safe Start partners worked to prioritize domestic violence–specific services that required the expertise and system knowledge and networks uniquely possessed by the advocates. The advocates then refocused their time in working with clients on these domestic violence–specific services and referrals (such as restraining order assistance and safety planning) and assisted clients in connecting with other service providers who could help meet other oftentimes intensive needs (such as housing, food stamps, and employment assistance). This program revision reportedly increased the availability of the advocates while still ensuring that families could continue to access advocacy-type services, if they chose to engage with the new provider. The Safe Start partners viewed this as a positive revision and felt it was critical to continuing to build and enhance the domestic violence–child welfare collaborative relationship.

A related issue arose around defining the end of advocacy services. The program chose to leave open the period of service and continued serving clients as long as needed. In practice, this resulted in high-need clients working with advocates for close to one year, sometimes well beyond the involvement of child welfare. As advocacy caseloads filled up, the partners determined that the advocates should more actively transition clients to other domestic violence service providers in the community, if they continued to need service beyond the close of child welfare involvement. The partners did not establish a firm timeline but rather allowed for flexibility in the advocate's decision about the appropriate point to help a Safe Start client transition to an appropriate community-based domestic violence provider.

#### *Child-Parent Psychotherapy*

Like advocacy, the therapy component of the program was initially slow in ramping up but eventually picked up to provide a sufficient caseload for the parent-child specialists delivering the sessions. Referrals primarily came through the domestic violence advocates, but eventually the parent-child specialist began receiving referrals directly from child welfare workers as they became more familiar with the goals and approach of the therapy. Services were provided by a single parent-child specialist. She was hired specifically for Safe Start by the Listen to Kids organization. She was co-located within child welfare after being trained by Listen to Kids staff in the CPP model. Initially, there was some uncertainty about delivering CPP to families involved with child welfare, because families sometimes disengage from services at the end of child welfare involvement. It was further complicated in situations where foster parents were temporarily caring for children and there was uncertainty about when/if children would be returned to live with their mothers. In these situations, staff reported that it was not clear how to appropriately work with the mother regarding her parenting and relationship with her children, and it was also unclear when CPP sessions should terminate with the mother if it appeared children would not be returned.

Unlike the manualized description of CPP, Multnomah County's implementation of CPP rarely focused on a dyad. Instead, the parent-child specialist reported that the work typically involved the mother and multiple children of varying ages and (occasionally) also a father. Thus, the parent-child specialist reported needing to modify strategies of the dyadic CPP approach for use within this larger or whole family context. The home-based delivery of the sessions was important to making participation manageable and consistent for many clients, but it also presented challenges. For example, there could be frequent distractions (such as telephone calls, visitors, television), and some mothers felt the need to "multitask" during sessions at home (such as doing dishes or caring for a small child). Overall, the parent-child specialist reported that, despite the implementation challenges, the modified CPP approach was a promising one for her clients.

#### *Case Coordination and Consultation*

As previously discussed, the case coordination and consultation were provided both as a direct service and as a way to promote system-level change. In terms of direct service, the case coordination meetings, or team decision meetings, were viewed by the providers as important and productive. In these meetings, service providers would discuss such issues as their individual, role-specific case plans; discuss their views on family needs and progress; and jointly coordinate services (to avoid duplication). Disagreements among the service providers were also discovered, discussed, and often resolved in these meetings.

In addition to serving the specific function of coordinating services in individual cases, the Safe Start partners reported that these meetings served to promote the system change goal. They deepened understanding of each provider's disciplinary perspective, constraints, motivations, and responsibilities. Along with the co-location of the Safe Start domestic violence service providers, these meetings were credited with helping to reduce some of the initial distrust between the domestic violence service providers and the child welfare workers.

The monthly meetings involving the domestic violence service providers, their supervisors, and representatives from the child welfare office also facilitated understanding and communication between these parties about program implementation and provided a forum for regular troubleshooting of challenges to implementation. These meetings were seen as indispensable to integrating Safe Start into the Gresham Child Welfare Office.

The parent-child specialist also provided ad hoc consultation on child development mental health issues to child welfare workers with increasing frequency, primarily focused on interpreting and addressing the behavior of children exposed to domestic violence in their caseloads. This form of informal consultation in the hallways of the office, along with the consultation offered by the domestic violence advocates, was also viewed by the interviewees as important to integrating Safe Start into the Child Welfare Office.

Our interviewees consistently reported that the Safe Start program was showing signs of success in terms of its system change goal. The domestic violence providers appeared to be fully integrated within the Child Welfare Office. Committed office leadership was cited as important to facilitating this progress. For example, the manager of the Gresham office intentionally located the Safe Start program staff just outside his office door. Thus, caseworkers would have to pass the Safe Start cubicles to come to his office. This physical location helped to elevate the status of the Safe Start program within the office as well as facilitate the informal conversations that were cited as key to relationship building.

With respect to system change, many interviewees mentioned the on-site training provided by a consultant with national stature (Sue Hubert) who was able to speak with considerable credibility to both child welfare workers and domestic violence service providers about strategies for recognizing and addressing the challenges surrounding collaboration and integration of the two service approaches. Several interviewees reported that these efforts, in combination with local trainings the Safe Start staff offered about their own services, helped to recruit several "core" child welfare workers to engage with the Safe Start program. Their participation and positive experiences then reportedly led to the engagement of many other workers in the office.

Locally, the partners reported that the Safe Start program in the Gresham Child Welfare Office came to be seen as a local success in creating system change, specifically in changing child welfare practice in cases involving children exposed to domestic violence. Accordingly, Safe Start staff members provided general domestic violence training to all new child welfare workers in the county as part of this general awareness and improved services effort, and Safe Start in the Gresham office was the focus of state-level attention as a potential model of collaboration for the rest of the state.

Although the program appears to have made significant strides toward its goal of system change, several continuing concerns were raised. The integration of the Safe Start program was limited to the Protective Services side of the child welfare office. The Permanency side of the office had not been targeted by Safe Start, although the leadership expressed an interest in doing so. In addition, concerns were raised that roles of the service providers could become blurred over time. In particular, as advocates were co-located within another agency, there was the potential for them to be "co-opted" by child welfare in their philosophy and function. The program found that regular oversight of co-located staff was needed to ensure firm grounding in the core domestic violence advocacy function.

There were other components of the Multnomah County's Safe Start program that helped shape the implementation. These are described the box titled "Multnomah County Safe Start Additional Program Components."

### Multnomah County Safe Start Additional Program Components

**Quality Assurance.** The domestic violence advocates, parent-child specialist, and child welfare workers had prior experience working with victims of domestic violence. Specific training on the intervention, the child welfare system, and implementation plans occurred early in the project. The domestic violence advocates were supervised during monthly meetings and ad hoc consultation with their respective agency supervisors. The advocates also participated in the monthly partner meetings to discuss their service provision overall. The parent-child specialist received clinical supervision once per week through her agency, augmented by weekly meetings with her direct supervisor to discuss her services and individual cases.

**Multnomah County Safe Start Additional Program Components (continued)**

**Training.** Over the course of the first two years of program implementation, Multnomah County Safe Start conducted or participated in 36 trainings. Most of these training sessions were focused on domestic violence (28%), child welfare (14%), and clinical intervention (14%) topics. Multnomah Safe Start spent training time with Sue Hubert, from the Massachusetts Department of Social Services, to improve collaboration between domestic violence and child welfare staff in working with children exposed to violence. This training is described earlier in this section.

**Policies and Protocols.** Multnomah County Safe Start has instituted and changed a number of policies and protocols to better serve its community and run more efficiently. For example, Multnomah County worked with a contracted child welfare agency to develop a protocol for identifying domestic violence cases; developed a new protocol to better facilitate the flow of appropriate information regarding domestic violence between the District Attorney's Office and Child Welfare Offices; developed a new procedure for reviewing and revising documentation practices for the team decision meetings to better protect the clients' safety and privacy; and created a new protocol for the Child Protective Services referral/cross-reporting for cases handled by the Domestic Violence Enhanced Response Team (DVERT).

**Program Advocacy.** Multnomah County's advocacy efforts included presentations to the community to gain support for Safe Start, meetings, presentations, and collaborations with other agencies to raise funding for programs that support the domestic violence community. The program also advocated for state funding to support the placement of domestic violence advocates in all Child Welfare Offices across the state. Also, Safe Start provided presentations and information about the overlap of domestic violence and child welfare issues and the co-location of domestic violence services for child welfare–involved families. Multnomah County's advocacy contributed to the proposal and passage of Oregon House Bill 3273, which encourages child welfare agencies to contract with domestic violence victim services to provide services to the victims with child welfare cases.

**Resources and Costs.** In the first two years of SSPA, Multnomah County Safe Start used less of their resources for staff salaries, relying on in-kind commitment not supported by OJJDP. However, they used funds for program implementation supplies and direct client assistance (e.g., basic needs such as food and travel).

## Summary

The Multnomah County Safe Start program developed an ongoing collaboration between the Oregon Department of Human Services Child Welfare Office, the Multnomah County Domestic Violence Coordinator's Office, and the service provider partner agencies. Co-location of the service providers (two domestic violence advocates and one parent-child specialist) in the Child Welfare Office appeared to play a central role in facilitating an understanding of staff's respective roles and responsibilities and communication between child welfare caseworkers and domestic violence service providers. This collaboration proved to be important to obtaining referrals from the caseworkers, working together on specific cases, and enco uraging caseworkers to seek out advocates for ad hoc consultation on domestic violence issues. In short, the program moved substantially toward its goals of institutionalizing the collaboration of domestic violence service providers (advocates and therapist) and child welfare workers.

Further case coordination was accomplished through monthly partners' meetings. These meetings appeared to serve a particularly valuable function by allowing partners to provide regular feedback about implementation and affording them an ongoing opportunity for troubleshooting and development of solutions. Moreover, the child welfare leadership's commitment to the program strongly reinforced the value of the program for the workers. However, the integration was limited to the Protective Services side of the office. It might take a similar investment of time and effort to build collaborative relationships with the Permanency side of the office.

**Data collection for this program summary included:**

- Key informant interviews with key program staff and community partners:
  - Safe Start project director and supervisor
  - Safe Start counselor and supervisor
  - Safe Start advocates and supervisors
  - Gresham Branch Child Welfare caseworkers and supervisors
  - Manager of Gresham Branch of the Child Welfare Office
  - Observations of service providers partner meetings
- Case review of randomly selected treatment group cases
- Quality assurance checklist completed by supervisor
- Quarterly activity reports on services, training, policies, and advocacy
- Grant application
- Green Light notes
- *Safe Start: Promising Approaches Communities Working Together to Help Children Exposed to Violence* (Safe Start Center, 2008).

## 10. Oakland Program Description

### Oakland Safe Start

- **Intervention type:** Case management integrated with dyadic caregiver/child psychotherapy
- **Intervention length:** 24 weekly sessions over 6 months
- **Intervention setting:** In-home, community, or agency setting
- **Target population:** Children residing in Oakland who have been exposed to domestic violence, community violence, and/or experienced abuse or neglect
- **Age range:** 0–5
- **Primary referral sources:** Family Paths, Inc. (formerly known as Parental Stress Services), Family Hotline, Oakland Police Department, Oakland Family Violence Intervention Unit, Alameda County Family Justice Center, Another Road to Safety, Children's Hospital-DOVES project, and early childhood education sites and community-based organizations

### Program and Community Setting

The Oakland Safe Start program was located in the City of Oakland, located in Alameda County, California. The population of the city was 399,484, according to the 2000 U.S. Census. About 7 percent of the population was younger than age 5; 31 percent of the population was white, 36 percent was black, 22 percent was Hispanic, 15 percent was Asian, and the remaining were other races. The income per capita for Oakland overall was $25,687;[17] 19 percent of the population was living under the federal poverty line.[18]

Prior to the development of the Oakland Safe Start program, there was no comprehensive source of data on the extent of CEV (East Bay Community Foundation Safe Passages Initiative, 2004). Sources (such as California Department of Justice and Oakland Police Department) indicated that the level of such exposure might be high. The Oakland Police Department, in a review of reported domestic violence incidents in 2000, found that 63 percent of the calls involved residences containing children ages 5 or younger (Safe Passages, 2004). The rate of violence in the City of Oakland was high overall compared to the rest of the cities in Alameda County and to the state of California. For example, the 2003 homicide rate in Oakland was 27 per 100,000, compared with slightly more than 9 for Alameda County and about 7 for the state as a whole (Federal Bureau of Investigation, 2006). This high level of violence was not equally distributed across the city. According to data from the Oakland Police Department, between 1999 and 2004 about 70 percent of violent incidents occurred in the Oakland neighborhoods of West Oakland, East Oakland, and San Antonio (Safe Passages, 2004). Thus, children living in these neighborhoods faced a particularly high risk of exposure to violence relative to those in other areas of the city.

Before the Safe Start program, several efforts had been made to identify and enhance the services available for children ages 0–5 exposed to violence in Oakland. Among these was the Early Childhood Policy Committee, which Safe Passages (the organization that would later lead the development of the Safe Start program) began convening in 2001. This committee brought together representatives from a host of agencies that frequently came into contact with or provided the types of services accessed by children exposed to violence. Among the

---

[17] This is the income per capita reported on the 2000 Census but converted into 2005 dollars.

[18] The information was all taken from the 2000 Census and can be found at the Census website (U.S. Census Bureau, no date).

numerous agencies were the Oakland Police Department, Oakland Head Start, the Oakland Unified School District, the Oakland Department of Human Services, and the Alameda County Social Service Agency. The committee's mission was to begin cataloging the existing services and identify key service gaps. In addition, in 2003 the Safe Passages organization launched a companion activity called the Safe Passages Oakland Early Childhood Initiative. This initiative began addressing some of the services gaps by implementing programs (such as a preschool program that provided a violence prevention curriculum) and providing access to mental health services for children exposed to violence.

Despite these efforts, Safe Passages and the Early Childhood Policy Committee continued to seek ways to address remaining service gaps. This commitment motivated Safe Passages to lead the development of an application to OJJDP for Safe Start program funding.

Specifically, the proposed Oakland Safe Start had three goals:

1. Increase identification of children ages 0–5 who have been exposed to violence.
2. Centralize intake and screening of these young children.
3. Provide culturally appropriate case management services for young children exposed to violence and their families.

Oakland's Safe Start proposal described how its program would address these three goals. Under the goal of increased identification, the project planned to identify and refer young children exposed to violence to agencies providing social services, particularly those collaborating with Safe Passages. The project intended to increase identification through public awareness campaigns, by training delivered to public and private organizations, and by adding additional staff to the Family Hotline. The hotline is a telephone-based service provided by Family Paths, Inc., to Alameda County residents seeking immediate assistance with parenting and care of children, including those exposed to violence.

The project also sought to create a new process for centralizing referrals of children exposed to violence and their families. This central location would be staffed by a single "intake coordinator," who would respond to calls from individuals and agencies across the city. The intent of this centralized model was to move away from a stovepiped process of screening and referrals, in which families were often offered only a subset of services available in the community, limited to those services that were available to the referring organization or agency.

The third goal of the proposed Safe Start project was to add to the services available in the community by offering longer-term, intensive case management to young children exposed to violence and their families. The proposed case management services had two distinctive features. First, in addition to helping families access needed services to address basic needs, the case management services would give priority to assisting families in accessing mental health services. Second, the case management emphasized culturally appropriate services, offered by staff that spoke the primary languages of underserved groups living in the city's high-violence areas, primarily speakers of Spanish, Chinese, and Vietnamese.

After the Oakland program was selected by OJJDP as a Safe Start site, Safe Passages led its partnership in further developing and refining its program and evaluation plans as part of OJJDP's Green Light process. During this process, the Oakland program leadership refined the formal integration of therapeutic services in the program. Thus, instead of case managers working with families to access therapists as a separate service (not provided by Safe Start), the program decided to integrate these two services—one individual would provide both case management and therapeutic services. This refinement was intended to implement the program's vision of building trust between the therapist and the family and helping to keep the family engaged in the services overall by reducing the number of individual service providers with whom families are asked to form relationships.

Also during the Green Light process, the Oakland Safe Start leadership conducted a series of meetings with potential referral agencies. The intention was to inform them about the Safe Start services and to train them to use the newly created web-based database for documenting children exposed to violence. The development of this database proceeded with support from Safe Start as well as the Violence Prevention and Public Safety Act of 2004, referred to as "Measure Y," a local ordinance that mandated resources for addressing CEV. Measure Y's age range included children up to age 17, so the focus expanded from young children to include all children for purposes of identification and intake coordinator services. The integrated case management and mental health services funded by Safe Start remained for young children, ages 0–5. Safe Start eligibility also required that the child reside in Oakland and that the child's primary caregiver needed multiple services, including basic needs such as food, clothing and housing, physical safety, as well as mental health services.

The box titled "Oakland Safe Start Partner Agencies" provides descriptions of the partnering agencies.

### Oakland Safe Start Partner Agencies

**Safe Passages.** Safe Passages is a nonprofit organization that functions as the research and development entity for public agencies within Alameda County, California. Founded in 1998, its focus is on developing, implementing, and evaluating prevention and intervention strategies for addressing needs of at-risk and vulnerable children and youth. It seeks to identify promising strategies to serve these needs as well as serve as a coordinating body to bring together the resources and insights of multiple private and government agencies at city, county, and state levels to implement them. Safe Passages was the lead organization in the Safe Start program. It managed the program, conducted the intake process, and provided leadership and support to the partner agencies delivering the intervention. The Early Childhood Policy Committee, the collaboration created by Safe Passages to address service gaps for children ages 0–5 exposed to violence and their families, convened bimonthly to discuss the implementation of the program.

**Oakland Department of Human Services (DHS).** Originating in the 1960s, the department is a local government agency that provides a range of social services to children, youth, adults, and seniors in Oakland. The department develops and delivers prevention and early intervention programs and participates in human service collaborations. The department's Early Childhood and Family Services Division contributes to the development of early childhood development and education, family support, and young children's readiness for school. The Oakland Department of Human Services was the coapplicant for the Safe Start program.

**Jewish Family and Children Services of East Bay.** This is a nonprofit, direct service organization that provides multilingual and multicultural case management and mental health services to underserved communities within Alameda and Contra Costa Counties. Founded in 1877, the organization houses 25 distinct programs that fall within the five areas of older adult services, parenting and youth services, counseling services, refugee and immigrant services, and volunteer services. In the Oakland Safe Start project, Jewish Family and Children Services staff provided the case management and therapy services for English- and Spanish-speaking clients.

### Oakland Safe Start Partner Agencies (continued)

**Asian Community Mental Health Services.** Established in 1974, this nonprofit, community-based organization provides multilingual and multicultural mental health and support services to Asian and Pacific Islander families in Alameda County. These services include case management, substance abuse treatment, services for the developmentally disabled, and behavioral health care services. The latter includes assessment, psychiatric evaluation, individual and family therapy, family education, clinical case management, and medication therapy, among other services. In the Oakland Safe Start project, Asian Community Mental Health Services staff provided the case management and therapy services for monolingual and bilingual Asian families.

**Family Paths, Inc.** This is a nonprofit organization targeting the prevention of child abuse and neglect in Alameda County. Formed in 1972, it provides a variety of services, including the Family Hotline (offering telephone-based crisis counseling, support, and referrals), respite child care, parent education classes, child and family therapy, telephone-based support and assistance for foster parents, and case management services. In the Oakland Safe Start project, Family Paths, Inc., participated in increasing capacity to identify children exposed to violence and in building the centralized referral process managed by Safe Passages.

## Intervention

Oakland's Safe Start program included a broad citywide effort to increase identification, screening, and referral of children ages 0–5 who had been exposed to violence. The program hired and trained the intake coordinator and established her office location in Alameda County's Family Justice Center located in Oakland. The intake coordinator's location was intended to increase referrals and provide easier access to the Safe Start program intake for children exposed to violence identified by agencies co-located at the Family Justice Center. Specifically, the intake coordinator

- obtained information about the child, family, and circumstances
- conducted a screening to determine the child and family's needs and eligibility for the Safe Start program
- referred eligible families (i.e., children ages 0–5) who were interested in participating in the Safe Start program
- provided uninterested or noneligible families with specific targeted referrals to community resources
- provided limited-term case management services to help families with urgent needs access community services.

The majority of referrals were expected to come from information entered by partner organizations and agencies into a web-based, password-protected database. Specifically, as these agencies encountered children exposed to violence, they were trained to inform the primary caregiver about the intake coordinator and seek consent to enter information about the child and family into this referral database. The intake coordinator would then regularly access this database and contact the family. Families who declined to be contacted for follow-up services would be asked if anonymous demographic information about the child and his/her violence exposure could be entered into the database for purposes of helping to compile descriptive data about the problem of CEV in Oakland. Families who agreed to be contacted for further information and were eligible for Safe Start were invited to participate in the program.

The Safe Start program consisted of integrated, intensive case management and mental health services provided by staff at one of two agencies. English- and Spanish-speaking clients were served by the Jewish Family and Children's Services of East Bay. Asian families (monolingual and bilingual) were served by at Asian Community Mental Health Services. Services at both agencies lasted for a minimum of 24 one-hour sessions delivered weekly over six months, but the specific content of the services and how they were implemented were not standardized. Each agency agreed to provide case management services along with therapy sessions, but the specific model of therapy was not closely coordinated across the two agencies. In addition, Asian Community Mental Health Services used a two-person case manager–therapist team for each family, whereas Jewish Family and Children's Services utilized therapists to provide both case management and mental health services. Both agencies conducted sessions either in the family's home or at another location convenient for the family. Also, staff at both agencies received domestic violence training and specialized cultural competency training in advance of implementation.

Therapists at both agencies received some initial training from Safe Passages staff on providing and integrating case management services. The case management services were expected to account for approximately half of the 24 weekly sessions. The total number of sessions offered by both agencies was extended as necessary to meet the family's needs both for therapy and for case management. Case management at both agencies included assistance to families in securing public and community services (such as legal, food, transportation, emergency financial assistance, medical care, housing support, child care, and employment) and collateral contact with other agencies to facilitate families' access to other services. Asian Community Mental Health Services' case management services are rooted in a strength-based empowerment model that draws on ethnic and cultural roots, and family and community assets. Services are also designed to address the various issues faced by young children and their families, such as translation and interpretation needs, and federal immigration assistance.

For the mental health services, the agencies implemented an approach referred to as "Dyadic Caregiver/Parent-Child/Infant Psychotherapy." This approach involves activities such as play therapy and includes the caregiver conveying empathy as well as interpreting child's behavior by commenting on the emotions and reactions of the child. It is a flexible, dyadic approach, targeted toward improving child social functioning, establishing or reestablishing positive parent/caregiver-child interaction and attachment, and identifying the root causes of mental health problems and maladaptive child behavior (such as anxiety, depression, or impulse control). Therapists already employed by both agencies were adequately trained in this approach prior to delivery. Safe Start therapists at Jewish Family and Children's Services were master's-level clinicians and either licensed or license eligible. Asian Community Mental Health Services therapists were master's-level licensed therapists. All therapists had received some training in early child mental health and in addressing trauma.

The intervention was conducted in the context of a rigorous evaluation as required by OJJDP (see the box titled "Oakland Safe Start Evaluation" for a description).[19]

---

[19] Because of differences in the implementation of the intervention at the two different program sites and challenges in obtaining multiple translations of evaluation assessments materials, only the Safe Start services provided through the Jewish Family and Children's Services were selected to be part of the outcome evaluation.

**Oakland Safe Start Evaluation**

**Design.** This randomized control effectiveness trial was focused on child outcomes.

**Treatment versus control group services.** Both groups received an initial intake and needs assessment, referral to existing community resources, and limited-term case management from the intake coordinator. Families randomized to the treatment group received integrated case management and dyadic therapy sessions from therapists at Jewish Family and Children's Services.

**Data collection.** Data were collected through longitudinal assessments of child-level outcomes.

**Enrollment.** The site originally planned to enroll 200 families over the four-year period (100 in each group). Funding for the National Evaluation ended prematurely. By the time it ended, enrollment had taken place over two years and three months and resulted in 41 families in the treatment group and 40 in the control group.

## Implementation

Figure B.10 shows Oakland's implementation of its intervention. The following description of the program implementation is the result of data collected for the national evaluation. See Appendix A for a full discussion of the data collection methodology employed at each of the Safe Start sites.

### Referrals

Under Oakland's Safe Start model, "referral" described both the identification referral of families to the Safe Start intake coordinator and the services referral by the intake coordinator to community resources, including the Safe Start program.

With the creation of the Safe Start intake coordinator position, the program hoped to create a citywide system of receiving and processing referrals of children exposed to violence to a centralized intake coordinator, who would in turn provide (1) screening and referrals to available community resources and (2) limited case management services, particularly to assist families in accessing the services to which they were referred. The intake coordinator then served as the source of family referrals to Safe Start–supported services of integrated case management/mental health services provided by Asian Family Community Mental Health Services and Jewish Family Services.

Eligibility for the Safe Start program was determined by the intake coordinator over the course of one or more in-person meetings with the family. A client's mental health, degree of abuse or exposure to violence, and basic needs were all assessed during the intake process. Because both the identification referrals to the intake coordinator and the service referrals from the intake coordinator to the case management/therapy component of the Safe Start program were coming through newly implemented processes, both types of referrals initially came in somewhat slowly. As a result, the intake coordinator engaged in a variety of training and outreach efforts to increase the referrals coming into the intake coordinator. By the second year of implementation, however, the pace of referrals had increased considerably to the intake coordinator and had approached the maximum capacity for a single individual to manage the duties of the role.

**Figure B.10**
**Model of Oakland Safe Start**

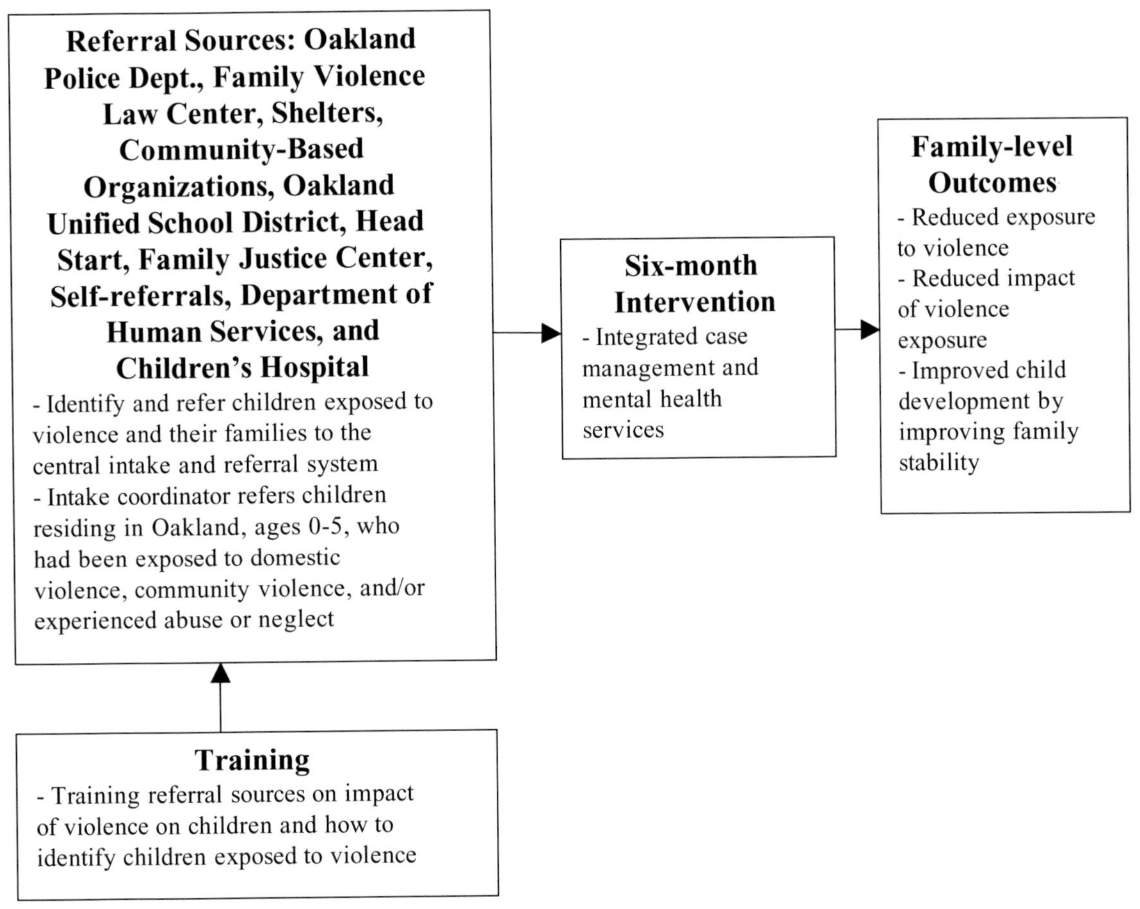


RAND *TR750-B.10*

The referrals and enrollments in the Safe Start intensive case management/therapy component remained somewhat under the pace anticipated. According to the Safe Start program staff, this may have been due to the eligibility criteria's focus on very young children, the potential concerns of families about being randomly assigned to a service, and stigma associated with receiving mental health services among families in the target population.

## Services

Table B.10 summarizes service delivery for the two agencies that delivered services through the Oakland Safe Start program. Jewish Family and Children Services had two to three providers during Year 1 and three to four providers during Year 2. In the first quarter of Year 3 (through March 2009), the program had 5 providers. The providers had an integrated role, with individual providers delivering both case management and mental health services. For Asian Community Mental Health Services, social workers and case managers provided the case management portion of the services and clinicians delivered the mental health services. Both types of providers made collateral contacts. Over the entire implementation period, Asian Community Mental Health Services had one mental health clinician and two providers delivering case management services.

**Table B.10**
**Service Delivery for Enrollees in the Oakland Safe Start Intervention**

| | Year 1 | Year 2 | Year 3 (3 mos) |
|---|---|---|---|
| Jewish Family and Children Services | | | |
| Average active quarterly caseload per staff member for providers | 3.8 | 4.6 | 4.2 |
| Total number of case management/mental health sessions | 303 | 569 | 219 |
| Total number of collateral contacts | 139 | 425 | 72 |
| Asian Community Mental Health Services | | | |
| Average active quarterly caseload per staff member for case management providers | 3.9 | 4.1 | 4.5 |
| Average active quarterly caseload per staff for the clinician | 1.8 | 2.3 | 2 |
| Total number of joint therapy sessions | 204 | 101 | 49 |
| Total number of case management meetings | 89 | 74 | 18 |
| Total number of collateral contacts | 70 | 73 | 15 |

### *Integrated Case Management/Mental Health Services Intervention*

English- and Spanish-speaking families were assigned to one of four Jewish Family and Children's Services therapists, each referred to as a case manager/mental health (CM/MH). These CM/MHs reported success in engaging families and establishing trusting relationships. Provision of immediately needed resources to the family was credited for the initial positive relations. Clinical staff sought to introduce the mental health component of the intervention as early as possible. However, family needs for housing, financial resources, medical services, and safety planning were reported by the staff as more pressing to the families than addressing child mental health needs. Thus, most time in family sessions focused on case management rather than therapy. Case management support included assisting families in completing such tasks as calling service providers to help them access needed resources.

Jewish Family and Children's Services staff reported great flexibility with implementing the clinical model. CM/MHs focused on supporting the parent/primary caregiver and providing education about the effects of domestic violence on children and about parent-child relationship building. Treatment submodalities included play therapy, psycho-education, and parent-child interactive therapy. CM/MHs described the typical case flow as follows:

- Parent/caregiver stabilization
- CM/MH-parent relationship building, focusing on addressing psychosocial issues experienced by parents/caregivers
- Joint development of a case plan containing both case management and therapeutic goals
- Termination of case when goals were met within six months.

CM/MHs reported difficulty keeping clients engaged. Program staff reported client transiency as a major impediment to retaining contact with clients. For example, many mothers who participated in the program were trying to separate themselves from a violent partner, so they sought housing in communities outside of the city of Oakland (and the program's service area). Also, as families' immediate social needs (e.g., housing, financial assistance) were addressed, they reportedly became less engaged in dealing with psychological issues. In fact, the staff reported that many families stopped participating in sessions with the CM/MH until they needed case management services. This start-stop-and-resume cycle caused the program to shift from an open-ended case flow to one that required the termination of cases in which the families repeatedly missed appointments.

The duality of the CM/MH role may have been difficult to implement. Program staff stated that clients typically pressed for the case manager role, and CM/MHs often emphasized the particular role in which they were most experienced. With ongoing training, CM/MHs reported learning how to better balance the two roles, yet they still delivered mental health services less frequently during sessions with families than anticipated because of the unmet basic needs of the families and requests from families to prioritize case management services to help stabilize their living conditions (i.e., the provision of housing, food, financial resources, medical services, and safety planning).

Families who were monolingual and bilingual Asian-speaking were referred to one of several two-person teams, comprising a case manager and therapist with the Asian Community Mental Health Services. The specific team was selected mostly based on the match between their language/cultural skills and that of the family to be served. As noted, Asian Community Mental Health Services implemented the services somewhat differently from Jewish Family and Children's Services.[20] The staff reported that, typically, they sought to dispatch a therapist and a case manager together to a session. The planned intervention length was hourly sessions once per week for six months. Each of these could be lengthened or made more frequent as client needs dictated. The staff reported that 40 sessions were typical for their clients.

These providers offered a positive impression overall of how the services were going with their client families. Primarily, staff reported that Safe Start was helping to identify more children exposed to violence and to expand service capacity for Asian families with children exposed to violence. The agency had already been providing case management and mental health services, but Safe Start enabled them to tailor their services more directly for families with children exposed to violence.

The program staff at the Asian Community Mental Health Services appreciated that the Safe Start model emphasized funding for case management. From the program staff's perspective, language and cultural barriers appeared to exacerbate the challenges that their families typically faced. Thus, the staff viewed case management assistance to be a particularly important service itself. They also viewed the home-based delivery of the services to be critical for engaging clients and informing how the services were provided. The staff reported that interacting with clients at their home helped provide a better understanding of the clients' needs for both case management and mental health services.

By the same token, home-based delivery and the intensity of the work with families to overcome language and cultural barriers also made the intervention very time consuming for the staff. From the program staff's perspective, this had several implications. First, the program staff were concerned about finding ways to guard against provider burnout. Second, the staff mentioned that they had very little time for attending larger Safe Start partner meetings, trainings, and case consultation meetings. So, although they reported appreciating the goals of these activities, the program staff at the Asian Community Mental Health Services could not fit these activities into their schedules without compromising client services.

---

[20] Because this organization was not providing services to clients included in the outcome evaluation, we did not devote equivalent resources to documenting the implementation of its services. The information described here was obtained during the second year of implementation from a single group interview with Asian Community Mental Health Services leadership and staff involved in providing services to Safe Start clients.

There were other components of the Oakland Safe Start program that helped shape the implementation (see the box titled "Oakland Safe Start Additional Program Components").

## Oakland Safe Start Additional Program Components

**Quality Assurance.** Oakland Safe Start selected clinicians who had experience delivering mental health services. In addition, clinicians were required to participate in a 40-hour certified training program on domestic violence; a training in child/caregiver dyadic therapy provided by the clinical supervisor of the lead service delivery agency, who had been trained in dyadic therapy; a cultural competency training; and an orientation to the Safe Start program, CEV, and community resources. The intake coordinator also participated in the domestic violence and cultural competency trainings. The clinicians engaged in on-site weekly case reviews for monitoring the application and delivery of services, and monthly supervision by a psychotherapist who was experienced in working with the target population and trained by a developer of a dyadic therapy model. The intake coordinator provided biweekly, group case management supervision to the clinicians, and individual supervision as needed.

**Training.** During the first two years of implementation, there were 44 training sessions. These sessions primarily focused on other intervention programs related to CEV (55%), the Safe Start referral processes (12%), and trauma-related issues (13%). Topics included intensive case management training, cultural competency, sexual assault advocate training, and general clinical or field supervision.

**Policies and Protocols.** Changes in policy and procedures at Oakland's Safe Start were made as the program developed to better serve the individuals, increase safety, and better track cases in the community. For example, zip codes were added to the CEV database to better map prevalence in the city of Oakland, and provisions for safe contacting were added to the electronic referral form for the safety of women in domestic violence cases when contact was made for referrals. Safe Start developed a protocol for the management of child abuse reporting and home-visiting safety for the intake coordinator. Also, Safe Start assisted with the development of diversion protocols for Oakland Police Officers, to better integrate systems of the Youth Intake Desk to align with their policies and procedures with CEV.

**Program Outreach.** The program's outreach efforts included various meetings, many to increase community awareness and support, and Safe Passages made a large number of posters, which were often accompanied by a short presentation on the topic of domestic violence, CEV, and Safe Start services. Dissemination of the posters and presentations was targeted at Head Start sites, doctors' offices, partner agencies, churches, and other community-based organizations that serve young children and their families. Safe Start also participated in community meetings to advocate for children exposed to violence and inform the community about the CEV database. To better reach the Latino community, a bilingual (Spanish and English) Master in Social Welfare intern was recruited to help conduct intakes at Alameda County Family Justice and assist in conducting public awareness presentations.

**Resources and Costs.** In the first two years of SSPA, Oakland Safe Start used most of their resources for their staff, including their project director as well as policy and program staff. Much of the time of these individuals also was given in kind to the project and not supported by OJJDP dollars. Other costs were incurred for office supplies and participant vouchers.

## Summary

The Oakland Safe Start program enabled development of processes to increase identification of children exposed to violence in Oakland, to help link those children and their families to existing services in the community, and to expand the capacity to provide services for very young children. Although the implementation of the new referral process was initially slower than expected, by the second year a single individual in the intake coordinator position was not sufficient to manage the high volume of referrals produced by the new citywide referral process. As the referral process becomes more institutionalized within Oakland, it appears that the position will need to expand to include additional staff or that the responsibilities of the single individual in this position be reduced to match the pace of referrals, should they continue to increase over time.

The integrated case management and mental health services were implemented somewhat differently than anticipated. Specifically, the staff reported that, due to the multiple needs of the families served, the focus of the intervention time in practice was heavily weighted toward case management rather than mental health services. Although the staff felt this was helping fulfill basic needs of the individual families (for such things as food, housing, and physical safety), the mental health needs of children were more difficult to address during the multipurpose sessions. Nonetheless, staff were committed to this blended service delivery model in seeking to address the needs of impoverished urban families exposed to violence.

**Data collection for this program summary included:**

- Key informant interviews with key program staff:
  - Safe Start program leadership
  - Safe Passages leadership
  - Staff from at Jewish Family and Children's Services and Asian Community Mental Health Services
  - Safe Passages research staff
- Case review of randomly selected treatment and control group cases
- Quality assurance checklist completed by the project director
- Quarterly activity reports on services, training, policies, and advocacy
- Grant application
- Green Light notes
- *Safe Start: Promising Approaches Communities Working Together to Help Children Exposed to Violence* (Safe Start Center, 2008).

# 11. Providence Program Description

## Providence Safe Start

### Tier 1

- **Intervention type:** Crisis intervention
- **Intervention length:** Initial contact and one follow-up contact
- **Intervention setting:** In-home
- **Target population:** Children exposed to domestic or community violence
- **Age range:** 0–18
- **Primary referral source:** Providence Police Department

### Tier 2

- **Intervention type:** Case management
- **Intervention length:** 24 months
- **Intervention setting:** Shelter and in-home post-shelter discharge
- **Target population:** Children exposed to domestic or community violence
- **Age range:** 0–18 for girls, 0–12 for boys
- **Primary referral source:** Domestic violence shelter

### Tier 3

- **Intervention type:** Child-Parent Psychotherapy (CPP) and case management
- **Intervention length:** 6 months
- **Intervention setting:** Clinic
- **Target population:** Children exposed to domestic or community violence
- **Age range:** 0–18
- **Primary referral source:** Family Service of Rhode Island

## Program and Community Setting

The Providence Safe Start program is located in Providence, Rhode Island. According to the 2000 Census, approximately 174,000 were living in the city of Providence; slightly more than 7 percent were children younger than age 5. The population was 55 percent white, 15 percent black, and nearly 18 percent marked "Other" as their race. There was a prominent Hispanic population that made up 30 percent of the population. At the time of the Census, the income per capita was $18,177,[21] with 29 percent of the population living below the poverty line.[22]

At the time of the Safe Start proposal to OJJDP, CEV consisted mainly of domestic violence, child maltreatment, and community violence. The Providence Police Department estimated that since 2001 there had been approximately 400 domestic violence incidents per year in homes were children were living. In the year prior to the proposal, the Rhode Island DCYF had nearly 600 cases of child abuse and neglect in Providence in which the investigation found that the child had been victimized. The Providence Police Department

[21] This is the 1999 per capita income converted into 2005 dollars. The 1999 per capita income that was recorded in the 2000 Census was $15,525.

[22] Information taken from the 2000 Census and can be found at the Census website (U.S. Census Bureau, no date).

also reported high levels of community violence, including shots fired, aggravated assaults, and drug offenses in the neighborhoods where many children live (Family Service of Rhode Island, 2004).

Prior to Safe Start, the resources in Providence for children exposed to domestic and community violence were somewhat limited and scattered. As described below, there were some resources for crisis intervention, shelter care, and treatment, but the community partners viewed the system as fragmented.

For crisis intervention for children exposed to domestic violence, Family Service of Rhode Island (FSRI) began working with the Providence Police Department in 2004 adhering to recommendations within the Child Development–Community Policing model developed at the Yale Child Study Center (Marans and Berkman, 1997). With Victims of Crime Act state-level formula funding through the Department of Justice's Office for Victims of Crime, FSRI developed a crisis intervention program to respond to families with children exposed to criminal or violent acts (called the GO-Team). An FSRI clinician was made available around the clock, seven days per week, to accompany the police who were responding to calls involving children exposed to violence and provide crisis intervention services, referral, and follow-up as a member of the GO-Team.

In serving women and children in domestic violence shelters, most of the service providers functioned independently of one another. The primary shelter serving the Providence area provided a variety of case management services to women, including assistance and support for employment, education, language services, welfare benefits, medical assistance, and housing. A child advocate provided case management to support school enrollment, day care issues, individualized education plans, and mental health needs. However, all of these services and supports ended upon discharge from the shelter.

Some mental health treatment options were also available, primarily through FSRI. With funds from the United Way, FSRI's Trauma and Loss Center provided support for children and families with trauma issues using a parent-child–based counseling model. The CPP model was being utilized at FSRI for children and families exposed to traumatic events in general, but not specifically for children exposed to violence.

To address the gaps in services and to provide a more systematic and coordinated approach, the Providence Safe Start project came together under the leadership of FSRI (see the box titled "Providence Safe Start Partner Agencies" for a brief description of each partner agency).

The Providence Safe Start program originally developed by FSRI was multitiered and it was possible for families to enter at any tier or to move between tiers:

- **Tier 1** was a crisis intervention program for children ages 0–18 who came into contact with the Providence Police Department because of exposure to domestic or community violence.
- **Tier 2** was a case management program for women with children (ages 0–18 for girls, 0–12 for boys) who entered a domestic violence shelter.
- **Tier 3** involved CPP and case management for children ages 0–18 exposed to domestic violence.

For each tier, Safe Start targeted children living in Providence who had been exposed to violence within the past two years. FSRI designed this program to attempt to fill in gaps in the existing service array and to improve continuity for those involved in the system. As originally conceived, families could enter Safe Start at any of these levels and move into other levels as necessary. However, the scope of services within each tier was fundamentally different.

### Providence Safe Start Partner Agencies

**Family Service of Rhode Island.** Founded in 1892, Family Service of Rhode Island (FSRI) is a nonprofit human services agency with state licenses for behavioral health services and substance abuse treatment. The Safe Start program was situated within FSRI's Trauma, Intake, and Emergency Services unit. This unit also included intake, the Emergency Response System, the Children's Crisis Assessment Team (see Department of Children, Youth and Families below), the Trauma and Loss Center, the GO-Team (see Police Department below), and the Critical Incident Stress Management Team.

**Women's Center of Rhode Island.** The Women's Center is a 13-room emergency shelter for women and children who have experienced domestic violence or become homeless. The shelter has the capacity to serve up to 8 mothers and 12 children at any given time. Families are allowed to stay for a maximum of three months, with the length of stay typically 45–90 days. Families at the shelter receive case management services through a Residential Advocate and a Child Advocate.

**Providence Police Department.** FSRI partnered with the Providence Police Department to develop a program based on the Child Development–Community Policing model developed at Yale University to enhance collaboration among law enforcement, juvenile justice, domestic violence, medical and mental health professionals, child welfare, schools and other community agencies. The resulting program was called the GO-Team. FSRI responded to police calls involving family violence by sending a clinician to the scene to provide crisis intervention services, referrals, and follow-up for families exposed to violence, particularly when children were involved.

**Rhode Island Department of Children, Youth, and Families (DCYF).** FSRI works with DCYF via the Children's Crisis Assessment Team. The Children's Crisis Assessment Team clinician partnered with DCYF staff to provide around-the-clock emergency clinical assessment and intervention.

In Tier 1, Safe Start was meant to reach families early with intervention services immediately following a domestic or community violence event. By partnering with the police department, FSRI would be able to identify families in need who might be missed through other referral mechanisms. In Tier 2, Safe Start envisioned creating an infrastructure to improve the case coordination of the children and families when they leave the larger shelter system. Eligible families would be identified at the domestic violence shelter, given case management services while in the shelter, and then given follow-up services by the family advocate upon exiting the shelter. This program would allow them to formalize a process in which to refer, serve, track, coordinate, and enhance delivery of services. In Tier 3, FSRI would be able to offer CPP and enhanced case management specifically for children and families with violence exposure.

The Providence Safe Start program was selected by OJJDP as one of 15 sites across the country. After receiving the grant, Providence went through the Green Light process to prepare for program implementation and evaluation. Because of the complexity of its multitiered program, Providence received intensive technical assistance from RAND, OJJDP, and the Association for the Study and Development of Communities to iron out the details of the intervention and evaluation strategy for each tier. The assistance resulted in agreement and clarification of the projected number of cases in each tier, the entrance criteria for each tier, the definition of the control or comparison group for Tiers 2 and 3, and the relationship between the three tiers of service.

## Intervention

The Providence Safe Start program involved three different tiers of services: (1) crisis intervention, (2) case management, and (3) CPP combined with case management.

### Tier 1: Crisis Intervention

In Tier 1, the site planned to identify families through the existing GO-Team program developed in partnership between FSRI and the Providence Police Department. The GO-Team is a crisis intervention program for families with children exposed to violence. Children eligible for Tier 1 services were ages 0–18 and had been exposed to violence, defined as any type of direct or indirect victimization that causes physical or psychological harm to the individual and that falls within one of the following three categories:

1. Community Violence: Violence between people who are not related, and who may or may not know each other (acquaintances and strangers).
2. Sexual Violence: Any sexual act, attempt to obtain a sexual act, sexual harassment, or act directed against a person's sexuality, using coercion, by any person regardless of his or her relationship to the victim, in any setting.
3. Family/Domestic Violence: Violence between family members, and intimate partners, including child abuse and elder abuse.

In Tier 1, eligible children and families were identified by the police department responding to a complaint. A police officer contacts the on-call clinician to come to the scene. The clinician provided crisis services, referrals, and follow-up care. The timing of the follow-up contact varied, depending on the family's circumstances. If necessary, the clinician linked the family to Tier 2 or Tier 3. With Tier 1, FSRI hoped to improve the case coordination of families who enter the larger system.

### Tier 2: Case Management

Tier 2 focused on case management for women in the Women's Center of Rhode Island domestic violence shelter. Eligible women were those residing in the domestic violence shelter accompanied by a child from birth to age 18. Because boys older than age 13 were not allowed to reside in the shelter, a common procedure for many domestic violence shelters, families including adolescent boys were not included.

The intervention case management was provided by the Safe Start family advocate. At the time of admission to the shelter, a general needs assessment would be completed by the Safe Start advocate. The family advocate also met with eligible mothers to assess her needs and the needs of her child or children. Once the assessment was complete, the family advocate met with the mother several times a week during her shelter stay to discuss goals and progress and other issues that may have arisen. The Safe Start family advocate participated in shelter team meetings with the shelter's residential advocate and child advocate to ensure continuity and consistency in service plans.

After the family's shelter stay, the advocate maintained weekly contact for the first two months and then monthly contact until the mother had been engaged with Safe Start for a total of 24 months (including her shelter stay). If the mother needed more intensive case management support during any time, then the advocate attempted to increase efforts to meet the mother's needs. The post-discharge services were similar to what was provided during the shelter stay but were more community based. The family advocate provided case management and linkage to existing community services. Transition services included assistance with housing and employment.

#### Tier 3: Child-Parent Psychotherapy Combined with Case Management

Tier 3 of the Providence Safe Start project consisted of parent-child dyadic therapy, specifically using CPP. CPP is a relationship-based intervention designed for use with children up to age 6. It can be used with any child whose relationship to his or her parent or other primary caregiver is impacted by negative circumstances, including family violence. CPP integrates psychodynamic, attachment, trauma, cognitive-behavioral, and social learning theories (NCTSN, 2008). There are two components in CPP: assessment and treatment, with information gained during the assessment used to inform the treatment component. In the intervention component, child-parent interactions were the focus of six intervention modalities aimed at restoring a sense of mastery, security, and growth and promoting congruence between bodily sensations, feelings, and thinking on the part of both child and parent and in their relationship with one another (NCTSN, 2008).

For Tier 3, eligible children included those between ages 0–18 who had been exposed to violence. Exposure to violence was defined in the same way as in Tier 1. Tier 3 also required that the client be a current resident of the greater Providence area at the time of intake into FSRI.

For children 13 and younger, the CPP was delivered by a clinician in one-hour sessions at the FSRI clinic (initially weekly, then every two weeks until termination). The therapist provided diagnostic assessments and clinical counseling using the CPP model. For children 14 and older, the clinician provided individual therapy, because the CPP model is not appropriate for older children. In addition, the therapists provided crisis intervention and assessment if needed and coordinated with case managers and other service providers. The families also received case management from case managers who made home visits to assist with housing, educational, and employment needs as needed. In addition, case managers would assist the parent with obtaining individual mental health services as needed.

The intervention period was planned to last approximately two to three months. During OJJDP's Green Light process, Providence specified that the intervention would be complete when approximately 12 sessions of CPP had been conducted. Based on the individual situation, there could be more or fewer sessions. The ending point was defined as when the sessions were completed and a wrap-up session had been delivered.

As with the other Safe Start sites, the intervention was conducted in the context of a rigorous evaluation as required by OJJDP (see the box titled "Providence Safe Start Evaluation" for a description). OJJDP, however, exempted Tier 1 from the outcome evaluation component because the implementation of an adequately rigorous research design proved to be infeasible with available resources.

### Providence Safe Start Evaluation

**Tier 2**

**Design.** A comparison group design was used.

**Treatment versus comparison group services.** In addition to receiving any services or supports from the referring agency, those who were assigned to the treatment group received case management from FSRI staff during and after their shelter stay. Those who were in the comparison group received the services and supports they were already receiving from the comparison shelter.

**Data collection.** Data were collected through longitudinal assessments of child-level outcomes.

**Enrollment.** The site originally planned to serve 200 families over the four-year period (100 in each group). Funding for the National Evaluation ended prematurely. By the time it ended, enrollment had taken place over one year and resulted in 15 families in the treatment group and 3 in the control group.

**Tier 3**

**Design.** This randomized control effectiveness trial was focused on child outcomes.

**Treatment versus control group services.** In addition to receiving any services or supports from the referring agency, those who were assigned to the treatment group received CPP and case management from FSRI staff. Those who were assigned to the control group received the services and supports they were already receiving from the referring agency and were offered a drop in support group for trauma and loss at FSRI.

**Data collection.** Data were collected through longitudinal assessments of child-level outcomes.

**Enrollment.** The site originally planned to serve 320 families over the four-year period (160 in each group). Funding for the National Evaluation ended prematurely. By the time it ended, enrollment had taken place over two years and five months and resulted in 35 families in the treatment group and 36 in the control group.

## Implementation

The following description of the program implementation is the result of data collected for the national evaluation. See Appendix A for a full discussion of the data collection methodology employed at each of the Safe Start sites.

### Tier 1: Crisis Intervention

Figure B.11a shows Providence's implementation of Tier 1 of its intervention.

#### *Referrals*

Referrals into the Tier 1 crisis intervention program came from the Providence Police Department. After police officers responded to a call involving violence where a child was present, they called the FSRI on-call clinician to respond to the scene. During the first two years of implementation, Safe Start received few calls from police officers to engage these Tier 1 services.

**Figure B.11a**
**Model of Providence Safe Start Tier 1**

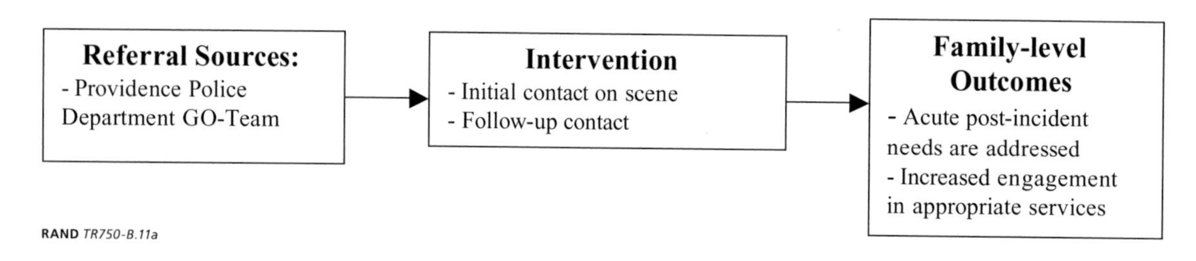


RAND *TR750-B.11a*

In an effort to increase referrals, Safe Start worked with the GO-Team to support outreach to victims of domestic violence within the city limits and used GO-Team as a referral source.

### *Services*

When clinicians did receive referrals, those who responded reported that most families were not interested in the program. In the first two years of implementation, Safe Start provided services to only seven families in the Tier 1 intervention. The Safe Start program staff felt that the families were dealing with the immediate crisis and had decisions that needed to be made immediately and thus were not interested in follow-up contact four to six weeks later, let alone participation in a two-year project.

Despite the limited use of Tier 1 services, the police department leadership appeared to view Tier 1 positively. According to police staff we interviewed, the ability to have a clinician on scene helped police be more responsive. It also allowed them to leave the scene earlier and move on to the next call, because they were not leaving the family alone and in crisis. Police staff also reported fewer calls back to the same address and attributed this to having clinical support at the time of the event. Given the positive feedback from the police department leadership, the reasons for the limited use of Tier 1 services remain unclear.

In addition, the Tier 1 crisis intervention approach allowed FSRI to work with the Rhode Island DCYF on a regular basis to maintain communication about particular families. The Safe Start program staff viewed this enhanced communication with DCYF as a benefit of the intervention.

## Tier 2: Case Management

Figure B.11b shows Providence's implementation of Tier 2 of its intervention.

The implementation of Tier 2 was delayed, as it took some time to develop a collaborative relationship with the domestic violence shelter and to work out the parameters of the services to be provided through Safe Start. The shelter also had difficulty hiring for the family advocate position and identifying a comparison shelter for outcome evaluation. Tier 2 began services in October of 2007.

### *Referrals*

Referrals into Tier 2 came from the domestic violence shelter. The shelter was supposed to identify mothers with children as they entered the shelter. The Safe Start program staff worked with the Women's Center to establish a protocol to facilitate after-hours enrollment for families. In this protocol, the advocate at the shelter sent out the Safe Start brochure along with the usual letters about shelter services that are routinely mailed by the shelter to victims of domestic violence.

**Figure B.11b**
**Model of Providence Safe Start Tier 2**

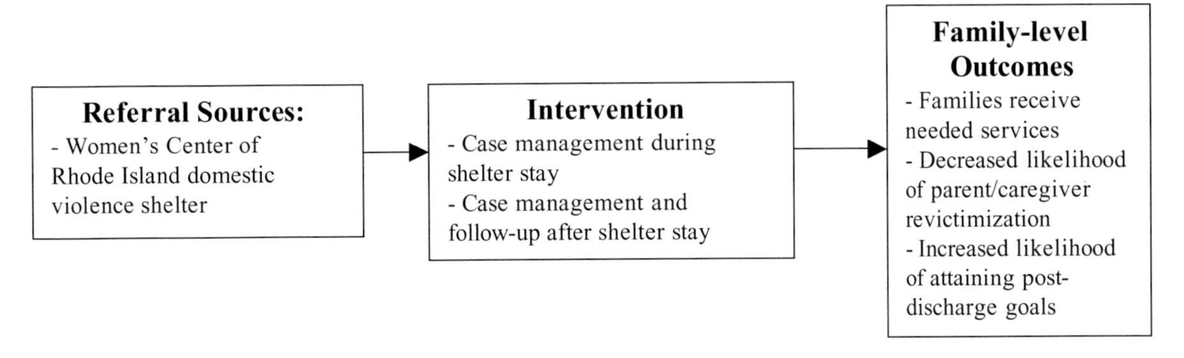


RAND *TR750-B.11b*

### *Services*

During its one year of operation, Safe Start served 19 families. The shelter staff reported that women rarely took advantage of transitional services offered by the Safe Start advocate. The staff speculated that this might have been due to lack of clarity about what services were offered and women being overwhelmed by their immediate circumstances (i.e., addressing crisis needs first). Safe Start program staff felt that the shelter staff did not make Safe Start a priority, and this contributed to the women not taking advantage of the services available through Safe Start. Both the shelter and Safe Start program staff indicated that there was confusion about coordination between the Safe Start advocate and the shelter staff (e.g., who was responsible for which function or service) in providing services to families, which contributed to a strained relationship among the staff of both organizations. Due to the slow pace of enrollment, OJJDP and FSRI mutually agreed to discontinue Tier 2 in the fall of 2008 after one year of operation and moved the project resources into Tier 3.

## Tier 3: Child-Parent Psychotherapy with Case Management

Figure B.11c shows Providence's implementation of Tier 3 of their intervention.

### *Referrals*

For Tier 3, referrals came from within FSRI, the partner agencies, and walk-ins. All of these referrals flowed through the intake unit of FSRI's Trauma, Intake, and Emergency Services unit. Partway through implementation, the eligibility criteria for Tier 3 were expanded to

**Figure B.11c**
**Model of Providence Safe Start Tier 3**

Referral Sources:
- FSRI Trauma, Intake and Emergency Services intake unit
Six-month Intervention
- Child-parent psychotherapy
- Case management
Family-level Outcomes
- Improvements in parent-child relationship
- Increased parent and child safety

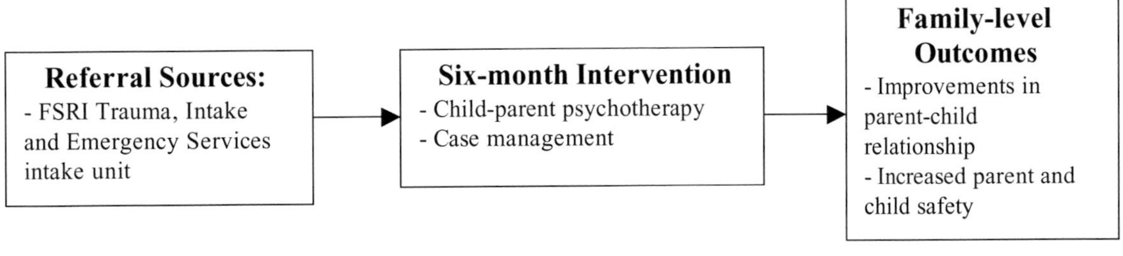

RAND *TR750-B.11c*

include several cities in the greater Providence area that had similar demographics and that FSRI already served. FSRI hoped to increase eligible referrals into Tier 3 by expanding the geographic areas served by Safe Start. They also conducted agency-wide training for all FSRI staff to increase the internal referrals to the Safe Start program.

### *Services*

Table B.11 summarizes service delivery for those who received services through Tier 3 of the Providence Safe Start program during the first three years of implementation (through March 2009). Providence had one to two therapists at any one time during the project. As enrollment increased from Year 1 to Year 2, the total number of therapy sessions and case management contacts increased. Starting in Year 2, the program started serving older children. Because CPP is not appropriate for those older than age 13, these children received individual therapy sessions.

A typical case flow for Tier 3 included engaging a case manager and clinician together initially to describe services to the family. The case manager worked with the clinician in the first three to four CPP sessions to build the relationship with the family. After these joint sessions, clinicians and case managers worked separately with families. Clinicians discussed therapeutic goals with the family, including issues such as children's nightmares and recurring thoughts about violence exposure. The CPP sessions entailed strengthening the child-parent relationship through play and other interactive activities and providing education to the parent about the effects of violence on children and its associated symptoms. Case reviews suggested that CPP seemed to have positive impacts for these individual families, but the case reviews also indicated that it was critical to address case management needs first for some families. For families with older children (e.g., teens), therapists exercised the flexibility of the model by setting aside time to meet with the adolescent alone.

The therapists participated in case review meetings facilitated by a CPP expert clinician and trainer. The details of the case and any questions from the clinician and caseworker were sent to the participants in advance. The case review meetings also included reviewing CPP treatment adherence checklists that incorporate both clinical and case management adherence to the model. Participants found these meetings valuable, because they were able to ask questions and propose alternative ideas and theories. The clinicians reported that the case review meetings were important for assessing how well the model was working and developing strategies to engage families.

After the case review discussion, the meeting was expanded to discuss the Safe Start program more broadly. This portion of the meeting included a community representative, the domestic violence center staff from Tier 2, the Providence Police Department, Family Court, and a member of the Coalition to End Domestic Violence (a statewide umbrella agency for domestic violence agencies). The purpose of this part of the meeting was to allow the different community partners to network, build support for Safe Start, and generate referrals.

**Table B.11**
**Service Delivery for Enrollees in the Providence Tier 3 Safe Start Intervention**

| | Year 1 | Year 2 | Year 3 (5 mos) |
|---|---|---|---|
| Average active caseload for therapists | 3.3 | 6.3 | 7 |
| Total number of CPP sessions | 37 | 118 | 123 |
| Total number of individual therapy sessions | — | 69 | 44 |
| Total number of case management contacts | 16 | 59 | 46 |

To promote continued participation in the program, FSRI revised various policies intended to keep families engaged and to support fairly regular contact. For example, there was a switch to in-person intakes instead of telephone intakes into the program. The program also increased the amount of phone, face-to-face, and postcard contact with program participants and sponsored a monthly Safe Start family night for families receiving Tier 3 services. These changes were made to increase family engagement in the therapeutic intervention.

There were other components of the Providence Safe Start program that helped shape the implementation (see the box titled "Providence Safe Start Additional Program Components").

### Providence Safe Start Additional Program Components

**Quality Assurance.** The site's training efforts included 100 hours of clinician training during the therapist's first month, followed by weekly booster sessions for new and current staff. The clinical supervisor provided on-site consultation as necessary. The therapists used an integrated checklist as a guide to each session. Each client's progress was noted in the progress notes.

**Training.** Over the initial two years of the program, Providence conducted or participated in 69 trainings (32% on issues related to Safe Start or systems of care, 23% on clinical services, 17% on child welfare, and 13% on domestic violence). Topics for training addressed issues such as domestic violence and children, how to work with the Providence Police Department (e.g., role playing), and several sessions on trauma and loss.

**Policies and Protocols.** The Providence Safe Start program implemented a number of new policies primarily focused on increasing the referral source and participation rate in the Safe Start program and spreading information regarding children and families exposed to violence.

**Program Outreach.** The site's advocacy efforts were primarily in the form of presentations to a number of groups and organizations in the community. The presentations introduced the Safe Start program, provided information about accessing and referring individuals to Safe Start, and aimed at gaining support for the start-up and continuation of the program. Providence also sought to implement regular trainings for police in the academy about CEV. The site also conducted informational/training sessions at a local children's hospital to increase awareness of the Safe Start Program and a training on CEV at the early childhood education program.

**Resources and Costs.** In the first two years of SSPA, Providence Safe Start used most of their funds for salary support. The rest was used for nominal expenses for supplies and other equipment.

## Summary

Providence Safe Start proposed and developed a multitiered program to address gaps in the system for children exposed to sexual, domestic, and community violence. The program employed multiple ways to identify and intervene with families. Yet, in implementing this ambitious intervention, the program faced several barriers.

Recruitment into the different levels of the intervention was challenging. For example, Tier 1 recruitment was difficult because families interacting with the police department were dealing with the immediate crisis and were often not interested in the longer-term intervention or participation in a two-year study. The police also did not provide many referrals into the program. Tier 2 recruitment was also an obstacle because it was difficult to engage the women at the shelter in the program and because the shelter staff were not fully invested in the Safe Start program. On the other hand, Tier 3 required an enhancement of in-house FSRI services, and thus it was somewhat easier to have staff recruit families. Nonetheless, the volume of referrals into Tier 3 fell short of expectations. Together, these recruitment challenges highlight that a multipronged approach requires more supports at each point of entry, such as more incentives for referrals and participation, more staff to engage families, and better communication processes.

Another challenge that spanned all three tiers was the case management needs of highly stressed families. For Tier 2, the women in the shelter did not take advantage of the transitional case management offered through Safe Start in part because the shelter staff did not prioritize Safe Start. In Tier 3, the therapist provided some case management during the therapy sessions at the clinic, whereas the case manager used home visits to help connect families to needed services.

In Providence, FSRI's relationships with community partners played an important role in its program development and implementation. In Tier 1, it strengthened an existing partnership with the Providence Police Department. Although enrollment did not meet expectations, the partners continued to work together toward improving service delivery immediately following a violent incident. For Tier 2, FSRI was unable to build a strong working relationship with the domestic violence shelter. The partnership was strained in part because of problems clarifying the goals and activities of the program.

**Data collection for this program summary included:**

- Key informant interviews with key program staff and community partners:
  - FSRI agency director and financial staff person
  - Safe Start program manager, counselor, and case managers
  - Department of Children, Youth, and Family staff
  - Women's Center of Rhode Island staff
  - Community representative
- Observation of a Providence Police Department Command Staff meeting
- Observation of a case consultation meeting
- Case review of randomly selected treatment and comparison/control group cases
- Quality assurance checklist completed by the clinical supervisor
- Quarterly activity reports on services, training, policies, and advocacy
- Grant application
- Green Light notes
- *Safe Start: Promising Approaches Communities Working Together to Help Children Exposed to Violence* (Safe Start Center, 2008).

## 12. San Diego Program Description

### San Diego Safe Start

- **Intervention type:** Trauma-focused cognitive-behavioral therapy, domestic violence–focused child advocacy, and case coordination
- **Intervention length:** Approximately 20 weekly sessions completed over 6 months for therapy services; 6 months or more for the advocacy and case coordination
- **Intervention setting:** Office-based for therapy services and case coordination; in-home or office-based for child advocacy
- **Target population:** Children exposed to domestic violence identified within a county child welfare population
- **Age range:** 3–12 years
- **Primary referral source:** Two regions of San Diego County's Child Welfare Services

### Program and Community Setting

The San Diego Safe Start Program serves children exposed to violence in San Diego County, California. According to the 2000 Census, the county's population was a little more than 2.81 million. The population was 67 percent white, 27 percent Hispanic, 9 percent Asian, and 6 percent black. There was a very small Native American population, and about 13 percent marked "Other" as their race. The income per capita in 1999 was $26,843,[23] and 12.4 percent of the population was living below the poverty line.[24]

In its 2004 application to OJJDP requesting Safe Start funding, San Diego County reported that each year there were more than 20,000 domestic violence–related 911 calls. Domestic violence fatality reviews conducted in the county between 1997 and 2003 found that 64 percent of adult victims had at least one minor child. And in 23 percent of the cases, a child witnessed the murder of his or her parent. Exposure to domestic violence was also a factor in many child welfare referrals. Because these cases were typically classified as "emotional abuse," however, the exact number of domestic violence–specific referrals could not be determined. Overall, emotional abuse cases made up about 20 percent of the new child welfare dependency petitions before county juvenile courts (County of San Diego, 2004).

Prior to Safe Start, San Diego County had been a national leader in the development of coordinated approaches to prevent and reduce domestic violence. In 1989, San Diego developed one of the country's first multiagency domestic violence coordinating councils and in 2002 developed its Family Justice Center. The center consisted of a co-located, multiagency "one-stop shop" for domestic violence victims and their children, providing access to a host of domestic violence–related services and support under one roof. The Family Justice Center has since been replicated in sites around the United States (some with federal funding) as well as in Mexico, Canada, and England (U.S. Department of Justice, Office of Violence Against Women, 2007).

---

[23] This represents 1999 income per capita in 2005 dollars; in 1999 dollars it was $22,926.

[24] Information was taken from the 2000 Census and can be found at the Census website (U.S. Census Bureau, no date).

Despite its high level of existing coordination around domestic violence, the county conducted a self-assessment and identified gaps in services available for children exposed to domestic violence and a lack of coordination of the services that were available. Families who had a child served within the county's Child Welfare Services agency were identified as the specific area of need. Thus, San Diego County proposed to OJJDP a Safe Start project that offered a family-level intervention program within the context of Child Welfare Services. But, as discussed in detail below, the proposed program also contained a broader countywide effort to raise awareness about the needs of children exposed to domestic violence and to improve system-level coordination and increase the capacity to provide appropriate services for this population.

The lead agency in the Safe Start project was the Office of Violence Prevention with San Diego County's Health and Human Services Agency. The development of the project concept involved representatives of numerous agencies with a long history of collaborating on domestic violence efforts. This included the San Diego Domestic Violence Council, consisting of more than 300 member agencies (San Diego Domestic Violence Council, 2009). Along with the Office of Violence Prevention, the core collaborators on the project design were Child Welfare Services, the Center for Community Solutions, the Chadwick Center for Children and Families, and the Child and Adolescent Service Research Center. (These organizations are described in the box titled "San Diego Safe Start Partner Agencies.") Clinical consultants were also involved through the management and leadership of the San Diego Treatment and Evaluation Resource Management program (TERM), housed within the county's Health and Human Service Agency. TERM managed a pool of more than 300 individual therapists who had been approved by and established contracts with San Diego County to provide mental health services to Child Welfare Services clients.

Initially, the partners envisioned Safe Start as a direct service program for families involved with Child Welfare Services, serving children ages 0–6 who were exposed to domestic violence. Families would be drawn from an existing caseload consisting mostly of involuntary (court-ordered) cases jointly involving Child Welfare Services and Adult Probation. Families in the treatment group would receive a multifaceted clinical assessment (that the Safe Start partners intended to develop) and then engage children in approximately 20 therapy sessions employing a number of therapeutic approaches and techniques, depending upon the assessed needs of the child. No specific therapy model was proposed. The families would also receive a "child advocate" (from the Center for Community Solutions), who would engage in child-focused safety planning, support and accompaniment, and general advocacy and support for the children and their primary caregivers. Regular case coordination meetings between the families' Safe Start therapist, child advocate, and Child Welfare social worker were also features of the proposed San Diego Safe Start program. The Child and Adolescent Services Research Center would provide local oversight of the evaluation plan, recruit families into the overall program, and execute data collection.

After San Diego's project was selected for funding by OJJDP, the project plans were thoroughly reviewed during OJJDP's Green Light process to prepare for program implementation and evaluation. Specifically, the Green Light process focused on the direct service portion of the planned project, because it would be the component tested in the outcome evaluation.

Leading up to the Green Light process, the site also formed its "Safe Start Steering Committee," consistent with its intention to build a program that represented a multiagency collaboration. This group consisted of key stakeholders in the Safe Start project and representatives from each of the agencies actively participating in the effort. During the Green Light process, the Safe Start Steering Committee was actively involved in reviewing and revising program plans leading up to implementation. This intensive collaborative effort served to lengthen the process, as key decisions were made by a multiagency group, rather than a single individual or agency. Overall, the process helped to develop a process of interagency communication and a deeper understanding among the partners of the evaluation-related need to adhere to the revised program design.

## San Diego Safe Start Partner Agencies

**Office of Violence Prevention.** The Office of Violence Prevention, within the Health and Human Services Agency of San Diego County, served as the lead agency in the Safe Start project. It was established in 1994. It coordinates and manages a number of the programs and initiatives, such as the county's Domestic Violence Fatality Review Team, Domestic Violence Response Teams, Domestic Violence Services for Families, Domestic Violence Safety Plan, and the domestic violence hotline. For the Safe Start program, this office served as the lead agency, providing program oversight, coordination, and overall leadership.

**Child Welfare Services.** Child Welfare Services is located within San Diego County's Health and Human Services Agency. It operates the county's child abuse reporting hotline and provides case management and services to children and families experiencing difficulties such as abuse, neglect, and domestic violence exposure. It provides assessment and services for families who have consented voluntarily and for those who are court ordered to engage with Child Welfare Services. The county is split geographically into six regions, with one or more individual Child Welfare Services offices providing services within each region. The Safe Start Program was implemented in the North Central and Central region Child Welfare Services offices.

**Center for Community Solutions.** Founded in 1969, the Center for Community Solutions focuses on domestic and sexual violence, both through prevention efforts and service provision. Its domestic violence services include legal clinic services, emergency shelter and transitional housing, advocacy, individual counseling and support groups, crisis hotline assistance, and culturally sensitive domestic violence prevention programming. For the Safe Start program, this organization provided trained domestic violence advocates to serve as the child advocates for program participants.

**Child and Adolescent Services Research Center.** Located within San Diego's Rady Children's Hospital, this is a National Institute of Mental Health–funded service center. It is a multidisciplinary research center with a specific focus on service delivery to children. By conducting interdisciplinary research, the center seeks to improve mental health care and service delivery to children, particularly those in the most vulnerable populations. For the Safe Start project, this organization provided local oversight of the evaluation plan, recruited families into the overall program, and execute data collection.

**Chadwick Center for Children and Families.** Located within San Diego's Rady Children's Hospital, Chadwick is staffed by more than 120 professionals and paraprofessionals in the fields of medicine, social work, psychology, psychiatry, child development, nursing, and education technology who offer family-centered care and a multidisciplinary approach to child abuse and neglect. Through a variety of services, including trauma counseling services, Chadwick seeks to promote the health and well-being of abused and traumatized children. For the Safe Start project, the Chadwick Center provided training and support to therapists providing mental health assessment and intervention.

The site made several key revisions and refinements to its direct service plans based on the Green Light review. The proposed program design had included an extensive clinical assessment that would identify the individual needs of children and then match those needs with any number of therapy models and techniques to address those needs. In the context of a rigorous evaluation of the overall program impact, it became clear there would not be an adequate number of children receiving any one type of therapeutic intervention or technique to test the relative efficacy of each therapeutic approach.

Thus, the site decided to select a single therapy model, Trauma-Focused Cognitive-Behavioral Therapy (TF-CBT), as the one to employ with all eligible children randomized to the treatment group. A set of comprehensive assessments would still be used to help inform the therapists' work with the child within the context of this single therapeutic approach.

This change also necessitated an increase in the target age range to ages 3–8, which was seen as a more appropriate age range for the model. (As discussed below, the age range was further expanded after implementation to 3–12 years.)

The site also determined that drawing from a specialized caseload within a single office of Child Welfare Services would likely produce an inadequate number of cases. An informal review of the numbers and characteristics of cases served by the whole of Child Welfare Services in the county suggested that more than one office would need to participate to obtain a sufficient pool of cases.

Thus, it selected two regions of Child Welfare Services, Central (containing two offices) and North Central (containing one office), to serve as the host of the Safe Start program and associated outcome evaluation. Eligible cases would be drawn from all referrals within these two Child Welfare Services regions.

## Intervention

The San Diego Safe Start direct services program involved three main components: (1) TF-CBT, (2) child advocacy, and (3) case coordination. The length of the intervention and the setting for the services will be discussed in turn below.

### Trauma-Focused Cognitive Behavioral Therapy

The therapy services were provided by county-contracted TERM therapists. (Their specific selection, training, and supervision will be discussed in a subsequent section.) The therapy model selected for use was TF-CBT. This model is a therapeutic intervention used for children, adolescents, and their parents or primary caregiver who have developed clinical levels of posttraumatic stress disorder (PTSD) as the result of a traumatic event such as child sexual or physical abuse, loss of a loved one, and exposure to domestic, school, or community violence.

The intervention is delivered by trained mental health professionals and can be offered in individual, family, and group sessions in outpatient settings. It targets symptoms of PTSD (i.e., re-experiencing the traumatic event, avoiding reminders of the event, heightened arousal or anxiety) and seeks to teach children skills to cope with the difficulties that this disorder creates. TF-CBT involves therapy sessions in which children work to build emotional skill training, and, later, with the help of trained therapists, children begin to confront the experience that initialized the PTSD symptoms (Cohen et al., 2003). As part of this process, the therapy includes the following:

- education about trauma and common reactions
- help with parenting and behavior problems
- relaxation/stress management training
- learning about feelings and ways to express them
- developing creative ways for children to gradually discuss their traumatic experience
- changing any unhelpful thoughts about the trauma
- family sessions to help the family talk together about the trauma
- learning and practicing safety skills.

The work with parents (or other primary caregiver) is generally focused on increasing their understanding of (1) the impacts of trauma on children's behavior and overall well-being and (2) appropriate strategies for supporting the process of addressing the impacts of trauma. This involves work on developing parenting skills and guiding parents to provide constructive support for the child undergoing therapy. This is done in part through working to address parental distress related to the child's traumatic event or exposure. To this end, parent involvement may include individual sessions with the therapist alone or joint sessions with both the therapist and child. Sessions may also include other family members, if their participation appears to the therapist to be of benefit in addressing the goals of treatment: reducing the impact of trauma and associated symptoms of PTSD.

For the San Diego Safe Start program, TF-CBT was used in combination with an extensive assessment of the child and primary caregiver, called the Trauma Assessment Pathway (TAP) model (Taylor et al., 2005). The TAP model used a multifaceted assessment process to assist clinicians in gaining a more in-depth understanding of the child, their developmental level, their traumatic experience, and the family, community, and cultural system in which the child lives. Developed at the Chadwick Center for Children and Families, the TAP model was designed to use this information as a tool to assist therapists with determining what type of therapeutic approach would best suit the needs of the assessed child.[25] Because the constraints of the outcome evaluation restricted the choice to only one model, the intended use of the TAP assessment process was to yield greater insight into the child's circumstances and functioning to assist in the TF-CBT treatment process.

The TAP assessment itself was expected to take up to three one-hour sessions to complete. That would be followed by the TF-CBT intervention consisting of approximately 20 sessions, delivered weekly at a therapist's office. If the goals of therapy had yet to be achieved, children could continue with additional sessions. Child Welfare typically maintains open voluntary cases for a six-month period, and, in some cases, the entire course of therapeutic treatment was limited to a six-month window because this is the maximum amount of time therapists could submit sessions for reimbursement from the county general funds as the payment source.

[25] For more information about the development, contents, and applications of the Trauma Assessment Pathway Model, see Chadwick Center for Children and Families (no date).

As noted, the Safe Start therapists were drawn from among the county's pool of more than 300 TERM therapists who had established contracts to provide mental health services to Child Welfare Services clients. Twelve TERM therapists were selected each year of Safe Start to receive TF-CBT training and to serve Safe Start clients. In addition to meeting TERM requirements and serving Safe Start's geographic area, the Safe Start therapists had experience working with young children exposed to domestic violence.

To participate in Safe Start, the therapists also needed to agree to

- complete a prerequisite TF-CBT online training course
- participate in three four-hour training sessions on TAP and TF-CBT
- participate in at least 8 out of 10 monthly Safe Start training and clinical support sessions offered by the Chadwick Center
- agree to follow a protocol for the Safe Start Intervention, including intervention format and case consultation.

### Child Advocacy

Advocacy services were provided in a client's home or other location, depending on the needs of the child and family. The child advocates were trained domestic violence advocates employed by the Center for Community Solutions and assigned to work with individual treatment group children and their families. The advocates were not "co-located" or stationed in close proximity to the Child Welfare Services offices. Instead, they traveled to the office and worked with families and staff as needed. The advocacy services were specifically focused on the child and family's domestic violence–related needs. For example, the child advocates assisted families in finding community resources available to victims of domestic violence and their children, such as support groups, housing assistance, and legal aid. They also provided emotional support and accompanied the family to court and appointments with agency service providers. The advocacy component varied in length depending on the level of family need but was expected to extend approximately six months.

### Case Coordination

The San Diego Safe Start program also planned to provide regular case coordination meetings (called "clinical case reviews") among all three key service providers who were independently, yet simultaneously, working with the child and family: the child welfare case manager, the Safe Start therapist, and the Safe Start advocate. Aside from participating in these case coordination meetings, the child welfare case managers were not trained to manage or serve Safe Start cases any differently from their other cases. (This issue will be discussed more fully in a subsequent section.) The purpose of the case coordination meetings was for the service providers to discuss their individual perspectives of the child and family's status, needs, and progress. The meetings served as forums for the three key service providers to jointly discuss any case difficulties, resolve any disagreements in service needs or provision, and jointly develop plans to help families achieve success in meeting goals in each of the three service domains: child welfare, advocacy, and therapy. The project planned to hold these case coordination meetings monthly.

The intervention was conducted in the context of a rigorous evaluation as required by OJJPD (see the box titled "San Diego Safe Start Evaluation" for a description).

**San Diego Safe Start Evaluation**

**Design.** This randomized control effectiveness trial was focused on child outcomes.

**Treatment versus control group services.** Children assigned to the control group received Child Welfare services as usual. Those assigned to the treatment group received Trauma-Focused Cognitive Behavioral Therapy, child advocacy, and case coordination among Child Welfare Services, Safe Start therapists, and Safe Start child advocates.

**Data collection.** Data were collected through longitudinal assessments of child-level outcomes.

**Enrollment.** The site originally planned to enroll 600 families over the four-year period (300 in each group). Funding for the National Evaluation ended prematurely. By the time it ended, enrollment had taken place over two years and one month and resulted in 52 families enrolled in the treatment group and 50 in the control group.

## Implementation

Figure B.12 provides a diagram to show San Diego Safe Start's planned implementation of its intervention. The following description of the program implementation is the result of data collected for the national evaluation. See Appendix A for a full discussion of the data collection methodology employed at each of the Safe Start sites.

**Figure B.12**
**Model of San Diego Safe Start**

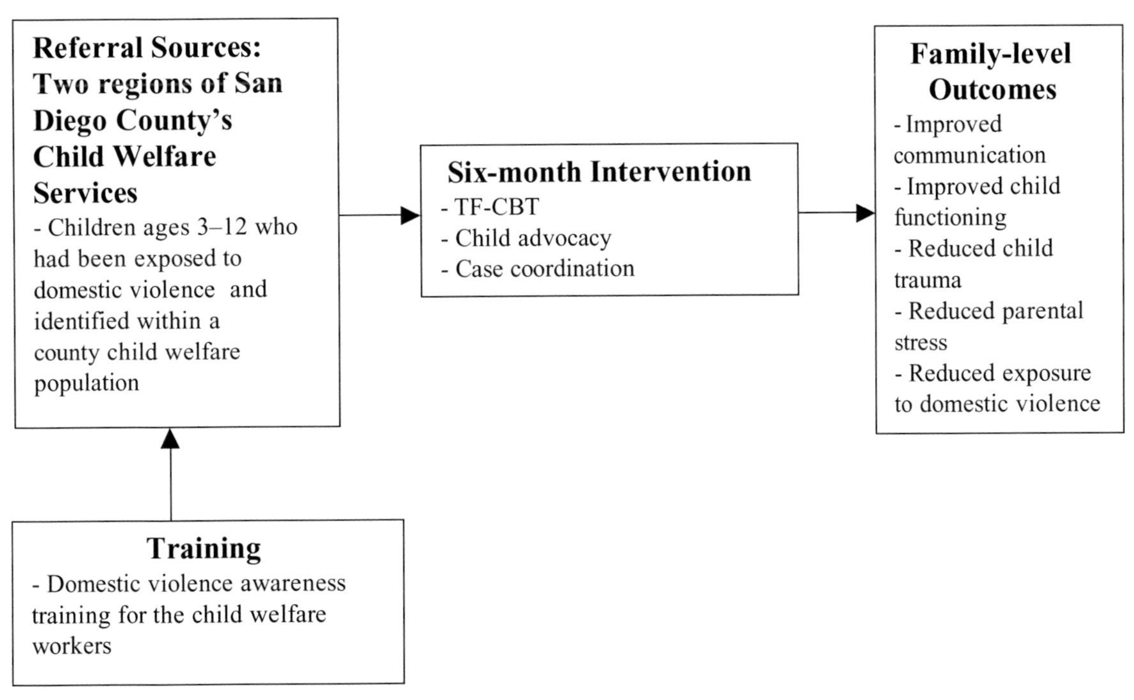

## Referrals

Referrals for the San Diego Safe Start program came exclusively from the caseloads of the North Central and Central regions of Child Welfare Services.

### *Standard Child Welfare Case Processing*

As part of standard operating procedure for Child Welfare Services, reports of suspected abuse and neglect of children are reported to the county's Child Abuse Hotline. These reports come from any number of sources throughout the community, including school staff, law enforcement officers, medical professionals, and therapists. Reports that are determined by hotline staff to present sufficient risk are forwarded to a Child Welfare Services staff for investigation and "initial services." This stage can last up to 30 days and is conducted for the purposes of the developing a case plan based on risk and safety factors.

If domestic violence exposure is identified in a child's family, it is documented in the case plan as an existing risk factor. The case plan describes all identified risk and protective factors in a child's home and related settings and then recommends appropriate services and one of three dispositions:

- Family maintenance (child remains in the care of parent; these cases can be either voluntary on the part of the parent or the result of court-ordered compliance with the case plan)
- Reunification (temporary removal with a plan for returning child to parent if the conditions of the case plan are met)
- Removal (child is made a dependent of the court and placed in foster care; reunification is not intended).

Some cases close completely without further Child Welfare Service involvement. The remainder are transferred to a permanent case manager, who then works with the family and monitors the case until the goals of the case plan are achieved or the Child Welfare Services case is otherwise closed.

### *Process of Identification and Referral of Safe Start–Eligible Children*

Child Welfare Services investigation supervisors of two selected regions identified and referred families to the Safe Start program. These supervisors oversaw the investigations and case plan development of the Child Welfare Services investigation workers. When a supervisor identified domestic violence as one of the identified risk factors in a case plan, the protocol was for him or her to call this to the attention of their office's Safe Start Program Supervisor. This point person would then evaluate the case against the program's eligibility criteria. These criteria were as follows:

- At least one child in the family is between the ages of 3 and 8 (expanded after one year up to age 12).
- Domestic violence exposure had occurred within six months of the family's referral to Child Welfare Services, as documented in the Child Welfare Services case plan.
- Only family maintenance cases were included, whether opened voluntarily or court ordered (to work toward compliance with the case plan).
- The family must be able to effectively communicate in either English or Spanish.
- A nonoffending caregiver must be available to participate in the child's treatment.

- The child and parent/primary caregiver must be free of significant cognitive impairment or severe mental illness.

All cases were screened by Child Welfare workers using the California Structured Decision Making Tool for documenting domestic exposure. No additional tools were employed for assessing trauma symptoms. Children in cases meeting inclusion criteria were considered by the program to have experienced a traumatic event.

For those determined to be eligible, a designated case manager then made an in-person contact with the family to provide information about the Safe Start program and offer them the opportunity to be contacted by the research team to hear more about the study and services. Those that declined to be contacted to hear more about the study and services were provided Child Welfare Services case management as usual. The project coordinator with the Office of Violence Prevention received all referral and signed consent forms and followed a secondary eligibility screening protocol.

Because of legal requirements, families had to agree to participate before Child Welfare Services could provide identifying information for eligible families to the local research team. Upon signed agreement, limited case information would be forwarded to the local research team at Child and Adolescent Services Research Center, which would then contact the family to explain the goals of the study and the experimental design, including the possibility of being assigned to the services-as-usual control group. Families who chose not to consent to the study, including the experimental design, received services as usual from Child Welfare Services (i.e., the Safe Start intervention services were available only to those who agreed to participate in the study).

#### *Pace of Referrals and Enrollments*

The San Diego Safe Start program expected to recruit approximately 150 families per year into the study, meaning about 75 families randomized into treatment group services per year. Instead, it enrolled 37 families in the first year and 58 in the second. Thus, the program had built up considerable service capacity that went unused, for lack of enrollment of eligible families. Over the first two years of implementation, the program worked to identify and address the causes of the slower-than-anticipated pace of enrollment. Over this period, several potential challenges were identified. Each is discussed in turn:

- Despite efforts during the Green Light process to streamline the referral process, it remained a two-stage procedure, required because of the context of Child Welfare Services. That is, Child Welfare Services had to obtain consent to refer clients to Safe Start, and then the Safe Start team at Child and Adolescent Services Research Center pursued consent for the program. Thus, program staff reported that some families might have been difficult to locate for the purpose of the two-stage consent process.
- Program staff also reported that many families resented or feared Child Welfare involvement in their lives. Many also may have felt overwhelmed by current circumstances. This might have led many of them to decline to participate in an optional activity in the context of Child Welfare (i.e., the Safe Start program), even though they might be required to participate in another form of therapeutic intervention as part of usual services.
- According to some Safe Start program staff, the program planners may have simply overestimated the number of potentially eligible cases within the Child Welfare population.

- Safe Start program staff also reported concerns that Child Welfare Services workers had not yet "bought in" to the Safe Start program and associated random assignment to services and thus were inconsistently following the referral protocols.

The program took several steps to address these potential problems:

- **Expand age range.** After about eight months of implementation, the Safe Start program expanded the upper age limit from 8 to 12 in an effort to identify more eligible cases.
- **Provide training to Child Welfare Services on referral process.** Within the first six months of implementation, the Safe Start program coordinator began meeting monthly with the Child Welfare staff at each of the offices, conducting active outreach and education for front end–line staff, and convening monthly leadership team meetings in an attempt to increase the identification of eligible cases.
- **Increase participation of Child Welfare Services offices.** One of the three offices in the two participating regions had initially agreed to participate only with those family maintenance cases that were voluntarily opened cases. The office cited concerns about whether it had the staff and capability to include court-involved cases as reasons for initially declining to fully participate. After approximately one year of implementation, however, this office agreed to expand its participation in the Safe Start recruiting and services for court-ordered family maintenance cases as well. This change was made specifically in hope of increasing enrollment.
- **Expand to another Child Welfare Services region.** The program also explored the possibility of expanding the recruitment to another region of Child Welfare Services. Implementation of this expansion, however, did not take place.

Overall, none of the changes made to the referral and recruiting process dramatically impacted enrollment, though the number of families served in the program did increase during the first two years of implementation.

### Services

Table B.12 summarizes the average active quarterly caseload per staff member over the first three years of the San Diego Safe Start program's implementation. Although San Diego maintained a pool of 12 therapists trained to provide services each year, the slow pace of referral meant that many of them never actually received a Safe Start case. Instead, there were four to seven active therapists and one to two child advocates at any one time during the first three years of implementation (through March 2009).

#### *Trauma-Focused Cognitive-Based Therapy*

During the initial contact with a family to discuss entry into treatment, the therapist explained the assessment and treatment process and gathered preliminary information about the family's concerns. When the family attended the first in-person session, the therapist collected the data needed to complete the TAP assessment. Two sessions were typically required to complete the TAP with the primary caregiver and the target child. During the third session, the therapist reviewed the TAP results with the family and developed a treatment plan. In some instances, the TAP results indicated lower than the expected level of trauma exposure. This presented a challenge to the implementation of TF-CBT, because the approach focuses on addressing PTSD symptoms and working with the child in the development of a trauma narrative.

**Table B.12**
**Service Delivery for Participants in San Diego County Safe Start**

| | Year 1 | Year 2 |
|---|---|---|
| Average active quarterly caseload per therapist | 1.5 | 2.3 |
| Average active quarterly caseload per child advocate | 10.6 | 10.5 |
| Total number of child individual therapy sessions | 44 | 105 |
| Total number of caregiver individual therapy sessions | 16 | 9 |
| Total number of joint therapy sessions | 88 | 58 |
| Total number of joint therapy sessions where child and caregiver are seen separately | 3 | 21 |
| Total number of therapy sessions involving additional members of the family | 41 | 93 |
| Total number of TAP assessments | 22 | 28 |
| Total number of case coordination meetings | 47 | 50 |
| Total number of child advocacy direct services | 390 | 252 |
| Total number of child advocacy indirect services/collateral contacts | 156 | 114 |

The therapists we interviewed indicated that they were uncertain about how to work with these children, because there did not seem to be an appropriate way to use the model. Some reported that they would use non–TF-CBT therapeutic methods in these situations. Alternatively, one therapist reported that she would identify whether a child had any kind of trauma (e.g., parent's divorce) and work to address that issue with TF-CBT, rather than domestic violence.

The Safe Start project team leaders acknowledged that there may have been a potential mismatch between the TF-CBT approach and the lack of trauma for some children. The program elected not to add a screen for trauma symptoms to eligibility criteria, in part due to concerns about further reducing the number of eligible children, which would have been problematic for the outcome evaluation component of the program. However, the Pediatric Emotional Distress Scale was implemented within the first two years to improve assessment for trauma symptoms and, when a family had multiple children in the eligible age range, to identify the targeted child with elevated trauma symptoms.

In implementing TF-CBT, the Safe Start therapist met with the child each week, either alone or jointly with the child's parent/caregiver. As noted, the therapist focused on educating the parent about the impacts of trauma, helping to reduce distress about the trauma exposure, and teaching her ways to help and support the child at home. The TF-CBT approach requires a level of support and involvement from parents that some may not be able to provide at the onset of treatment. Thus, the therapists reported a need to refer parents to individual counseling to address their own mental health needs. The therapists felt that it was important for many parents they encountered to be receiving individual counseling at the same time that their child was receiving TF-CBT.

Another implementation issue arose from the county's existing therapy reimbursement arrangements that were also used to reimburse the therapists participating in the Safe Start program. Specifically, therapy services were eligible for reimbursement only for six months from the point of the referral, with some variation depending on the source of funding covering the services for that particular family. Even though the Safe Start therapy was intended to last for six months, occasionally, families did not engage in therapy services for some time after the referral was made. For example, when the Safe Start program was first launched, referred families were responsible for initiating contact with the therapist. If the family did not follow up for a long time, then the window available for the therapy services to be reimbursed was shorter than for families who engaged in services right away.

Another challenge was that the county's funding structure for all therapists (not just those participating in Safe Start) limited each therapy session to 50 minutes. TF-CBT was initially designed for 60 to 90 minute sessions, which could be spent involving the child, parent, or other family members alone or together. The Safe Start therapists reported that they often felt they had inadequate time to work with each family.

#### *Child Advocacy*

The child advocates for the Safe Start program were trained domestic violence advocates from the Center for Community Solutions and had been previously working as advocates with adult female victims of domestic violence. The Safe Start program assigned the term *child advocate* to the role because there was more emphasis on parenting and the specific needs and behavior of children than is typical of adult-oriented domestic violence advocacy. This advocacy generally took the form of helping to educate mothers about the effects of CEV and working with the therapists and child welfare workers in the case coordination meetings to develop strategies for addressing the needs of children.

The advocates reported experiencing some difficulty in getting used to working with victims of domestic violence in a child welfare setting, due to the organizational orientation toward the child, rather than the mother. Advocates emphasized the importance of establishing trust with the families and differentiating themselves from the Child Welfare staff. Engagement in advocacy services depended largely on building rapport and trust with each client. This was accomplished by allowing the mother to determine the nature and focus of advocacy services she was willing to engage in, and by providing nonjudgmental emotional support. The domestic violence advocacy framework often described a client's perspective of Child Welfare involvement as punitive. Thus, in establishing client trust and building a working relationship, this advocacy team felt it important that clients understand that advocacy services were related to, but not an extension of, the Child Welfare system.

The advocates described their role as supporting the caregiver's choices. There was some conflict between the child welfare workers and the advocates, as the child welfare workers were mostly attentive to protecting the children in the home. Conflicts reportedly could arise when child welfare workers would refer the mother to a service that she was not interested in or felt unable to participate in. Child welfare workers reported making these referrals for the benefit of the child, but advocates felt these requirements could be punitive and disempowering to mothers. Moreover, the advocates felt that nonabusive mothers were often compelled to participate in services at the direction of Child Welfare, whereas abusive fathers without custody of the children faced no requirements at all. The child welfare workers we interviewed recognized that this situation sometimes occurred but stated that they had no authority over a parent who was not living with the children or was not actively seeking to reunite with them.

#### *Case Coordination*

The therapist, child advocate, and child welfare workers met monthly to discuss the cases they had in common. At these meetings, the participants discussed the progress and ongoing needs of the family from their own service perspective. They also discussed continuing service plans and strategies for jointly working with the family to address continuing concerns.

Overall, our interviewees indicated that, because of the Safe Start training and coordination meetings, the communication and coordination efforts improved. In some cases, however, communication between the service providers was limited and challenging because of turnover, differing views on family needs, and unavailability of some therapists for meetings. The advocates indicated that they viewed the meetings as more productive and constructive when therapists attended. They reported that the caseworkers seemed to be more open to collaboration with the advocates when the therapists participated. The therapists reported finding the meetings very helpful and valuable. The biggest obstacle for them was finding mutually workable meeting times.

The program offered cross-training and team meetings to address divergent views of family needs. The participants reported that these trainings were helpful but did not eliminate the challenges inherent in working to integrate the differing approaches to families used by child welfare workers, advocates, and therapists.

There were other components of the San Diego Safe Start program that helped shape the implementation (see the box titled "San Diego Safe Start Additional Program Components").

### San Diego Safe Start Additional Program Components

**Quality Assurance.** Twelve therapists were selected each program year from the county of San Diego's TERM panel of approved providers. TERM therapists possessed expertise in child maltreatment and delinquency cases. Before providing services to clients, therapists were trained in the TAP and TF-CBT models, as well as program implementation protocols. Clinical supervision for the therapists was provided by the Chadwick Center, in the form of monthly clinical supervision and support meetings. The clinical consultants were additionally available to therapists on an as-needed basis by phone or email. In addition, numerous strategies to monitor model fidelity were implemented from the outset of the program (e.g., face-to-face case consultation for all therapists for each active Safe Start case, a therapist-administered TF-CBT self-assessment fidelity tool). In addition, assessment of therapist competencies and monitoring of treatment and discharge plans for all county clients was provided by the county. Oversight of the child advocates was provided by their agency supervisor in regular meetings and in case-specific consultation on an as-needed basis. Monthly case management meetings including Child Welfare and Advocacy line staff were implemented early in the project to add an additional layer of quality assurance for all Safe Start cases.

**Training.** San Diego participated in or conducted 42 trainings in the first two years of Safe Start. As described in more detail in Appendix C, the two key trainings were clinical training in TF-CBT for Safe Start clinicians and the Safe Futures program to educate community agencies about issues for children exposed to violence. Approximately 40 percent of trainings were about clinical approaches, 29 percent were about Safe Start, and 14 percent were about domestic violence.

**Policies and Protocols.** San Diego implemented and changed a number of protocols, primarily with the goal of increasing referrals. These efforts included simplifying the referral form, adding a program description to the Center for Community Solutions' standard agency training, and having the Domestic Violence Response Team recommend Safe Start referrals to the Child Protective Hotline intake workers. The site also revised Child Welfare Services social workers' procedure to encourage them to make referrals of eligible families and, in conjunction with a larger agency

**San Diego Safe Start Additional Program Components (continued)**

restructure, assigned two Safe Start workers to a newly implemented Domestic Violence Specialty Unit. The site also standardized the documentation of Safe Start clinical reviews, the screening for family violence of all clients seen by Public Health Nurses, and the law enforcement's domestic violence reporting protocol to be uniform across San Diego County.

**Program Advocacy.** Advocacy efforts included disseminating information about the Safe Start program, educating various populations and organizations on domestic violence and the impacts of CEV, and increased funding and support requests for their target population. Presentations to increase awareness of issues related to children's exposure to domestic violence and support of San Diego Safe Start were given to the various child welfare entities and community coalitions in various regions of the county. To increase support and funding for CEV, the Safe Start project manager engaged in proposal writing activities. Additionally, Safe Start began to work with a military advocacy center to review the existing policy and protocols related to CEV in military families in an effort to develop and update an intake protocol for caseworkers. The site also advanced its effort to expand into East County.

**Resources and Costs.** In the first two years of SSPA, San Diego Safe Start devoted most of its resources to labor costs, specifically salaries for its child advocates, data collection coordinator, and clinical consultants. Other funds were used for office supplies to support running the program.

## Summary

The San Diego Safe Start program offered an opportunity for the community to use its expertise in multiagency coordination to address a gap in services and service coordination for children exposed to violence. In addition to improving system-level coordination, the program sought to increase awareness of the needs of children exposed to domestic violence and increase the capacity to provide appropriate services for this population.

San Diego Safe Start appeared to be successful in bringing together service providers from the child welfare, advocacy, and therapy sectors. Although it was difficult at times for the providers to agree on the shared goals for the families and to clearly define and understand each other's roles, the service providers reported that their relationships improved, particularly in terms of increased understanding and communication, over the first two years of the program. Child welfare workers, advocates, and therapists expressed appreciation for the opportunity to meet regularly to discuss their shared cases and to learn more about each other's roles.

Despite the improvements in communication, however, it was clear that tensions still remained regarding the contrasting philosophies and approaches of the child welfare workers and the advocates. In short, the philosophy of the advocates was that helping the mother results in help for the child and that mothers should be empowered to select the type of help they require and to decline, without consequence, services they do not want. The child welfare workers, however, were oriented toward the needs of the child, separate from (yet still related to) the needs of the mother and rest of the family. Working to address the needs of the child directly often meant that child welfare workers were directing mothers to services that they did not want. This continuing conflict in philosophy and approach was a challenge apparent to the Safe Start leadership, including the Safe Start Steering Committee, which remained committed to working to integrate the two approaches by continuing to facilitate communication and cross-trainings between the two sets of providers.

In addition, the Safe Start program faced difficulty in the fit between its target population and TF-CBT as the single intervention selection. TF-CBT was designed to address trauma symptoms, yet therapists reported that these were not present in some of the children enrolled in the Safe Start program. This suggests that future attempts to replicate the program should screen for trauma symptoms before enrolling children in TF-CBT services or offer alternate therapy models more closely matched to the needs of the child. This was the original intent of the San Diego Safe Start program, but the needs of the outcome evaluation for a relatively large sample size in both the treatment and control group led the program to select a single therapy model.

**Data collection for this program summary included:**

- Key informant interviews with key program staff and community partners:
  - Safe Start project directors
  - Safe Start therapists
  - Safe Start advocates
  - Child Welfare Services social workers
  - Local evaluation director
  - Fiscal and grant management staff
  - Group interview with and observation of a meeting of the Safe Start Steering Committee
- Case review of randomly selected treatment and control group cases
- Quality assurance checklist completed by the clinical supervisor
- Quarterly activity reports on services, training, policies, and advocacy
- Grant application
- Green Light notes
- *Safe Start: Promising Approaches Communities Working Together to Help Children Exposed to Violence* (Safe Start Center, 2008).

## 13. San Mateo County Program Description

### San Mateo County Safe Start

- **Intervention type:** Child-Parent Psychotherapy (CPP)
- **Intervention length:** 12 months
- **Intervention setting:** In-home, office, or other community setting
- **Target population:** Children who reside with their grandparents or other relatives (i.e., kinship care) and have been exposed to domestic violence, community violence, and/or experienced abuse or neglect
- **Age range:** 0–7
- **Primary referral sources:** San Mateo County Kinship Support Network

### Program and Community Setting

The San Mateo Safe Start Program was located in San Mateo County, California, adjacent to but not including the City and County of San Francisco. The population of the county was slightly more than 707,000, according to the 2000 U.S. Census. About 7 percent of the population was younger than age 5, and the population was nearly 60 percent white, 20 percent Asian, 22 percent Hispanic, 4 percent Black, and 12 percent other racial/ethnic groups. The income per capita for the county overall was $42,204, reflecting its location within California's relatively prosperous Silicon Valley. The program operated out of two city locations, South San Francisco and East Palo Alto, where per capita incomes were much lower, $27,588 and $16,128, respectively.[26] The percentage of the population living under the federal poverty line was 6 for the county overall; however, it was 5 percent in South San Francisco and 16 percent in East Palo Alto.[27]

The San Mateo County Safe Start program was specifically focused on serving "kinship families," referring to families where children live in the care of grandparents or other relatives. Approximately 7 percent of the county's children live in such family arrangements, compared with an estimated 5 percent of children nationally (Edgewood Center for Children and Families, 2004). Kinship children were more likely to live in low-income households in San Mateo County than other children, and as such were at elevated risk for a host of difficulties associated with poverty, such as poor health, lack of food, and difficulties in school (Edgewood Center for Children and Families, 2004). Edgewood Center Children and Families is the San Francisco Bay area's primary provider of services to kinship children and their families. In a 2004 review of its existing cases, Edgewood found in 72 percent of their kinship families that children had experienced abuse and neglect and about 50 percent had witnessed family violence (Edgewood Center for Children and Families, 2004).

The Kinship Support Network was established by the Edgewood Center for Children and Families in 1999 (a description of the network is provided in the box titled "San Mateo

---

[26] This is the income per capita reported on the 2000 Census but converted into 2005 dollars. The income per capita for San Mateo County, South San Francisco, and East Palo Alto in 1999 dollars, as reported in the census, was $36,045, $23,562, and $13,774, respectively.

[27] The information was all taken from the 2000 Census and can be found at the Census website (U.S. Census Bureau, no date).

> ### San Mateo Safe Start Partner Agencies
>
> **Edgewood Center for Children and Families.** Edgewood is a nonprofit, multiservice agency focused on serving the needs of children who face significant challenges, such as abuse, neglect, mental health, and family crises. Operating in the San Francisco Bay area, it operates two central locations in San Francisco and one in San Mateo County. It provides direct services to children and families, training, advocacy, and research. Its direct service programs include case management and support for kinship families, school-based programs, behavioral and mental health services, medical services, and residential and day treatment programs, among other prevention and intervention activities. Edgewood is the lead agency for the San Mateo Safe Start program. It provides the staffing, leadership, support, and oversight. Numerous other public and private organizations provide referrals to Edgewood's Kinship Support Network, which in turn serves as the source of families referred to and recruited for participation in the Safe Start program.

Safe Start Partner Agencies"). The intent of the Kinship Support Network was to fill the gaps in public social services available to kinship families within San Mateo County. Prior to the network's advent, only kinship families formally involved in the county's child welfare system (less than an estimated 5 percent of such families in the county) received coordinated services. These services were not tailored to the unique needs of kinship families, who are often headed by older or elderly caregivers (most often grandmothers) facing a host of physical and financial difficulties and other challenges (Edgewood Center for Children and Families, 2004).

To address these needs, the Kinship Support Network developed a range of services available to the entire kinship family (caregivers and children). The services included home-based case management along with a needs assessment and case plan, community health nursing, caregiver support groups, trainings and workshops for caregivers, family and youth recreational activities, and tutoring and educational advocacy. For its services overall, the Kinship Support Network typically serves about 350 kinship families, including about 600 children each year (Edgewood Center for Children and Families, 2004). In addition, Edgewood, through the Kinship Support Network, works with both public and private agencies to make social and community services more accessible to kinship families and to increase the range of kinship-specific services available in the community.

Prior to the Safe Start partnership, Edgewood staff providing Kinship Support Network case management services (called "community workers") were aware that many kinship children had been exposed to violence, but this exposure was not systematically assessed as part of the case planning process. When it was identified in individual cases, Kinship Support Network providers reported being very limited in the resources they could offer to kinship families. In proposing the Safe Start project to OJJDP, Edgewood indicated that mental health services for young children exposed to violence were a significant need in the San Mateo community, and particularly lacking were services tailored to the unique needs of children in kinship families.

To address this need, Edgewood proposed to build on its existing Kinship Support Network services by developing a process for routine violence-exposure screening of young children (ages 0–6) in the kinship families it served. Violence was defined as domestic violence, abuse, and neglect, as well as community violence. Children identified as having such exposure would be eligible for participation in the Safe Start intervention, in addition to continuing to receive the home-based case management and support services of the Kinship Support

Network. For the Safe Start intervention, CPP was selected as the intervention model because it was thought to offer the most promise for addressing the needs of the target population. Edgewood proposed to adapt CPP for use with kinship families, with the consultation, direct training, and ongoing clinical supervision by one of the CPP "Preschool Witness to Violence Program" model developers, Patricia Van Horn.

After the San Mateo program was selected by OJJDP as a Safe Start site, it worked to further develop and refine its program and evaluation plans as part of OJJDP's Green Light process. The program leaders reported that the Green Light process was productive because it helped them think through their plans for implementation. During this process, San Mateo focused on refining the eligibility criteria to include recruitment from the existing Kinship Support Network (rather than only new cases) to increase the pool of potentially eligible participants. The program also selected a violence-screening tool. The program also decided to expand eligibility to kinship families having some contact with the Kinship Support Network and receiving some services but who were not receiving active case management services. During the Green Light period, the site prepared for and facilitated training for the master's-level mental health clinicians who would be delivering the Safe Start intervention.

## Intervention

The San Mateo County Safe Start model consisted of therapeutic intervention for kinship children ages 0–7 that have been exposed to violence. The selected model, CPP, was delivered by master's- and doctorate-level clinicians in the client's home, community, or one of Edgewood's offices, typically on a weekly basis for one year.

### Child-Parent Psychotherapy

CPP is a relationship-based intervention designed for use with children up to age 6. It can be used with children whose relationship with a parent or other primary caregiver is impacted by negative circumstances, including family violence. CPP integrates psychodynamic, attachment, trauma, cognitive-behavioral, and social learning theories (NCTSN, 2008). There are two components in CPP: assessment and treatment, with information gained during the assessment used to inform the treatment component. In the intervention component, child-parent interactions are the focus of six intervention modalities aimed at restoring a sense of mastery, security, and growth and promoting congruence between bodily sensations, feelings, and thinking on the part of both child and parent and in their relationship with one another (NCTSN, 2008).

Although the CPP model is relatively flexible, the San Mateo Safe Start anticipated some need for modification of the model for the kinship context. A key reason for this expectation was that the model was designed for a parent-child dyad, most commonly a mother and child. In the San Mateo kinship setting, however, the primary caregiver was not a parent but most often a grandparent. Thus, the site anticipated at least several complications coming from these unique kinship circumstances. For example, grandparents or other kin may view themselves as only temporary caretakers of kinship children and resist an intervention approach that casts them in a permanent parent-like role. Moreover, birth parents may cycle in and out of the kinship household for varying periods of time. This can create complicated relationship dynamics surrounding parental authority, involving the child and their birth parent but also the birth parent and the primary kinship caregiver (most commonly birth parent's own mother or father). Thus, the site expected that it would need guidance on the appropriate strategies for adapting the CPP model to address these unique dynamics. To that end, it retained one of the model developers to provide initial training for the clinical staff to deliver the model and also provide ongoing, in-person weekly clinical supervision. The site's intention was to ensure that the model was modified for the target population in a way that would not detract from the key clinical features of the model.

In the planned delivery of the model, the therapists would use the first one to three therapy sessions as a time to establish a treatment plan. The treatment plan contained the areas of concern or issues that would serve as a particular focus of the therapy sessions and outlined the family-specific goals of treatment. In this process, the therapists also identified other needs of the family, such as individual therapy for the primary caregiver, legal assistance or assistance obtaining food stamps, and the like. For these needs, therapists would connect families to Kinship Support Network community workers or services to assist them.

The length of the Safe Start intervention was intended to be 12 months, with weekly sessions lasting approximately one hour. The program did expect that family need could require longer and more frequent sessions initially and fewer sessions nearer the conclusion of the course of treatment.

The intervention was conducted in the context of a rigorous evaluation as required by OJJDP (see the box titled "San Mateo Safe Start Evaluation" for a description).

### San Mateo Safe Start Evaluation

**Design.** This randomized control effectiveness trial was focused on child outcomes.

**Treatment versus control group services.** Both groups received the services and supports available through the Kinship Support Network, including home-based case management, health care services, support groups, and advocacy services. In addition, the treatment group families received home-based CPP sessions.

**Data collection.** Data were collected through longitudinal assessments of child-level outcomes.

**Enrollment.** The site originally planned to enroll 220 families over the four-year period (110 in each group). Funding for the National Evaluation ended prematurely. By the time it ended, enrollment had taken place over two years and ten months and resulted in 26 families in the treatment group and 28 in the control group.

## Implementation

Figure B.13 shows San Mateo's implementation of their intervention. The following description of the program implementation is the result of data collected for the national evaluation. See Appendix A for a full discussion of the data collection methodology employed at each of the Safe Start sites.

**Figure B.13**
**Model of San Mateo Safe Start**

Referral Sources: Kinship Support Network
- Refer kinship families whose children, ages 0–7, had been physically or sexually abused, witnessed domestic violence, or witnessed any violent crime
12-month Intervention
- Child-parent psychotherapy
Family-level Outcomes
- Increased caregiver knowledge of how to reduce impact of a child's exposure to violence
- Reduce child symptoms of post-traumatic stress
- Improve child's cognitive, language & motor development
- Reduced risk of re-exposure to violence

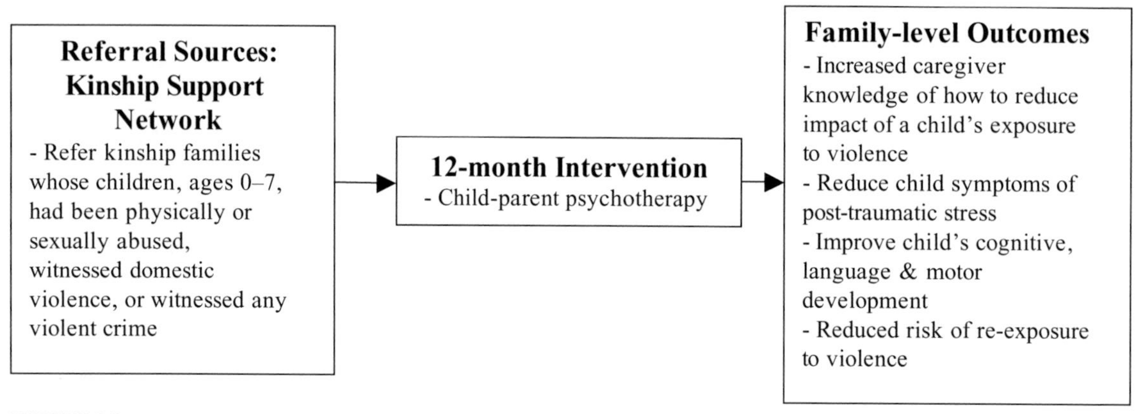

RAND *TR750-B.13*

## Referrals

The specific eligibility criteria for the Safe Start program were as follows:

- kinship families living in San Mateo County
- at least one child ages birth to age 7 who had been exposed to violence, as determined by the caregiver, answering yes to any one of the screening questions.

The San Mateo Safe Start program established a procedure for eligibility screening and referrals that built on the existing procedures of the Kinship Support Network. As part of their usual practice for all newly referred families to the Kinship Support Network, community workers conducted an intake process, offered families available services, and began working with the family on accessing the services in which they may be interested. For Safe Start, the community workers would not introduce the program to families until after two months of involvement with the Kinship Support Network, giving the family time to become more stabilized and obtain knowledge and access to available community services. This period also allowed time to assist kinship caregivers with determining and/or obtaining legal guardianship status over the children in their care.

After the two-month period had passed for kinship families with children in the target age range, the community worker would introduce the Safe Start program, explain the evaluation research context, and ask whether the family was interested in being screened for participation in the study and program. When families expressed an interest, the community services worker would administer a six-item trauma-screening inventory, containing questions about the child's exposure to domestic violence, community violence, and abuse. If there was a positive answer to any item, the kinship family would be scheduled to meet with Edgewood research staff, who would provide a detailed explanation of the Safe Start study and services, including the random assignment of the treatment services; confirm legal guardianship; obtain consent; confirm eligibility; and conduct a baseline assessment interview (for evaluation research purposes). Families were then randomly assigned to either the Safe Start treatment group (receiving the CPP intervention) or to the control group, receiving services as usual provided through the Kinship Support Network. Treatment group families also received the usual whole-family case management and other supportive services provided through the Kinship Support Network, designed to help meet the broader needs of kinship families.

In May 2006, San Mateo Safe Start received OJJDP's Green Light approval to begin receiving clients. The program anticipated it would soon begin receiving referrals from Kinship Support Network community workers. Instead, the pace of enrollment was quite a bit lower than anticipated. The first Safe Start family was seen in July 2006. The Safe Start program staff reported that this appeared to be due to hesitation on the part of the community workers to introduce the Safe Start program to kinship families. Program staff cited several reasons for this hesitation. First, initial buy-in of the community workers to the concept of random assignment was low. Community workers were hesitant to offer "their" families an intervention that they might not ultimately receive, should they be randomized to the control group. Second, community workers were said to have low interest in referring families to the Safe Start program because of the perception that it would be available only on a temporary basis, as a grant-funded experiment. Community workers were described as preferring to engage "their" families in services they regarded as more permanent in the community. Third, turnover among community workers was a challenge, requiring training and retraining of new staff on the Safe Start referral and screening process.

When community workers did introduce Safe Start to families, there were challenges in engaging kinship families in the intervention. One factor reducing interest was the experimental component, but the continuing stigma of receiving mental health services reportedly also served to depress interest in the program. Safe Start program staff explained that elderly caregivers who often head kinship families were particularly likely to hold negative views of mental health interventions generally and to express concern about being stigmatized (e.g., considered "crazy") for participation.

In response, the Safe Start program staff undertook a series of activities and steps to address factors thought to be suppressing enrollment. Key among these were ongoing trainings and informal discussions between the Safe Start therapists and the community workers. These activities were undertaken to increase the community workers' familiarity and comfort level with the intervention model as well as to increase their appreciation of the value of the research component. Also, the program eliminated the two-month window of kinship services before seeking to recruit families into Safe Start. They also worked collaboratively on refining the manner in which the program was presented to the kinship families during recruitment, with the goal of identifying language that would minimize caregiver concerns about stigmatization and avoid the caregivers thinking of their families as being "experimented on." Kinship Support Network supervisors also began to regularly check with community workers to confirm whether they had been following the Safe Start recruitment protocol with their individual cases.

Within six months of implementation, the program also increased its target age range by one year (to age 7 at the time of referral) in an attempt to boost enrollment. In addition, Safe Start therapists engaged in a variety of outreach activities in the community. These included raising awareness and distributing materials to agencies that regularly interact with kinship families (such as child welfare) who may not have already been involved in the Kinship Network. These outreach activities were targeted toward increasing referrals of eligible kinship directly to the Safe Start program. Any kinship families who directly contacted Safe Start therapists as a result of these outreach efforts would then be connected with the Kinship Support Network, contacted by a community worker, and screened for eligibility and enrollment in the Safe Start intervention.

Despite these multiple efforts, the pace of referrals remained slower than expected over the first two years of implementation. Yet, the project staff continued to seek to promote the program and to overcome a general resistance to mental health interventions among its target population.

### Services

Table B.13 summarizes average quarterly caseload per staff member for the San Mateo Safe Start program during the first three years of implementation (through March 2009). The program involved two therapists. It intended for each to carry a caseload of 10 families in the first year and increase to 15 families each in the subsequent years. The lighter initial caseloads were to allow time for more intensive training and clinical supervision at the outset of the intervention.

#### *Child-Parent Psychotherapy*

For those families randomized into the treatment group, the family was assigned one of two therapists for CPP. In general, the therapists reported that they felt confident in the strengths of the model for use with a kinship population. They appreciated the broad flexibility of the model to use a variety of therapeutic techniques and approaches, such as play therapy, to accomplish the broad goals of improving child-caregiver relationship and strengthening attachments.

However, the therapists did report a need to work closely with one of the CPP model developers to expand the therapy's focus beyond a child-caregiver dyad. In the context of kinship families, they described the intervention as constituting more of a family model, because kinship families often contain several adults, each with some type of relationship with the child. These adults may include biological parent(s), adult extended-family members, and siblings. Thus, in the course of working with the family, the therapists held a number of collateral sessions with other household members and made referrals for them to specific services, such as for individual counseling or for substance-abuse treatment programs. In short, the therapists reported engaging in a significant amount of case management–type activities for all the household members in addition to delivering sessions targeted toward child-caregiver relationships. The therapists were able to work with Kinship Support Network community workers to help reduce the amount of their time spent on case management. Nonetheless, because the therapists were more intimately involved with the family, they felt that they were more likely to uncover a pressing family need, and thus they needed to work intensively with the family to help address it. To help facilitate and coordinate the identification of need and delivery of services, the Safe Start therapists found that participating in meetings with community workers helped increase communication and coordinate services.

**Table B.13**
**Service Delivery for the San Mateo Safe Start Intervention**

| | Year 1 | Year 2 | Year 3 (10 mos) |
|---|---|---|---|
| Average active quarterly caseload per therapist | 3.6 | 5.4 | 4.8 |
| Total number of CPP sessions | 155 | 220 | 184 |
| Total number of collateral contacts made by therapists | 92 | 306 | 268 |

In the first year of implementation, the Safe Start therapists reported that the slow pace of referrals and enrollment was the biggest challenge. As their caseload increased, however, the provision of services in each case proved to be more time intensive for the therapists than anticipated. Thus, even though caseloads did not reach the full planned capacity of 15 new kinship families per year, the therapists expressed concern that they would be unable to keep pace with the caseload, particularly given the home-based nature of the intervention. Further, the size and traffic conditions of San Mateo County meant that therapists could spend a considerable amount of time in transit to client homes, limiting the number of sessions that could be scheduled in a given day.

In response, during the second year of implementation the Safe Start staff decided that home-based sessions would not be automatically started with each new kinship family. Instead, individual circumstances would be reviewed to determine whether the family could come to the Edgewood office for some or all of the CPP sessions. The therapists viewed this as a partial solution to the logistical challenges of providing in-home services but remained unconvinced that they would be able to continue to provide the same level of service to all families should the program ever reach its intended capacity. During the period of implementation covered by this report, however, the enrollment did not increase sufficiently to observe the program's operation at its intended capacity.

There were other components of the San Mateo Safe Start program that helped shape the implementation (see the box titled "San Mateo Safe Start Additional Program Components").

### San Mateo Safe Start Additional Program Components

**Quality Assurance.** At the outset of the project, the Safe Start program hired therapists who were then training in the intervention model by one of the model developers. During program implementation, the therapists and their supervisor participated in weekly two-hour clinical supervision sessions with the CPP model developer. In addition, each clinician received an in-person, individual, one-hour weekly session of clinical supervision with a trained member of the developer's staff. They also received in-person clinical supervision and case consultation with their agency supervisor at other points as needed. In addition, the therapists had access to materials that described the treatment model, the Safe Start program, and the implementation plans.

**Training.** Over the course of the first two years of program implementation, San Mateo Safe Start conducted and/or participated in 41 other trainings. Of these, 46 percent focused on Safe Start procedures and/or intervention issues. The remainder of the training focused on related issues, such as cultural diversity, and general professional skills, such as boundary setting.

**Policies and Protocols.** Changes to policy were made by the San Mateo Safe Start program, primarily to give better feedback to those in the treatment and control groups. Specifically, clinicians began to review the scored assessment measures for their use in treatment planning as part of their work with families receiving the CPP intervention. For families in the control group, clinicians provided feedback on their completed assessments if their scores reflected clinical or subclinical levels of concern.

**Program Outreach.** The site's outreach efforts included a number of presentations on the Safe Start program to gain community support, reform policy, and, in a few cases, funding, as well as two testimonies to advocate for policy change. Presentations to increase awareness and

**San Mateo Safe Start Additional Program Components (continued)**

understanding of the program were given to a domestic violence survivor group, middle and high school counselors and parents, churches, pediatricians, community health nurses, human service agencies, and domestic violence agencies. Program staff also made presentations that were more targeted toward gaining funding to various groups.

**Resources and Costs.** In the first two years of SSPA, San Mateo Safe Start devoted most of their resources for labor costs, specifically, the program director, kinship safety specialists, and the data coordinator. Other costs were for instrumentation to be used with the therapy and incentives for clients.

## Summary

The San Mateo Safe Start program allowed Edgewood to expand the services provided by the existing Kinship Support Network to include a therapeutic intervention for young children in kinship care who had experienced abuse and neglect or who had been exposed to family violence. With the assistance of one of the model developers, the Safe Start program customized the CPP intervention treatment to better suit the unique needs of kinship families. Primarily, this involved expansion of the CPP model from a focus on a parent-child dyad to working with all family/household members surrounding the target child. This modification addressed the living situations of the often-multigenerational, blended families served by the program.

Overall, this program was implemented as initially proposed; however, the program made some early revisions to refine the recruitment and screening process and to increase the pool of eligible families. The Safe Start program had planned to be fully integrated into the Kinship Support Network's mix of services offered to families. With the launch of the program, community service workers were trained to work in collaboration with the Safe Start program clinicians to conduct the initial family assessments and recruit eligible families for Safe Start Services. Early in the implementation phase, however, the Safe Start program learned that the community workers were not completely "bought in" to the idea of offering the Safe Start program to their clients. This was reportedly due to several factors, including the research context (with the possibility that clients might be assigned to the control group) and a view of Safe Start as a service destined to end at the conclusion of its grant funding. This reportedly led some community workers to feel hesitant about accepting the program model and actively recruiting families in their caseloads to participate.

Another challenge facing Safe Start was the stigma associated with receiving mental health services. According to the program staff, particularly for the elderly caregivers common in the Kinship population, this negative perception of mental health services contributed to some families choosing not to participate in Safe Start.

Over the period of implementation, the program's leadership was aware of these challenges and undertook a number of steps to overcome them. These steps included conducting additional trainings with the community service workers to assist them in overcoming hesitation in recruiting families and providing them with ways to talk about the intervention that reduced the potential stigma surrounding the mental health component. The program also actively engaged in external community outreach to raise awareness about the availability of

Safe Start in the context of the Kinship Services Network. Although the number of participants did not reach the intended capacity for the program, it nonetheless appeared to provide an intervention within San Mateo County that was previously unavailable for serving the unique needs of children exposed to violence living in kinship families.

**Data collection for this program summary included:**

- Key informant interviews with key program staff:
  - Safe Start program leadership
  - Edgewood Center for Children and Families leadership
  - Safe Start therapists
  - Kinship Support Network community workers
  - Kinship Support Network supervisors
  - Edgewood research staff
- Case review of randomly selected treatment and control group cases
- Quality assurance checklist completed by the project director
- Quarterly activity reports on services, training, policies, and advocacy
- Grant application
- Green Light notes
- *Safe Start: Promising Approaches Communities Working Together to Help Children Exposed to Violence* (Safe Start Center, 2008).

# 14. Toledo Program Description

**Toledo Safe Start**

- **Intervention type:** Child-Parent Psychotherapy (CPP)
- **Intervention length:** Up to 12 months
- **Intervention setting:** Clinic
- **Target population:** Children exposed to domestic violence
- **Age range:** 0–5
- **Primary referral source:** Help Me Grow

## Program and Community Setting

The Toledo Safe Start program is located in the city of Toledo, Ohio, which, according to the 2000 Census, had a population slightly more than 313,600 people, 7 percent of whom were younger than age 5. Approximately 70 percent of the population was white, 24 percent was black, less than 2 percent Native American or Asian, and 6 percent Hispanic. The 1999 per capita income was $20,359,[28] and about 18 percent of the population was living below the poverty line at that time.[29]

According to Toledo's original proposal for the Safe Start initiative, Lucas County law enforcement responded to more than 8,000 calls related to domestic incidents during 2003. Nearly 1,500 of these resulted in domestic violence charges, and 315 resulted in arrests for domestic violence (Toledo Hospital, 2004).

Prior to Safe Start, Toledo had limited resources for young children exposed to domestic violence. In particular, developmental assessments and evidence-based treatment for children exposed to violence were not available in the community. To address this need, the Toledo Safe Start project was created as a collaborative endeavor of several organizations. The Cullen Center of Toledo Children's Hospital provided the Safe Start project's leadership and oversight. The Cullen Center provides support and counseling for children and families suffering from different types of trauma. The other collaborating organizations were several of the Help Me Grow program sites. Help Me Grow is Ohio's statewide early identification program for at-risk families with children ages 0–3 (see the box titled "Toledo Safe Start Partner Agencies" for a brief description of each agency).

The planned Safe Start project included four Help Me Grow sites, three of which were within service agencies that could provide treatment services. In the fourth site, which did not have an on-site therapist, the Cullen Center planned to provide therapy for the referred families. With Safe Start, the project sought to develop their relationships with the Help Me Grow programs and build capacity within the community for providing evidence-based mental health treatment for children exposed to domestic violence.

[28] This is the 1999 income per capita reported in 2005 dollars. The 1999 income per capita as originally reported in the 2000 Census is $17,388.

[29] The information was taken from the 2000 Census and can be found at the Census website (U.S. Census Bureau, no date).

The program that was originally developed targeted children ages 0–3 who had been exposed to domestic violence. Evidence of exposure to violence was expected to be based on caregiver self-report, child protective services reports, screening assessment results, police reports, intake information from domestic violence shelters, or other mental health history.

The Toledo program was selected by OJJDP as one of 15 sites across the country. After receiving the grant, Toledo went through the OJJDP's Green Light process to prepare for program implementation and evaluation. Toledo used the Green Light period to expand their age range from the 0 to 3 range originally proposed to include 0-to-5-year-old children exposed to domestic violence in an attempt to increase the number of possible referrals. It took the Toledo program almost 10 months to complete the Green Light process, largely because of the need to bring the Help Me Grow programs on board with the implementation procedures and the evaluation component. Despite the long start-up time, the project was successful in keeping the community partners engaged and committed.

### Toledo Safe Start Partner Agencies

**Cullen Center, Toledo Children's Hospital.** Established in 2002, the Cullen Center is a collaborative partnership between the Toledo Children's Hospital and Family and Child Abuse Prevention Center. The center provides counseling and group support to children and their families who have experienced any type of trauma, including child abuse, witnessing violence, serious illness or injuries, loss of a family member of friend, serious accidents, fires, or other traumatic events. As one of the initial community treatment sites for the National Child Traumatic Stress Initiative, the Cullen Center has provided Trauma-Focused Cognitive-Behavioral Therapy for traumatized children since 2001. As the lead agency, the Cullen Center provided project leadership and oversight. Also, the center contributed a therapist to provide therapy to families who were enrolled from one of the Help Me Grow sites that did not have an on-site therapist.

**Help Me Grow.** Help Me Grow is Ohio's statewide early identification program for at-risk families with children ages 0–3. Through a centralized intake process, eligible families are linked with community-based providers and receive home visitation and other supports from a community service worker who follows the Help Me Grow protocols. Four Help Me Grow sites in Lucas County served as referral sources for the Safe Start program, and three of the four also provided therapeutic services during the Safe Start implementation.

## Intervention

The Toledo Safe Start program involved CPP in a clinic setting. The intervention period lasted up to one year.

### Child-Parent Psychotherapy

The therapy component involved parent-child dyadic therapy using the Lieberman model for CPP. CPP is a relationship-based intervention designed for use with children up to age 6.

It can be used with any child whose relationship to his or her parent or other primary caregiver is impacted by negative circumstances, including family violence. CPP integrates psychodynamic, attachment, trauma, cognitive-behavioral, and social learning theories (NCTSN, 2008). There are two components in CPP: assessment and treatment, with information gained during the assessment used to inform the treatment component. In the intervention component, child-parent interactions are the focus of six intervention modalities aimed at restoring a sense of mastery, security, and growth and promoting congruence between bodily sensations, feelings, and thinking on the part of both child and parent and in their relationship with one another (NCTSN, 2008).

Eligible children included those ages 0–5 who had been exposed to domestic violence. Evidence of exposure to violence might include self-report by family, results of screening tools, reports to child protective services, police reports, emergency room medical data, domestic violence shelter intake data, or history as reported by a professional.

Toledo delivered CPP for domestic violence in weekly one-hour clinic sessions at one of the four treatment sites. During the Safe Start Green Light process, Toledo specified that the therapy would continue until there was mutual agreement between the family and the clinician that treatment goals had been met and the clinician determined that affect regulation was stable and the relationship was "pleasing" for both the parent and child.

The intervention was conducted in the context of a rigorous evaluation as required by OJJDP (see the box titled "Toledo Safe Start Evaluation" for a description).

### Toledo Safe Start Evaluation

**Design.** This randomized control effectiveness trial was focused on child outcomes.

**Treatment versus control group services.** In addition to receiving any services or supports from the referring agency, those who were assigned to the treatment group received CPP. Those who were assigned to the control group received only the services and supports they were already receiving from the referring agency and referrals to local mental health services, if needed, in accordance with standard practices at the referring agencies.

**Data collection.** Data were collected through longitudinal assessments of child-level outcomes.

**Enrollment.** The site originally planned to enroll 160 families over the four-year period (80 in each group). Funding for the National Evaluation ended prematurely. By the time it ended, enrollment had taken place over two years and four months and resulted in 15 families in the treatment group and 16 in the control group.

## Implementation

Figure B.14 shows Toledo's implementation of the intervention. The following description of the program implementation is the result of data collected for the national evaluation. See Appendix A for a full discussion of the data collection methodology employed at each of the Safe Start sites.

**Figure B.14**
**Model of Toledo Safe Start**

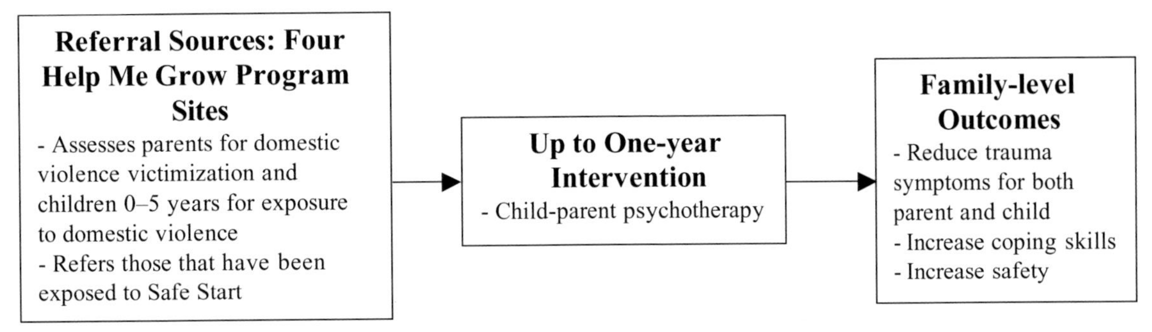


RAND *TR750-B.14*

## Referrals

From the program's inception in the fall of 2006 until November of 2007, Toledo received all of its referrals from the four local Help Me Grow programs. As originally envisioned, the Help Me Grow service coordinators, who conduct home visits with the at-risk families, would identify women within their caseloads who had been victimized by domestic violence and refer them to Safe Start. Many of the referrals came from the existing caseloads of the service coordinators, which meant that the service coordinators may not have been actively engaged with the family at the time of the referral. Early on, Toledo developed a fax referral form for the service coordinators to use when they made referrals. Later, the program switched to a telephone intake process. The referring party directed the caregiver to call the Cullen Center. The intake person would then complete a telephone intake form with the caregiver to make sure that the family met the eligibility criteria.

Once a referral was received, the Safe Start project director at the Cullen Center screened the caregiver for eligibility via phone. At that time, the screening information provided by the referring agency was discussed with the parent and documented on an intake form. The parent had the opportunity to provide additional information regarding the family's exposure to violence. The Safe Start project director then made the final determination of the family's eligibility for the study. If there were multiple eligible children, the target child to serve as the focus of the intervention was selected by the mother based on which child she felt had the greatest need.

When the eligibility had been established and the intake form completed, the project director scheduled the baseline assessment at the Cullen Center. After the assessment, the project director implemented the random assignment procedures and informed the family and the Help Me Grow Service Coordinator about the results. The project director then assigned the family to a therapist at one of the Help Me Grow sites or at the Cullen Center on a rotating basis, although family preferences related to accessibility and comfort with the location were taken into consideration when making case assignments.

From the beginning, Toledo received very few referrals from the Help Me Grow service coordinators. There were several reasons identified by Safe Start and Help Me Grow program staff for the slower-than-expected rate of referrals:

- **Client readiness.** The service coordinators found that because their clients were often overwhelmed with their situation (as young mothers with few resources), they were focused on the basics of daily living. According to the service coordinators, the young mothers did not recognize domestic violence as a problem that was having an impact on their children.

- **Domestic violence and program knowledge.** The service coordinators were not all experienced in recognizing or assessing clients for domestic violence, which made them hesitant to even broach the topic with their clients. The service coordinators reported that they did not feel confident explaining domestic violence or the Safe Start program to their clients.
- **Research design.** The research design also posed challenges to maintaining a steady flow of referrals from the service coordinators. The service coordinators indicated that they did not want to refer their clients to the program, because their client might be assigned to the control group instead of the treatment group. Even though the treatment group was receiving an intervention that was not proven effective, service coordinators perceived the treatment group as receiving better and more effective services.

In an attempt to remedy these problems, the Safe Start project director (who worked at the Cullen Center) met regularly with the service coordinators, provided more client-friendly materials about the Safe Start program, and provided a packet of materials on domestic violence and trauma for the service coordinators to integrate into their curriculum. Although the service coordinators found the materials useful, the slow pace of referrals continued and the program began to explore options for expanding its referral sources.

In November of 2007, Toledo Safe Start added Lucas County Children's Services, Toledo Children's Hospital, and battered women's shelters and transitional houses as referral sources. All these additional referring agencies or programs were involved in serving families with children in the target age range and had already made referrals to the Cullen Center for other programs and services.

- **Lucas County Children's Services.** Lucas County Children's Services is the county's child protective services agency. Prior to Safe Start, it was the Cullen Center's primary referral source, so it was aware of Safe Start. The Safe Start project director met with the Children's Services staff to further educate them about the program and the referral process. To add them as a referral source, the Cullen Center intake coordinator screened all referrals from Children's Services for eligibility for Safe Start.
- **Toledo Children's Hospital.** Prior to Safe Start, the Cullen Center regularly received referrals from various departments within the hospital system. The Safe Start project director met with the hospital's pediatricians to educate them about Safe Start and the referral process. To add the hospital system as a Safe Start referral source, the Cullen Center flagged all internal referrals and screened them for their eligibility for Safe Start.
- **Battered women's shelters and transitional houses.** The battered women's shelter and transitional houses provide services to the women and children attempting to leave violent relationships. They operate three facilities, including one short-term facility and two long-term facilities for women and children. Prior to adding these organizations as a referral source, the Safe Start project director met with the director and service providers to discuss Safe Start and the referral process. Starting in January of 2008, the battered women's shelters and transitional houses began making referrals to Safe Start. According to Safe Start program staff, the families who were referred from this source were more likely to continue with the program because they were women who had moved beyond the immediate crisis situation and because the shelter staff established and maintained contact with the women after making the Safe Start referral.

### Services

Table B.14 summarizes service delivery for those who received services through the Toledo Safe Start program. During the first year of implementation, one to two therapists provided services as part of the intervention, and in the second and third years of implementation, three to four therapists provided services. Although Safe Start had therapists lined up to deliver CPP at all four of the treatment sites, because of the lack of referrals there was always at least one therapist with no active caseload.

#### *Child-Parent Psychotherapy*

Services were provided by a therapist at one of the four treatment sites. Toledo Safe Start sent a clinician from each of the four treatment sites to San Francisco to be trained in the use of CPP by the model developer. Despite the slow pace of referrals, the program staff maintained the involvement of the clinicians through regular clinical supervision, also provided by the model developer. Given the relatively low service numbers, our assessment of the implementation process has been somewhat limited because we only visited the program once, and that was early in the implementation process.

During the Safe Start program's first year of implementation, the therapists all appeared positive about the project and were eager to receive more cases. Even with the low caseloads, they met twice a month, with one of the sessions reserved for external clinical consultation. The therapists viewed the clinical consultation as particularly helpful, because quite a bit of time had passed between their initial CPP training and receiving their first case.

The assigned therapist contacted the family to set up the first appointment within a few days of receiving the case. According to Safe Start program staff, this response time represented an improvement over the wait time for other mental health services, which sometimes spanned several weeks. Nonetheless, the therapists noted that there were a lot of steps in the process before the case reached them. Furthermore, because the therapists would not have had any prior involvement with the Help Me Grow service coordinators or other referral sources, they were often coming into the initial contact and appointment without much contextual information about the family circumstances. This meant that they had to orient themselves to the family's situation during the first appointment.

The therapists reported doing some case management with families who were not actively involved with Help Me Grow either because they came from one of the other referral sources or because some of the referrals from Help Me Grow came from existing caseloads, which included cases that were no longer active with Help Me Grow. Case management typically happened near the beginning of their involvement with the family and reportedly helped to build trust. For families who were actively involved with Help Me Grow, the therapist worked with the service coordinator on the case management issues.

**Table B.14**
**Service Delivery for Enrollees in the Toledo Safe Start Intervention**

| | Year 1 | Year 2 | Year 3 (4 mos) |
|---|---|---|---|
| Average quarterly caseload per therapist | 1 | 1.2 | 2.8 |
| Total number of joint therapy sessions | 18 | 79 | 46 |

According to the therapists, the families appeared excited about the therapy. Once they engaged the family, it was a positive experience, but the therapists felt they had to work hard at the beginning to gain the families' trust. The therapists found that families with a family or community support system already in place were easier to engage, whereas those who did not had more difficulty establishing a trusting relationship with the therapist. The therapists found the younger teenage mothers to be difficult to retain in treatment. They noted that some of the mothers who had left the initial violent relationship later got involved in another unhealthy relationship. Therapists also found that some mothers had multiple stressors, such as severe financial stress, relocation, or reunification with their children's fathers. Because they had often been in longer-term relationships, these mothers had been exposed to more chronic abuse and seemed to be more tired and mentally exhausted.

There were other components of the Toledo Safe Start program that helped shape the implementation (see the box titled "Toledo Safe Start Additional Program Components").

## Toledo Safe Start Additional Program Components

**Quality Assurance.** The site's training efforts included initial clinician training for the project director of the Cullen Center and the Help Me Grow program therapists provided by one of the CPP model developers. The therapists also received "booster" training sessions, had access to materials about the model, and received monthly telephone-based clinical supervision from one of the model developers.

**Training.** Over the course of the first two years of Safe Start, Toledo Safe Start participated in five trainings. Two were focused on child welfare issues, one on domestic violence, and the remaining two focused on clinical interventions. The main training was CPP for the clinicians.

**Policies and Protocols.** Toledo had few new or changed policies during the course of the Safe Start project. However, there was one policy change made in an attempt to increase efficiency and engagement of new enrollees. During the transition to a new project coordinator, the system of case tracking for new referrals was redesigned to improve communication. Through a shared and comprehensive database, the Safe Start support coordinator was able to assist with scheduling, reminders and updates, particularly as follow-up assessments came due. As a result, there have been additional efforts to engage families and increase the number of baseline and follow-up assessments completed.

**Program Outreach.** Toledo's primary outreach efforts were presentations on the Safe Start program that were meant to increase community support and gain referrals. Presentations were given to various county agencies, human services agencies, domestic violence organizations, and other community-based groups with an interest in the project and its goals. In addition to presentations, Toledo also created a brochure to disseminate to potential referral sources that explained the project.

**Resources and Costs.** In the first two years of SSPA, Toledo Safe Start devoted most of its resources for labor costs, particularly salaries for the project manager and a clinical therapist. In addition, the majority of the remaining resources were used for supplies to support the intervention, including therapeutic and clinical assessment tools.

## Summary

Toledo Safe Start selected established therapeutic intervention and trained community-based agency clinicians to deliver the intervention. In doing so, the program aimed to increase the community's capacity to serve young children who witnessed domestic violence. The Safe Start project also integrated domestic violence awareness and assessment into the Help Me Grow curriculum. By making domestic violence part of the curriculum, the service coordinators were able to broach the topic of domestic violence in a systematic way that may have helped women disclose their situations and agree to a referral for services.

Toledo struggled for referrals throughout the project. The Help Me Grow service coordinators did not provide the anticipated level of referrals to Safe Start. Despite the persistent efforts of the Cullen Center program coordinator, the Help Me Grow program's pace of referrals remained very low, for reasons that remain unclear. Even adding three additional referral sources did not substantially increase the number of referrals, again for reasons that remain unclear. Ultimately, Toledo Safe Start's low enrollment numbers meant that it was unable to fully utilize the increased capacity and training to provide an evidence-based intervention to children exposed to domestic violence in their community.

**Data collection for this program summary included:**

- Key informant interviews with key program staff and community partners:
  - Cullen Center agency director and project director
  - Clinical therapists from four treatment sites
  - Help Me Grow service coordinator from one of the referral sites
  - Data collector
  - Brighter Futures director, coordinator, supervisors and nurses
  - Artemis therapist for the KIDS program
  - Cullen Center financial director
- Observation of Help Me Grow service coordinator meeting
- Observation of Safe Start steering committee meeting
- Case review of randomly selected treatment group cases
- Quality assurance checklist completed by the clinical supervisor
- Quarterly activity reports on services, training, policies, and advocacy
- Grant application
- Green Light notes
- *Safe Start: Promising Approaches Communities Working Together to Help Children Exposed to Violence* (Safe Start Center, 2008).

# 15. Washington Heights/Inwood Safe Start Program Description

**Washington Heights/Inwood Safe Start**

- **Intervention types:** Child-Parent Psychotherapy (CPP), Kids' Club and Reflective Functioning Parent Group
- **Intervention length:** CPP: approximately 1 year. Kids' Club and Reflective Functioning Parent Group: 12 weeks
- **Intervention setting:** Outpatient hospital clinic-based services
- **Target population**: Children exposed to domestic violence
- **Age range:** 0–5: Child-Parent Psychotherapy
  6–12: Kids' Club and Reflective Functioning Parent Group
- **Primary referral sources:** Domestic and Other Violence Emergencies (DOVE), Administration for Children's Services (ACS), Mayor's Office to Combat Domestic Violence (OCDV), New York District Attorney's Office of Family Violence and Child Abuse Bureau, CONNECT's Family Violence Prevention Program, Manhattan/Harlem Legal Services, HELP USA, Northern Manhattan Improvement Corporation (NMIC), Columbia Head Start, and medical and social work professionals from New York Presbyterian Hospital

## Program and Community Setting

The Washington Heights/Inwood Safe Start Program, called the Family PEACE (Promoting, Educating, Advocacy, Collaboration, and Empowerment) Program, was designed to provide services to children exposed to domestic violence in the Community District 12 of Northern Manhattan, which consists of the neighborhoods of Washington Heights and Inwood. As of the 2000 Census, the population was almost 209,000, nearly 7 percent of which were children younger than age 5. The population was predominantly Hispanic (74%); 13 percent was white and 8 percent was black. There were very small Asian and Native American populations. In 1999, the median family income was $35,054,[30] approximately 60 percent of the median family income of Manhattan, and 30 percent of the population was living below the poverty line.[31]

High rates of poverty, low educational attainment, high unemployment, and high rates of domestic violence were evident in this community prior to the beginning of the Safe Start program. In 2002, half of Manhattan's reported incidents of domestic violence came from the Washington Heights/Inwood community, with more than 5,000 Domestic Incident Reports filed (New York Presbyterian Hospital, 2004). The Administration for Children's Services (ACS) and New York Presbyterian Hospital both conducted needs assessments and found the issue of domestic violence at the top of the list of priorities for this community. Data from the needs assessment indicated that 5 percent of pediatric primary care patients had been exposed to domestic violence (New York Presbyterian Hospital, 2004). Further, 19 percent of children in the ACS system had a history of exposure to domestic violence (New York Presbyterian Hospital, 2004). This recognition spurred the development of several programs targeting domestic violence prior to the advent of Safe Start, but few of them focused on the well-being of children.

---

[30] This is the 1999 median family income reported in 2005 dollars. In 1999 dollars, the median family income was $29,084.

[31] The information is from the 2000 Census (U.S. Census Bureau, no date).

Thus, the Safe Start collaboration was formed to address this gap, with New York Presbyterian Hospital's Ambulatory Care Network as the lead agency, in partnership with the other key agencies serving the community, including Domestic and Other Violence Emergencies (DOVE), the New York Police Department, the ACS, the Mayor's Office to Combat Domestic Violence, the New York District Attorney's Office of Family Violence and Child Abuse Bureau, CONNECT's Family Violence Prevention Program, Manhattan/Harlem Legal Services, the Dominican Women's Development Center, and the Northern Manhattan Improvement Corporation (NMIC). The Ambulatory Care Network contained a Child Advocacy Center and a Women, Infants, and Children (WIC) Center that is also engaged with the Safe Start program. These referral sources were adjusted over time, as will be described below, and the ultimate partnering agencies are described in the box titled "Washington Heights/Inwood Safe Start Program Partner Agencies."

The Safe Start program set out to create a more coordinated community approach to children exposed to domestic violence by increasing identification and access to interventions and by implementing evidence-based interventions for these children and their mothers. Planned activities toward this goal included outreach efforts with community partners, training sessions, providing resources to law enforcement, developing cross-agency referral protocols, and providing assessments and intervention within the program. The evidence-based programs would include CPP for young children (ages 0–5) and a group-based intervention for older children and their mothers (ages 6–12). Outcomes expected included improved parent-child communication, strengthening of the parent-child bond, reduced isolation, improved coping, and better conflict resolution among older children. The ultimate impacts of the program were expected to be stronger infrastructure for addressing child exposure to domestic violence within the community, a reduction in child internalizing (e.g., sadness, anxiety) and externalizing (e.g., conduct) symptoms, a decrease in mothers' negative outcomes, and a reduction in family violence.

Within the program, children's exposure to domestic violence was defined broadly to include all types of exposure (intervening, being victimized, participating in the violence, seeing or hearing the assault, observing the initial effects, experiencing the aftermath of violence, or overhearing conversations about the assault). Domestic violence was defined more narrowly, however, as a pattern of assaultive and coercive behaviors (physical aggression, psychological abuse, intimidation, threats, controlling behavior, and forced sexual acts) committed against a mother by her current or former partner. In the proposal, families would be excluded if (1) the domestic violence included assault with a deadly weapon or injury of the victim to the point of lost consciousness within the past six months and the partners had not separated or (2) the mother or child were determined to have a serious mental health condition requiring more intensive mental health treatment, although this second criterion was changed somewhat when the program was implemented (as described below).

### Washington Heights/Inwood Safe Start Program Partner Agencies

**New York Presbyterian Hospital's Ambulatory Care Network (ACN):** The ACN is a network of community health centers (within the hospital or stand-alone) that emphasizes preventive health care and promote wellness through health education. It includes 21 primary care and 75 specialty and subspecialty services, including the Family PEACE Program. The ACN was the lead agency for the Washington Heights/Inwood Safe Start project.

**Washington Heights/Inwood Safe Start Program Partner Agencies (continued)**

**Domestic and Other Violence Emergencies (DOVE):** DOVE is part of New York Presbyterian Hospital's Social Work Department and is funded by the New York State and the hospital. It offers to victims of violence crisis intervention and accompaniment during emergency medical treatment, counseling, and support and offers community outreach. This agency provided referrals into the Safe Start project.

**The Mayor's Office to Combat Domestic Violence (OCDV):** OCDV formulates policies and programs, monitors the citywide delivery of domestic violence services, and works with diverse communities to increase awareness of domestic violence. OCDV works closely with community leaders, health care providers, city agencies, and representatives from the criminal justice system to hold batterers accountable and to create solutions that are critical to preventing domestic violence in New York City. This agency provided referrals into the Safe Start project, particularly in the first two years of the project.

**Northern Manhattan Improvement Corporation (NMIC):** NMIC has been providing the poor, mostly immigrant residents of Washington Heights and Inwood (Manhattan Community District 12) with critically needed community development services for nearly 30 years. NMIC's Domestic Violence Project provides holistic, bilingual, and bicultural social and legal services to victims and survivors of domestic violence, the majority of whom are immigrant Latinas. The Domestic Violence Project serves approximately 300 clients per year from more than 20 different countries. This agency provided referrals into the Safe Start project.

**HELP USA:** Founded in 1986, HELP USA is one of the largest builders and operators of service-enriched transitional and low-income permanent housing for homeless populations in the United States. The organization has 19 residential communities in the New York metropolitan area and is expanding to Philadelphia, Las Vegas, Buffalo, Newark, and Houston. Programs and services include jobs, housing, domestic violence, veteran affairs, homeless prevention, case management, youth services, HIV/AID, and more. This agency provided referrals into the Safe Start project, particularly in the later phases.

**Manhattan Legal Services and Harlem Legal Services of Legal Services NYC:** Both of these agencies are part of Legal Services NYC. For more than 40 years, they have provided free civil legal services, such as advice, brief services, and full representation to low-income residents of their respective boroughs. Specifically, they provide assistance in the following areas: tenant advocacy, welfare claims, unemployment hearings, claims against Social Security Administration, victims of domestic violence, people living with AIDS or HIV, and some consumer and employment issues. This agency provided referrals into the Safe Start project, particularly in the later phases.

After the program was selected by OJJDP as one of the 15 Safe Start Promising Approaches program sites, program staff made some changes to the original program design as part of OJJDP's required Green Light process. First, they were concerned about including a control group from the same community for the evaluation component, because they feared that other agencies would not refer families into the program if some families would not receive services. After considering other options, such as recruiting a control group from a different community, they ultimately decided on the six-month wait-list design, which would allow them to offer services to all eligible families, though on different timelines.

In addition, they planned to augment the control group during the waiting period by offering limited case management for urgent matters and a drop-in weekly support group during the waiting period. During implementation, these services were expanded somewhat, as will be discussed below. The Green Light planning period was seen as necessary, but it took longer than was hoped for by the site, since community partners were eager to start making referrals and program staff were eager to begin serving clients.

## Intervention

All families referred to Safe Start received an intake interview to assess for biological, social, and psychological functioning as well as eligibility for the program, safety, and need for intervention. The Safe Start intervention model included two main components: CPP for children ages 0–5, and Kids' Club Group and concurrent Reflective Functioning Parent Group for children ages 6–12. The intervention period lasted approximately one year for CPP and 12 weeks for the kid and parent groups. All services were provided by Safe Start staff at the Charles B. Rangel Community Health Center of New York Presbyterian Hospital, one of the hospital's community health clinics. Since individuals in the community were 90–95 percent Spanish speakers, intervention staff were bilingual and intervention services were offered in either English or Spanish.

### Child-Parent Psychotherapy

CPP is a relationship-based intervention designed for use with children up to age 6. It can be used with any child whose relationship to their parent or other primary caregiver is impacted by negative circumstances, including family violence. CPP integrates psychodynamic, attachment, trauma, cognitive-behavioral, and social learning theories (NCTSN, 2008). There are two components in CPP: assessment and treatment, with information gained during the assessment used to inform the treatment component. In the intervention component, child-parent interactions are the focus of six intervention modalities aimed at restoring a sense of mastery, security, and growth and promoting congruence between bodily sensations, feelings, and thinking on the part of both child and parent and in their relationship with one another (NCTSN, 2008).

For children ages 0–5, the therapy was planned to be held weekly for 52 weeks (one hour per session), and families would be considered to have completed treatment if they attended at least 25 sessions in total and/or the treatment goals were met. Therapy could be extended beyond 52 weeks if clinically indicated.

### Kids' Club

This group treatment for children exposed to domestic violence was designed to reduce its impact on children as well as to reduce the risk of repeated violence. The program was developed in 1992 by Sandra Graham-Bermann and includes 10 group sessions based on three theoretical frameworks: social learning theory, attachment theory, and trauma theory (Graham-Bermann, 2000). The sessions targeted children's knowledge about domestic violence; their attitudes and beliefs about families, relationships, and family violence; their emotional adjustment; and their social behavior. Safe Start program staff had permission to use the program and to train others in its use, and they made a few modifications to the program. They extended it to 12 sessions, adding content on body reactions to events (e.g., how the body feels when emotions are experienced, such as headaches and stomach aches) and content on coping skills, including safety skills, in relation to domestic violence. In addition, they reduced content related to gender that was in the original manual, feeling that this content was too abstract and didn't work well with the younger children. Instead, they included issues of gender throughout the program. They documented these changes in an updated manual used within the program.

In the Safe Start program, Kids' Club was offered for children ages 6–12. Groups were planned separately for children ages 6–7 and those ages 8–12. For families with more than one child in this age range, all were invited to attend. The Kids' Club sessions were planned to take place once per week for 90 minutes over 12 weeks. Successful completion of the program was defined as attendance of nine or more sessions. In addition, for some children ages 13–16, a different 12-week psycho-educational group was provided. Mainly, these were siblings of target children who received Kids' Club, but in one case was a control target child who aged out of Kids' Club. This group focused on developing healthy relationships.

#### Reflective Functioning Parent Group

While children attended the Kids' Club, their mothers attended the Reflective Functioning Parent Group. A commitment to attendance of both kids and parents was a prerequisite for these groups. While children or parents may have missed one or two sessions for reasons such as illness, overall the kids and parents met concurrently. The meetings were held at the same time, on the same schedule, also consisting of 12 weekly 90-minute sessions. This model, designed by John Grienenberger, is designed to provide a step-by-step method for enhancing the parent-child attachment relationship in the context of specific parenting issues (Grienenberger et al., 2005; Slade, 2006). A combination of didactic information and activities, its primary goal was to help parents understand and respect their children's own independence and point of view, and guide parents to understand their children's behavior as a response to underlying feelings, thoughts, and attitudes. Parents were taught how to consider the child's perspective or "be in his shoes" in interpreting and reacting to things related to domestic violence, such as witnessing the violence itself, having visits from the father, and so forth. This understanding was intended to then help guide the parent's response to the child's behavior. The group goals were tailored to better fit the domestic violence context, using examples from domestic violence situations, so that the mothers in the group would share their personal stories, discuss their own children's exposure to domestic violence, and attempt to understand the child's feelings and relationship to the other parent. The groups also sought to teach parents to attend to safety for themselves and their children to enhance the child's sense of safety.

The intervention was conducted in the context of a rigorous evaluation as required by the funder (see the box titled "Washington Heights/Inwood Safe Start Evaluation" for a description).

### Washington Heights/Inwood Safe Start Evaluation

**Design.** This was planned as a randomized control effectiveness trial with a six-month wait-list control group, focused on child outcomes. However, services within the randomization were not always implemented as planned.

**Treatment versus control group services.** The treatment group received CPP (ages 0–5) or Kids' Club/Reflective Functioning Parent Groups (ages 6–12), as well as case management, individual treatment, and family sessions according to need. Control group families could attend drop-in

**Washington Heights/Inwood Safe Start Evaluation (continued)**

support groups during the waiting period of six months and were also offered other services, such as case management, individual treatment, and family sessions according to need. During implementation, the waiting period was not always adhered to, so some children received intervention services during the six-month waiting period even though they were assigned to the control group.

**Data collection.** Data were collected through longitudinal assessments of child-level outcomes.

**Enrollment.** The site originally planned to serve 240 families over the four-year period (120 in each age group). Funding for the National Evaluation ended prematurely. By the time it ended, enrollment had taken place over two years and nine months and resulted in 62 assigned to the treatment group and 54 assigned to the control group.

### Implementation

Figure B.15 shows the Family PEACE Program's implementation of its intervention. The following description of the program implementation is the result of data collected for the national evaluation. See Appendix A for a full discussion of the data collection methodology employed at each of the Safe Start sites.

### Referrals

As planned in the proposal for this project, several community agencies referred children exposed to domestic violence to the Washington Heights/Inwood Safe Start Program. These included ACS, domestic violence shelters, pediatricians and psychologists within

**Figure B.15**
**Model of Washington Heights/Inwood Safe Start Program**

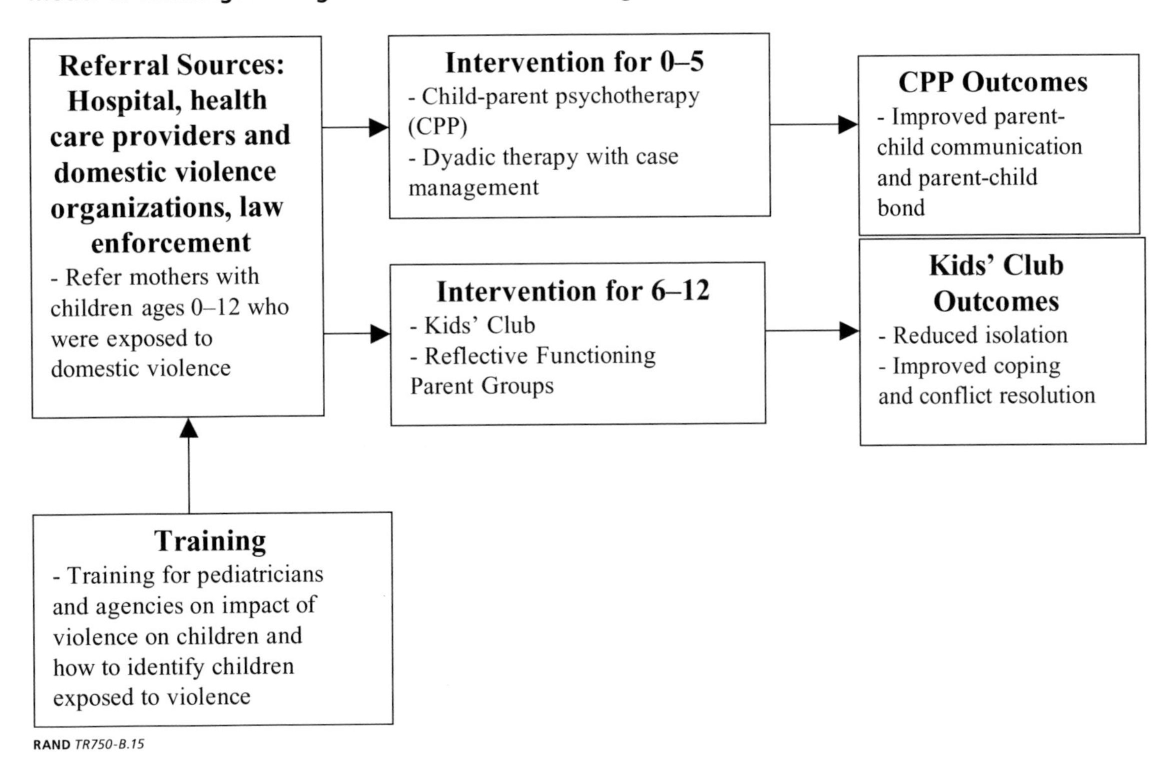


RAND *TR750-B.15*

the Ambulatory Care Network as well as outside of the hospital, NMIC, local Head Start programs, DOVE, infant mental health specialists, and social workers at legal advocacy agencies. The program staff reported that part of the success in gaining referrals was due to the partnerships existing prior to funding of the Safe Start program and levels of trust established with the community by specific program staff members who were leading this specialty program within the Ambulatory Care Network. The Safe Start program maintained regular involvement in the Northern Manhattan Coalition Against Domestic Violence, which made monthly contact with the referring partner agencies to maintain the flow of referrals as well as training opportunities.

One exception to this successful recruitment was that the New York Police Department did not refer as many families as expected. The original plan had been to train police officers on how to respond to domestic violence incidents when children were present and about the Safe Start program, so that they could refer the family directly to the Safe Start program. However, any police officer in a patrol unit might respond to 911 calls related to domestic violence, not just those who were in the specialized domestic violence unit. Whereas the staff were able to conduct trainings with the domestic violence specialty units, it was much harder to reach the larger number of police officers who might respond to a call, given different shifts and competing priorities. In addition, police officers who were trained were more likely to refer families to a domestic violence agency such as the Northern Manhattan Improvement Corporation than to Safe Start directly. The police department was reportedly working on training more of its officers. These training efforts had not yet been completed when the Safe Start program was being implemented. However, many families referred by domestic violence partners were involved with the police, indicating that referrals were coming to them through the domestic violence agencies as an intermediate step.

The program also saw opportunities to continue expansion to other referral sources, such as an agency that worked with clergy within the community, but had not solidified that relationship during the first two years of implementation. However, in the third year of implementation, the program began to receive steady referrals from two agencies, Help USA and Manhattan Legal Services/Harlem Legal Services. In addition, the program received referrals from the Child Advocacy Center.

The site modified its criteria for admission to the program slightly, to focus on safety and potential need for more intensive mental health services rather than specific forms of violence exposure. The family was provided with a referral to an appropriate service provider that could address their needs. For instance, a psychiatrist on staff and co-located with the program one day per week was able to conduct a psychiatric evaluation of the mother and/or the child on an as-needed basis, and either refer them to services or recommend that they continue with the Safe Start program. One reported challenge was the high level of need that some families had upon referral. In addition to concerns about the child, women were entering with ongoing domestic violence and safety issues, as well as mental health issues. Thus, program staff had the sense that some referrals were being made for case management services rather than child mental health. These issues led to some changes in policies within the program, such as requiring women in unsafe relationships to also have a domestic violence advocate outside of the Safe Start Program and ensuring that mental health problems were stabilized prior to beginning the intervention. This allowed the program to focus on the planned intervention, while still ensuring that the families' other needs were met.

Thus, in general, the program received referrals as planned from local shelters and community partners, and this success created the challenge of ensuring adequate capacity to serve the many families in need.

### Services

Table B.15 summarizes service delivery for those who received services through the Washington Heights/Inwood Safe Start program during the first three years of implementation (through March 2009). New York started with one psychologist and two social workers and increased to two psychologists and two social workers by the end of the second year of implementation in June of 2008, in order to meet the demand for treatment. During the third year of the program (through March 2009), program staff included two to three psychologists and one to two social workers.

After referral, each family was assessed at the beginning of the project for eligibility, safety, and appropriateness of services, and families were enrolled as patients in the hospital's Ambulatory Care Network. At this stage, the mother was asked to identify the child she was most concerned about. If that child was in the 0–5 age range, the family assigned to the intervention was offered CPP (and randomized to the immediate treatment or delayed intervention control group). Older siblings were also allowed to participate in Kids' Club if desired. If the mother identified a child in the 6–12 age range as the one she was most concerned about, the child and mother were assigned to the group treatments (Kids' Club and Reflective Functioning Parent Group) and randomized to receive those services immediately or in six months. Because more than one child per family could be treated at a time via the Kids' Club, the intervention could include just the mother and one child, or the mother and multiple children. Some older siblings of children in the control group, and one control target child who aged out of Kid's Club, attended a different psycho-educational group for teens. At the outset of the project, the plan was for families assigned to the control group to wait six months for the intervention to begin, and to be invited to attend drop-in support groups to obtain case management during that time. However, in reality, children in the control group were occasionally offered, and took part in, more intensive services, including CPP, Kids' Club, and individual therapy by intervention staff. If the mother was worried about all children or did not choose one child she was most concerned about, the youngest child was chosen as the target child for intervention services.

Program staff appeared to struggle to find appropriate ways to balance the many basic needs of the families across their caseloads and found that families needed to link with domestic violence advocates to handle domestic violence issues so that they could focus on the child's mental health as planned. Program staff reported having a sense that the families occasionally

**Table B.15**
**Service Delivery for Enrollees in the Washington Heights/Inwood Safe Start Intervention**

| | Year 1 | Year 2 | Year 3 (9 months) |
|---|---|---|---|
| Average quarterly caseload per therapist | 3.8 | 3.6 | 3.7 |
| Average quarterly caseload per social worker | 6.8 | 4.2 | 9.3 |
| Total number of CPP sessions | 174 | 351 | 264 |
| Total number of child group therapy sessions | 27 | 44 | 25 |
| Total number of parent group therapy sessions | 27 | 44 | 35 |

stopped coming to the program when their immediate needs were met, rather than finishing the therapy or group; in some cases, they would return to the program again when there was a new problem. Thus, some families may have been using the Safe Start Program more as a means to obtain case management for help with meeting their basic needs than as a specialty service for child mental health.

Staffing changes also may have contributed to the inconsistencies between the plan for the project and its actual implementation. Staff turnover (social work clinician, social work intake coordinator, psychologist) was an issue. The program relied to some degree on graduate interns and research assistants to help with program logistics (such as intake assessments), and those staff turn over yearly or biyearly. The project director was on leave for a portion of the project and the principal investigator left his position and was replaced, creating other challenges in continuity of operations and training.

#### *Child-Parent Psychotherapy*

Following training by one of the model developers (Van Horn) in May of 2006, the primary Safe Start therapist began to implement CPP within the program, supported by an on-site supervisor who had previously been trained and had several years of experience with CPP. Before therapy could begin, there were challenges in helping families solve real-life problems, such as safety from domestic violence and housing issues. Although case management is part of the CPP model, in some cases the intake coordinator provided crisis intervention before services started. Once therapy began, the families still faced multiple issues. Mothers reportedly wanted help with their children's behavior, but also had problems with literacy, housing, mental health, and other needs. Thus, the therapists tried to address both child mental health and other issues in the therapy sessions. The therapist worked with each family on a case-by-case basis to ensure that the family's basic needs were being met while also addressing their therapeutic needs in session.

#### *Kids' Club*

The Safe Start project director had been trained in Kids' Club and had received permission from Graham-Bermann to train others. The program included siblings of the outcome evaluation's targeted child in these groups, whether this identified target child was in therapy or the Kids' Club. There were generally about seven children in each group, with one or two groups running concurrently in the late afternoon after school. Implementation challenges included families coming late to the groups or missing groups, particularly during holidays. Program staff said this was particularly true when school was out, and that some families came to groups about twice per month on average rather than once a week.

#### *Reflective Functioning Parent Groups*

The parent groups ran on the same schedule as the Kids' Club, with two groups running with about four mothers in each (one English group and one Spanish group). The developer of this model gave permission for the use of the program but did not formally train staff on the project at the outset of the project. The program used the model's standard curriculum, but in a more flexible way to accommodate the mothers' needs. The mental health director created a curriculum that incorporated domestic violence and trained others to implement the model. The group sessions allowed time to discuss difficulties the mothers were currently facing, for support to be offered and received among group members, and to discuss particular incidents with their children. Challenges in implementation were similar to those in the Kids' Club—with parents missing groups or coming late. In the third year of the project, formal training in the model did occur.

There were other components of the Safe Start Program that helped shape the implementation (see the box titled "Washington Heights/Inwood Safe Start Additional Program Components").

### Washington Heights/Inwood Safe Start Additional Program Components

**Quality Assurance.** Therapists and staff running the groups were trained in the intervention practices at the beginning of the project. For CPP, the therapists were trained by the developer. Individual and group supervision was provided by an on-site supervisor who had prior training and experience in delivering this model and later augmented by consultation with the developer as needed. Some supervision was conducted jointly with the Bronx Safe Start site three times per month. Additionally, the program participated in a National Learning Collaborative provided by the developers of the intervention. For Kids' Club, the program manager had prior experience with this model and conducted the training and supervision for the staff running the groups. For the Reflective Functioning Parent Groups, the mental health director provided training for staff using a curriculum that incorporated domestic violence and reflective functioning. The program manager was trained by Grienenberger in the third year of the project.

**Training.** Over the course of the first two years, the Washington Heights/Inwood program conducted and/or participated in 81 trainings, which were mostly focused on domestic violence issues (61%), followed by clinical services (12%) and child welfare–focused sessions (7%). Topics for training included the criminal justice issues concerning domestic violence perpetrators, addressing domestic violence in a pediatric setting, and PCC.

**Policies and Protocols.** Washington Heights/Inwood's policies and protocols mainly focused on establishing the protocols for referrals, assessments, and intake procedures as well as adjusting those protocols for changes in staffing and to improve procedures. For example, the site adjusted the intake protocol to improve the accuracy of reporting services and improve the quality of care provided; documented family visits in order to better track services being provided; and recommended that in addition to taking part in Family PEACE services, women work with a domestic violence advocacy agency to help them take steps toward legally distancing themselves from their batterer.

**Program Outreach.** The site's advocacy and outreach efforts consisted of two meetings to obtain funding to expand and improve the Safe Start Program. Safe Start staff met with a foundation for funding to better link Safe Start with day care centers, preschools, and Head Start and to fund a part-time psychologist to provide CPP. The site also met with another funder for funding to expand services to teenagers ages 13–18.

**Resources and Costs.** Washington Heights/Inwood Safe Start did not provide information about program resources or costs for the purposes of our cost analysis.

## Summary

The Safe Start Program delivered a combination of services designed for mothers and their children who were exposed to domestic violence, which primarily included CPP, Kids' Club, and Reflective Functioning Parent Groups. The program received many referrals from community partners and from within their own hospital system, making it possible to enroll families relatively easily. The large private hospital is located in a high-need community and strives to maintain solid relationships with the community. Whereas some program staff believed there were some hurdles relating to families feeling distrustful of the hospital, particularly in relation to disclosure of violence, others disagreed and felt the hospital provided a safe way for domestic violence victims to seek help with the stigma of going to a social service agency.

Program staff also reported struggling with some families that were referred to them in a high degree of stress and in need of multiple services in addition to the child mental health program. Indeed, program staff found that they needed to spend much more time than anticipated assisting families in times of stress and with related domestic violence case management issues. This was true for families in both the immediate treatment and the delayed intervention control groups. Thus, some children in the control group received services during the six-month waiting period and, overall, children and families were provided additional services based on overwhelming need. Over time, the program also instituted new policies to help mothers to be involved with a domestic violence advocate in another program, to allow the Safe Start Program to focus more on child mental health.

The heavier-than-anticipated workload required hiring of additional staff, some of whom were graduate interns, and therefore continual training was needed and staff operated under heavy supervision loads. Staff reported that families felt at home at the Safe Start Program, but attended the program intervention services more regularly in times of crisis than in times of stability. Thus, families occasionally stopped coming to services once their life circumstances were stabilized, but before all treatment goals had been met.

**Data collection for this program summary included:**

- Key informant interviews with key program staff and community partners:
  - Project director and mental health director
  - Therapists, social work interns
  - Chief Medical Officer of the Ambulatory Care Network
  - Data collectors
- Case review of randomly selected treatment and control group cases
- Quality assurance checklist completed by the clinical supervisor
- Quarterly activity reports on services, training, policies, and advocacy
- Grant application
- Green Light notes
- *Safe Start: Promising Approaches Communities Working Together to Help Children Exposed to Violence* (Safe Start Center, 2008).

APPENDIX C

# SSPA Training Evaluation

## Contents

## 1. Training Evaluation Overview

The SSPA sites conducted or participated in several trainings related to improving awareness, knowledge, and practice for children exposed to violence and working with families to address these issues. In order to describe and track the impact of these trainings, the national Safe Start evaluation included a component to assess whether and how some of these trainings changed program staff perspectives in working with these children. In particular, the evaluation examined program staff *knowledge* of how to work with children who are experiencing trauma or other mental heath difficulties as a result of witnessing domestic, family, or community violence. The evaluation also explored the extent to which these trainings changed staff *perspectives* on the needs of children and increased awareness about best practices and community resources to aid families.

There were two components to the training evaluation. First, we evaluated a select number of trainings for which we were able to obtain the planned training materials in advance, develop a survey, and survey the participants before and immediately after the training and three months later. Second, we conducted short interviews of training participants to obtain their perspectives on the sessions. We include exemplar quotes from these participant interviews throughout this appendix where appropriate. The training evaluation components and methods are described further in Appendix A.

In conducting the training evaluation, we attempted to capture trainings across sites within the first two years of Safe Start, to the extent that sites were willing to participate in this part of the evaluation and could participate in the planning necessary to carry it out. We worked with trainers and their training materials to develop surveys collaboratively to ensure that survey content was appropriate to the planned training curriculum. While most training opportunities were site-specific and tailored to the needs of that program, all sites participated in the Safe Start Center–funded training on engaging families in mental health services.

In the next section, we summarize findings from the engaging families training conducted with each site. Then, we describe the content of site-specific trainings; provide site-specific data on participant characteristics and changes in knowledge and perspectives where appropriate; and briefly summarize pooled data across sites, with attention to changes in attitudes and practice in working with children exposed to violence.

It should be noted that some sites started training sessions that were not fully completed; thus, we only have three-month follow-up surveys on a subset of trainings (further described in the next sections). Further, we provided gift card incentives to improve trainee retention at follow-up; however, in some cases, our retention rates were low. The retention issues, coupled with generally small sample sizes, precluded tests of statistical significance, but we report trends that highlight changes in knowledge and attitudes over time.

## 2. All-Site Engagement Training

As described earlier, the training for staff on strategies for engaging families in mental health services ("engagement training") was sponsored by the Safe Start Center and conducted individually with all Safe Start program sites. The evaluation of this training effort sought to track the knowledge gained from this training and to determine how staff practices changed with respect to recruiting and retaining families in the Safe Start programs.

### Overview of Training Content

The goal of the engagement training was to improve the recruitment and retention of families in the Safe Start services. The Providence Safe Start program was the first to participate in the training, led by Mary McKay and Richard Hibbert (two experts in engaging families in mental health services), and the other 14 sites followed with financial support from the Safe Start Center (13 are included in this evaluation). All trainings were conducted by Mary McKay or Richard Hibbert. Each of the Safe Start sites had some challenges with involving their families in their interventions, particularly over the course of treatment, and this training focused on various strategies to overcome barriers to engagement. These barriers included logistical obstacles (e.g., time, transportation, money) and perceptual barriers (e.g., negative attitudes about mental health services).

The engagement training included several sections related to telephone-based strategies to improve engagement and active problem-solving with the family. The staff participants were led through a telephone engagement intervention, a process that was designed to start during the first telephone contact. This contact focused on clarification with the caregiver/parent regarding the need for mental health services to increase caregiver investment and self-efficacy as it relates to ability to seek and obtain services. The telephone engagement training also instructed trainees to include questions such as "What could stand in the way of getting to the appointment?" and "How hopeful do you feel that this treatment will help?"

The engagement training also covered four elements to the engagement process:

1. Participants were instructed on how to explain how mental health services works and the process of intervention participation for the client. This included clarifying expectations about the intake process and services.
2. Participants were instructed about how to develop the foundation for a collaborative working relationship with a client by balancing the need to obtain intake data with the opportunity for families to share their personal narratives, thus fostering trust.
3. A focus on immediate and practical concerns was emphasized. This mainly centered on helping parents to negotiate other system barriers and working to schedule a second appointment as early as possible rather than waiting for long lag times between appointments.
4. Problem-solving about barriers was a cornerstone of the training. This included discussion of an "obstacle checklist" and strategizing with a parent or caregiver on how to overcome each obstacle to ongoing participation.

## Survey Results

### Participant Characteristics

For the engagement training evaluation, data from 14 of the 15 sites were included (we were unable to evaluate the training at the 15th site because of logistical difficulties). Because this training was standard across the sites, we present the results for all the sites combined rather than individual site results. Across the 14 sites, 231 participants attended the engagement training and completed at least the baseline (pre-training) survey. As discussed above, two post-training follow-up surveys were conducted, one immediately at the conclusion of the training and one three months after the training. Of the 231 participants who completed the pre-training survey, 220 (95%) completed the first post-training survey and 92 (40%) completed the follow-up survey three months later. The 40 percent retention rate at the follow-up was not ideal; the rate was low despite a number of attempts to contact participants and use of the bookstore gift card incentive.

Figure C.1 summarizes the occupation of the baseline survey participants. Most participants were social workers (23%) or clinical social workers (16%). Over half of the participants had a master's degree (51%), and 16 percent had a master's degree in social work.

The participants had a range of experience in therapeutic approaches and case management. Approximately 46 percent had conducted individual therapy with parents, 48 percent had joint parent-child therapy experience, and 74 percent had experience with case management or family advocacy. Further, most participants had at least some experience working with children (69% with preschool, 70% with elementary age, 71% with middle school, 74% with high school age youth) and 79% with adults.

### Pre-Training Experience

Prior to the engagement training, we queried participants about their experience recruiting and engaging families and their understanding of strategies to better retain families in mental health services. On the pre-training survey, 30 percent of participants reported knowing a

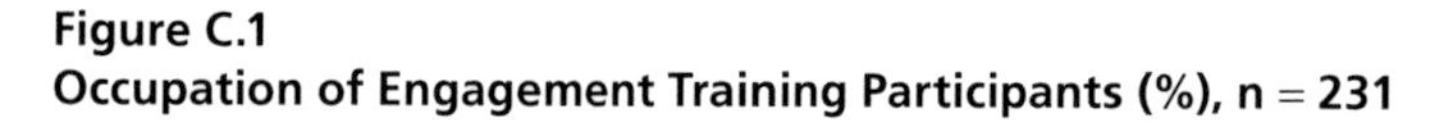

**Figure C.1**
**Occupation of Engagement Training Participants (%), n = 231**

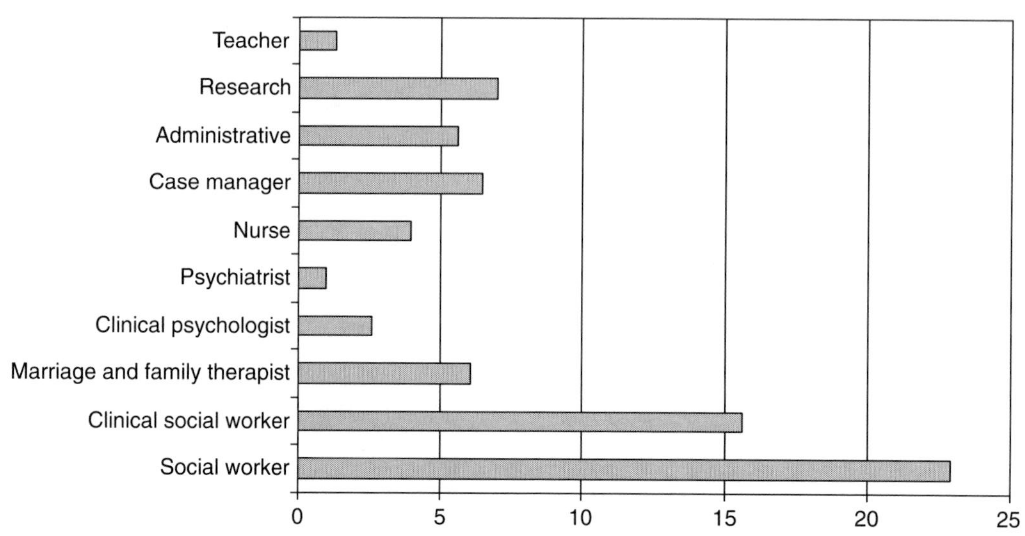


RAND *TR750-C.1*

great deal about engaging families in mental health services, and over half (51%) reported using engagement strategies to involve families in their services.

### Changes in Knowledge

We asked participants to answer a series of true/false questions about family engagement strategies. Pre-post change in knowledge by item is summarized in Table C.1. This table presents data only for the 220 participants who completed both the pre- and the post-training survey. In general, knowledge increased directly after the assessment, except for one item: "Each intake call should be treated as a crisis."

Since a much smaller sample completed all three waves of the survey, we present the results for these 92 individuals separately. Among those completing a follow-up assessment, knowledge remained generally unchanged from the post-training test but did not markedly improve (Table C.2).

**Table C.1**
**Changes in Engagement Training Knowledge, for Pre- and Post-Training Only (n = 220)**

| | % Correct | |
|---|---|---|
| Item | Pre | Post |
| Common perceptual barriers for families are intelligence and mental health stigma. (False) | 19 | 23 |
| Common concrete barriers for families are fear, time, and money. (False; fear is not a *concrete* barrier) | 3 | 8 |
| Concrete barriers keep more families from engaging in mental health treatment than perceptual barriers. (False) | 34 | 53 |
| The goals of telephone engagement include clarifying the need for mental health care and verifying insurance coverage. (False) | 43 | 61 |
| During the first phone contact, you should avoid asking things that might upset the parent. (False) | 27 | 48 |
| Each intake call should be treated as crisis. (False) | 36 | 26 |
| Defining the concern helps to clarify the need for mental health care. (True) | 89 | 97 |
| Increasing caregiver investment and efficacy involves asking parents to sign a treatment contract. (False) | 23 | 48 |
| Problem solving is essential to engaging families. (True) | 86 | 97 |

**Table C.2**
**Changes in Engagement Training Knowledge, for All Three Waves (n = 92)**

| | % Correct | | |
|---|---|---|---|
| Item | Pre | Post | Follow-up |
| Common perceptual barriers for families are intelligence and mental health stigma. (False) | 23 | 23 | 32 |
| Common concrete barriers for families are fear, time, and money. (False; fear is not a *concrete* barrier) | 8 | 8 | 3 |
| Concrete barriers keep more families from engaging in mental health treatment than perceptual barriers. (False) | 46 | 54 | 54 |
| The goals of telephone engagement include clarifying the need for mental health care and verifying insurance coverage. (False) | 54 | 54 | 54 |
| During the first phone contact, you should avoid asking things that might upset the parent. (False) | 43 | 45 | 43 |
| Each intake call should be treated as crisis. (False) | 38 | 38 | 32 |
| Defining the concern helps to clarify the need for mental health care. (True) | 92 | 97 | 97 |
| Increasing caregiver investment and efficacy involves asking parents to sign a treatment contract. (False) | 22 | 33 | 22 |
| Problem solving is essential to engaging families. (True) | 97 | 97 | 96 |

**Table C.3**
**Change in Average Knowledge, by Occupation, Among Individuals Completing All Three Survey Waves (n = 92)**

| Occupation | Average Number Correct | | |
|---|---|---|---|
| | Pre | Post | Follow-up |
| Social worker (master's-level social worker or licensed clinical social worker) | 3.5 | 4.7 | 4.3 |
| Other clinician (e.g., psychologist) | 4.1 | 4.6 | 4.2 |
| Other | 3.6 | 4.5 | 4.2 |

We also analyzed how much knowledge changed over time among those who completed all three waves of the survey (n = 92), with attention to differences by occupation: master's-level social worker or licensed clinical social worker, other clinician (e.g., psychologist), or other participants (including administrative staff) (Table C.3). We organized analyses by these occupations because of the unique roles and approaches to using the training content that may be employed by social workers (e.g., as part of case management) and clinicians (e.g., in treatment), compared with other staff, such as administrative staff (e.g., phone calls for appointments). Overall, participants responded correctly to less than half of the items prior to the training, but this knowledge improved at the immediate post-training assessment. Clinicians scored higher before the training, but their knowledge matched the other participants at the post-training and follow-up time points. Across all occupations, knowledge slightly declined at the three-month follow-up survey from what it was immediately after the training. Differences in mean knowledge by occupation were not statistically significant.

In addition to conducting an objective assessment of knowledge, we also examined whether participants felt that their understanding of how to engage families in mental health service improved over time. In this case, reported knowledge increased immediately post-training, but was tempered at the three-month follow-up. Figure C.2 provides an aggregate assessment of reported knowledge change over time among those who completed all three survey waves. As noted, three-month follow-up knowledge decreased for all occupations, but the relative decrease in the percentage of social workers who felt they had a great deal of knowledge about engaging families from before the training to three months after (39% pre-training to 79% post to 46% at follow-up) was much greater than other clinicians who generally reported similar levels of knowledge at follow-up ($p < 0.05$).

### Changes in Attitude and Reported Practice

We queried participants about their *comfort level* in their ability to use engagement strategies and their *actual use* of the engagement strategies in working with families. Figure C.3 summarizes how respondents perceived their ability to engage families in mental health services as a result of the training. Prior to the training, clinicians (26%) and social workers (24%) reported more ability than social workers and administrative and other staff (12%) ($p < 0.05$) to engage families in services. At follow-up, clinicians still reported more ability to engage families, while administrative and other staff continued to report the least comfort with these strategies. All respondents reported an increase in ability immediately after the training. While the perceived ability level had dropped at follow-up, particularly for social workers (49% at follow-up versus 72% for clinicians and 39% for other staff, $p < 0.05$), it was still greater than baseline levels.

We also assessed the use of engagement strategies by occupation type. Prior to the training, approximately 40 percent of administrative and other staff reported using the engagement

**Figure C.2**
**Participants Reporting "a Great Deal of Knowledge" About Engagement Strategies, by Occupation (n = 92)**

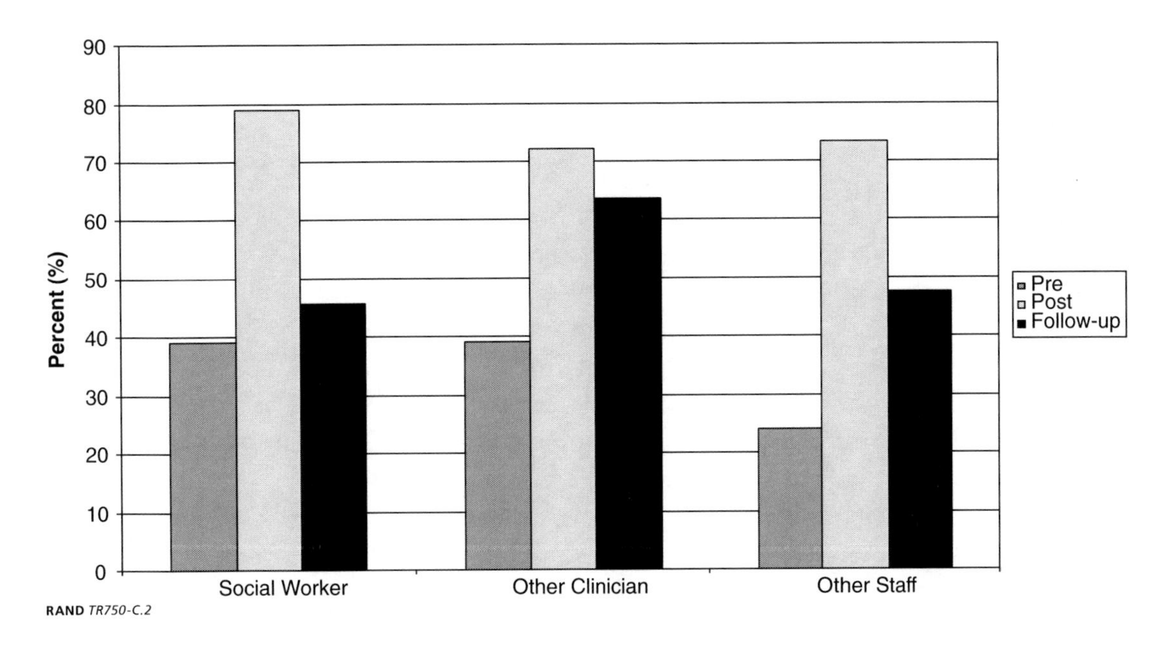


RAND *TR750-C.2*

**Figure C.3**
**Participants Reporting "a Great Deal" of Comfort/Ability to Engage Families in Services, by Occupation (n = 92)**

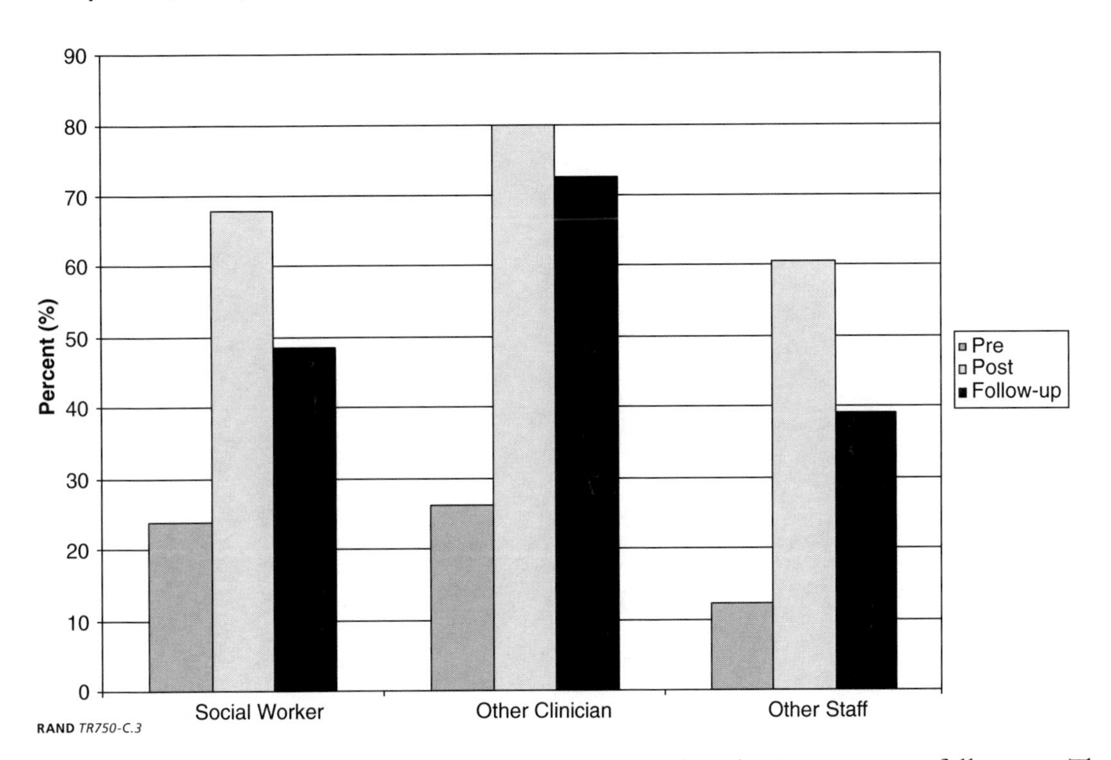


RAND *TR750-C.3*

strategies that were the focus of the training, compared with 60 percent at follow-up. The impact of the training was less pronounced among social workers and clinicians. This would be expected, as the latter two groups were more likely to have been trained and had more opportunity to use these sorts of strategies in the course of their work, relative to other staff such as administrative workers. About 60 to 70 percent of these participants who completed the follow-up survey reported using the engagement strategies in most encounters with clients.

## Perspectives on Training

A random sample of ten training participants from 14 sites was contacted and asked to participate in a semi-structured interview regarding the training content. The semi-structure interview protocol contained questions about the participants' satisfaction with training, their suggestions for improvement of the training, and how they had used the training content in their work since participating in the engagement training. Overall, the respondents indicated that the training was useful. The main criticisms arose from participants who worked in nontraditional, nonclinical settings and the difficulty applying the strategies in those contexts. Many participants described how they had used the content of the training in their work, primarily related to problem-solving with families to overcome logistical barriers. For instance, training participants reported that they learned how to use more flexible scheduling around family needs and to have better understanding of the socioeconomic and cultural factors that may drive family decisionmaking about mental health services. As one participant shared,

> At the end of each session, I process the client's feelings and experience of that session. I take more time on the phone with my clients. I call to remind my clients about their appointments at least the day before.

## 3. Site-Specific Trainings

In addition to the engagement training that took place at all sites, each site undertook its own series of trainings based on their own local needs and interests. These individual site trainings varied in scope and length and were focused on such issues as educating staff and community partners about working with children and families exposed to violence, improving community services and service coordination for families, and increasing capacity for how to treat children exposed to violence using evidence-based interventions.

In order to assess the impact of these training sessions on staff awareness, attitudes, and reported practice, we surveyed participants before and after the trainings using a core set of items that we could employ uniformly across all site training sessions, regardless of the specific topic. In addition, we created unique knowledge items tailored to the content of each site's specific training. Where possible, we conducted brief interviews with a sample of participants from selected training sessions to obtain more qualitative perspectives on training content. As described earlier, we do not have follow-up surveys on all participants, due to retention issues, or for all trainings sessions, because the sites' plans for their training sessions sometimes changed too rapidly for inclusion.

In the remainder of this section, we describe the content of each site-specific training opportunity. We also include information on the change in knowledge scores for each site-specific session, for which we at least have pre-post data. Finally, we provide pooled data on changes in attitudes and comfort in working with children exposed to violence across all site trainings.

### Chelsea: Attachment, Self-Regulation, and Competency (ARC) Framework

One of the key components of the Chelsea Safe Start program was use of the Attachment, Self-Regulation, and Competency (ARC) framework, which guides mental health intervention for traumatized youth (Kinniburgh et al., 2005). ARC is a translation of clinical principles that focuses on three domains (attachment, regulation, competence). The ARC framework includes key concepts, a therapist "toolbox" (e.g., in-session implementation tools), and information about developmental and system considerations in real-world therapy (Kinniburgh et al., 2005). The goal of the **attachment** domain is to focus on attachment as a dyadic process between parent and child (i.e., the connection between the two). The goal of the **self-regulation** domain is to work with children to build ways to identify (e.g., feeling faces, use of stories), modulate (e.g., breathing, muscle relaxation), and share emotional experiences safely (e.g., initiating communication, self-expression). The third domain is **competency**, and the goal of this area is to build skills for ongoing resilience.

#### Participant Characteristics

In the initial training session, 14 staff participants completed pre- and post-surveys, with 11 of them completing surveys at the three-month follow-up. Three of the participants at baseline were social workers, six were clinical social workers, and the rest were clinical (psychology, social work) interns. Approximately 65 percent reported having experience with individual child therapy, group child therapy experience, and joint therapy. Most of the sample (79%) had worked with children of all age ranges (elementary, middle, and high school). The training itself was delivered by an outside consultant who had developed the framework.

**Table C.4**
**Pre-Post and Follow-Up Knowledge from the ARC Training (n = 11)**

| Item | % Correct | | |
|---|---|---|---|
| | Pre | Post | Follow-up |
| One of the building blocks of the ARC framework is affect modulation. (True) | 87 | 92 | 100 |
| One example of up-regulation is progressive muscle relaxation. (False) | 7 | 62 | 91 |
| One intervention to help caregivers with consistent responding is behavioral parent training. (True) | 57 | 88 | 92 |
| Trauma is associated with chaos and a lack of predictability. (True) | 100 | 100 | 100 |
| Tools in a feeling toolbox are generally interchangeable. (False) | 29 | 29 | 55 |
| A goal for caregiver attunement skills is to build the caregiver's ability to support child self-regulation skills. (True) | 100 | 86 | 100 |
| A goal of affect expression is to support children in learning to effectively share emotional experience with others in order to meet emotional or practical needs. (True) | 100 | 93 | 100 |
| One principle of competency is to build child executive function skills. (True) | 64 | 93 | 100 |

### Changes in Knowledge

On the baseline survey, 21 percent reported any knowledge (on a scale of no knowledge to a little, some, or a great deal) of the ARC framework before the training, and by the three-month follow-up, nearly 43 percent of the 11 participants reported a great deal of knowledge about the ARC framework. Table C.4 summarizes change in knowledge on questions related to the ARC training, among those who completed all three surveys (n = 11). In general, knowledge increased both immediately after the training, and this knowledge was retained even at the three-month follow-up.

#### Perspectives on Training

Two months after the training, we conducted brief semi-structured telephone interviews with three participants in the training. These participants commented that the training was useful because it reminded them of behaviors that can be affected by violence exposure. Participants wanted more tools and strategies for implementing the principles but believed that this guidance would come over time as they became more familiar with the ARC framework.

## Toledo: Child Parent Psychotherapy (CPP)

The Toledo Safe Start program incorporated CPP as its core intervention (Lieberman and Van Horn, 2005). The training covered the following principles:

- tasks of early childhood development
- the importance of relationships in helping children accomplish those tasks
- understanding that the child and caregiver shape each other
- understanding how stress and trauma change meanings for the dyadic relationship.

One core CPP principle is the importance of facilitating the parent's role in guiding the child through trauma. CPP employs play, physical contact, and language in order to achieve developmental goals. In addition, CPP focuses on unstructured developmental guidance (e.g., helping children cope with strong feelings), modeling protective behavior (e.g., restoring parent to role of protector), emotional support (e.g., allowing parents to bring problem interactions into sessions), and assistance with basic needs and case management (e.g., helping the family access needed food, housing, medical care).

The other cornerstone of CPP is that it is flexible and finds therapeutic opportunities in multiple "ports of entry," including the parent-child interaction, the child-therapist relationship, and the parent-therapist relationship. There are many domains of intervention that were covered in the CPP training, including

- using play to help reveal the child's experience
- supporting a parent to address a child's fearful behavior
- working with a parent to confront a child's aggression toward him or her by helping the child express anger in a non-hurtful way
- addressing the relationship with the absent parent, particularly if that parent perpetrated violence.

### Participant Characteristics

In the initial training session, all five of the training participants completed the pre-training survey. Four of those five completed the three-month follow-up survey. The participants were clinical social workers, counselors, or clinical psychologists. All participants reported having experience with individual child therapy, and the majority had experience with joint therapy. Most of the sample had worked with children of all age ranges (elementary, middle, and high school). The training itself was delivered by Patricia Van Horn.

### Changes in Knowledge

All participants reported at least a little knowledge of CPP prior to the training, and all had used dyadic techniques (non-CPP) with children exposed to violence prior to the training. After the training at the three-month follow-up, most participants reported a little or some comfort with using CPP for children exposed to violence, but none of the four reported great capacity to employ the therapeutic approach. Table C.5 summarizes change in knowledge on questions related to the CPP training. In general, knowledge increased during the post-training survey and maintained at three-month follow-up, among those who completed all three surveys (n = 4).

**Table C.5**
**Pre-Post and Follow-Up Knowledge from the CPP Training (n = 4)**

| | % Correct | | |
|---|---|---|---|
| **Item** | **Pre** | **Post** | **Follow-up** |
| Children's behavior has meaning and may be related to earlier experiences. (True) | 100 | 100 | 100 |
| One of the six intervention modalities in CPP is structured reflective developmental guidance. (False) | 0 | 0 | 25 |
| CPP uses behavioral methods to train the caregiver to be a more effective parent. (False) | 20 | 100 | 100 |
| One of the features that makes CPP unique is the selection of each intervention modality to change the mental representations that child and parent have of each other. (True) | 75 | 75 | 75 |
| Child-parent psychotherapy is not recommended in cases of ongoing domestic violence. (True) | 50 | 50 | 75 |

**Table C.5—Continued**

| Item | % Correct | | |
|---|---|---|---|
| | Pre | Post | Follow-up |
| Children under five understand the events around them and are able to develop their own narrative about events. (False) | 25 | 25 | 50 |
| In CPP, the clinician models the most effective way for the parent to play with the child, and the parent follows the clinician's lead. (False) | 25 | 25 | 50 |
| The use of flooding is one technique that can be used with CPP. (False) | 75 | 100 | 100 |
| After a traumatic event, a parent may view an infant as threatening and dangerous. (True) | 100 | 100 | 100 |

### Perspectives on Training

We conducted brief interviews with two staff members who had participated in the training approximately two months afterwards. These participants reported that the content of the training was interesting, but they did not feel that they would integrate all principles of CPP into their current practice. At the time of the interview, only one clinician had actually used CPP with a client, but this was mostly due to the low recruitment rates at the Toledo Safe Start site. Participants also felt that the training needed to be longer with booster sessions while they were actually implementing CPP.

## Miami: Infant Mental Health

A core component of the Miami Safe Start program was training clinicians in the principles of Infant Mental Health (IMH), including a parent-child assessment. These trainings were conducted on a monthly basis by Joy Osofsky, one of the developers of IMH. In order to assess training impact, we were able to conduct two sets of pre-post assessments on two training sessions that occurred in the first two months of the program's implementation.

The first training was focused on introducing the concept of IMH. *Infant mental health* is defined as the developing capacity of the child (from birth to 3 years) to experience, regulate, and express emotions as well as the ability to form close and secure relationships. Guiding assumptions of IMH are that babies and toddlers function in the context of a relationship and that understanding the child and the relationship helps to optimize social and emotional functioning. The training session also examined the key concepts of interaction (interaction with others helps young children develop a sense of competence to engage in relationships), mastery motivation (the inborn drive to explore and master one's environment), and attachment (infant's ability to bond with the primary caregiver). Participants were also instructed that IMH is a relational construct and combines both psychodynamic and family systems perspectives.

In the second training session, participants were introduced to the IMH status assessment and infant observations. The goal of the assessment was to work with caregivers to identify problems and to design appropriate treatment strategies. The session covered the common reasons that infants are referred for treatment, including dysregulation of psychological function (feeding or sleeping problems). Reasons for toddlers are usually behavioral issues (aggression, defiance, impulsivity). A mental health status evaluation involves examining how the child looks and acts, with attention to physical appearance, motor functioning, self-regulation ability, and speech and language. The assessment also includes gathering data on thoughts (e.g., nightmares, fears), affect and mood, play, intellectual functioning, and how the child relates to his/her caregiver. Participants were provided the global assessment scale for the parent-infant relationship, in which high scores translated to being well-adapted and low scores signaled some distress or impairment in the relationship.

Our evaluation included participants in these first two training sessions; however, the IMH training program consisted of many more sessions, lasting a total of six months. Subsequent content included more detail on assessing the parent-child relationship, how to create a developmental profile for infants and toddlers, healing the child within the juvenile court system, and research on kinship care.

### Participant Characteristics

We assessed pre-post change in knowledge for each of the two training sessions. Three-month follow-up was not included for IMH because the trainings were organized month to month. We attempted to evaluate others, but did not have materials in time. For the first training session, eight participants completed surveys. Four of these eight were master's-level therapists, and the remainder had a mix of counseling backgrounds but not at the master's level. All but one participant had experience with individual child therapy, six of them with group child therapy, six of them with individual parent therapy, and seven of them with joint therapy. Four of the participants had experience working with infants.

### Changes in Knowledge

Prior to the first training session, only two of the eight participants felt they knew a great deal about infant mental health (on a scale of no knowledge to a little, some, or a great deal), but after the first training session, all but one reported a great deal of knowledge. As noted in the table below, most knowledge improved at the end of the first session, but some improvements were more modest, particularly regarding the concepts of affect attunement and stranger anxiety (Table C.6).

**Table C.6**
**Pre-Post Knowledge from the Introduction to Infant Mental Health Session (n = 8)**

| | % Correct | |
|---|---|---|
| Item | Pre | Post |
| One of the behaviors to observe in infant observations is how the mother holds the baby. (True) | 100 | 100 |
| Mastery motivation is the internal drive to explore one's environment. (True) | 13 | 86 |
| Infant mental health is explained theoretically as developmental using psychodynamic and behavioral perspectives. (True) | 75 | 50 |
| Assessing infant mental health includes looking at physical appearance. (True) | 75 | 100 |
| Most of the referral concerns for infants are based on behavioral disturbances such as aggression and impulsivity. (False) | 0 | 25 |
| In an infant assessment, the interaction between infant and caregiver is critical but the interaction between infant and evaluator is not important. (False) | 88 | 88 |
| The awakening of sociability happens during the 2–7 month range. (True) | 75 | 100 |
| The focus for affect attunement is the behavior you can observe, not the internal state of the individual. (False) | 13 | 25 |
| Stranger anxiety generally begins around 8 months. (True) | 63 | 88 |
| Symbolic play generally begins around 13 months. (False) | 50 | 0 |
| Some of the problems that can emerge in how an infant relates to parents or other adults include a sense of defiance, hyperactivity, and impulsive hyperactivity. (True) | 88 | 88 |

**Table C.7**
**Pre-Post Knowledge from the Infant Mental Health Assessment Session (n = 9)**

| Item | % Correct | |
|---|---|---|
| | Pre | Post |
| While you observe clean-up time during an assessment, aspects to pay attention to include the level of compliance and cooperation. (True) | 89 | 100 |
| An authoritarian parent is a parent who is both high on warmth and high on firmness with a child. (False) | 67 | 78 |
| During the reunion step of an infant-caregiver assessment, a poor reunion is when a parent returns to the child and does not reference the child at all. (True) | 79 | 100 |
| Components to include in a write-up of a relationship assessment include the overall emotional tone and how the dyad relate to each other. (True) | 100 | 100 |
| In the Crowell procedure for infant-caregiver assessment, you should spend 15-20 minutes in free play. (False) | 33 | 89 |
| When you set up the playroom for an infant-parent assessment, you should have lots of toys in the room. (False) | 56 | 100 |
| The toys to use in the playroom should promote cooperative play, but should not include soothing items. (True) | 11 | 78 |
| The purpose of using bubbles in an assessment is to help the child who may have had a stressful time during free play. (False) | 11 | 11 |
| During floor time, you open the circle of communication to assess the child's style and mood. (True) | 44 | 78 |
| When rating how well a caregiver helps a child to achieve developmental tasks, ratings should include the caregiver's use of praise and age-appropriate assistance. (True) | 100 | 100 |

Nine participants completed surveys for the second training session. Prior to the second training session, one of the nine participants reported a great deal of knowledge about infant-parent relationship assessments, but after the training all of them reported this level of knowledge. Table C.7 summarizes changes in knowledge after this session; improvements were noted across all concepts except for one item, where knowledge remained the same.

## Multnomah County: Collaborations between Child Welfare and Domestic Violence Staff

The Multnomah County Safe Start site-specific trainings we evaluated focused on bridging the working relationship between child welfare and domestic violence staff. The training was delivered by Susan Hubert, a nationally known subject matter expert from the Massachusetts Department of Social Services. While Hubert led a series of training sessions, only the initial training session was included in the training evaluation because of scheduling issues. The initial training session was nontraditional in that it was less didactic or instructional and more focused on bringing child welfare and domestic violence staff together to discuss their current working relationship and their attitudes about working with children exposed to violence. The following sections describe the participants in the initial training session and their changes in attitudes and reported practice.

### Participant Characteristics

Twenty-two staff members participated in this initial training session, and all completed the baseline and post-training surveys. Approximately 64 percent of the 22 participants were child welfare workers, and the remaining participants were domestic violence staff. Fifteen participants completed the three-month follow-up survey.

Based on the pre-training survey, half of the participants reported working in their current position for three years or less. Most of the participants had experience working with children of all ages (86% elementary, 77% middle school, 82% high school) and adults (90%). Prior to the training, 69 percent of staff reported a great deal of work with children exposed to violence.

### Changes in Reported Knowledge and Practice

Participants were also queried about the extent to which they worked with staff in the other field (domestic violence or child welfare) to help children exposed to violence. Prior to the training, 37 percent reported a great deal of collaboration. Of the 15 staff members who completed the three-month follow-up surveys (representing 47% child welfare, 53% domestic violence staff), approximately 60 percent reported a great deal of collaboration with their counterparts in the other field.

The post-training survey mainly assessed reported knowledge immediately after the training and offered an opportunity for input on training quality. Immediately after the training, the proportion reporting a great deal of knowledge about collaboration increased from 22 percent to 37 percent.

Figures C.4 and C.5 show changes in reported collaborations between the pre-training survey and the three-month follow-up with respect to working with children exposed to violence. Since most questions were focused on reporting changes in collaborative practice, the

**Figure C.4**
**Child Welfare Staff Reported Practice Changes in Working with Domestic Violence Staff (n = 15 who completed all three survey waves)**

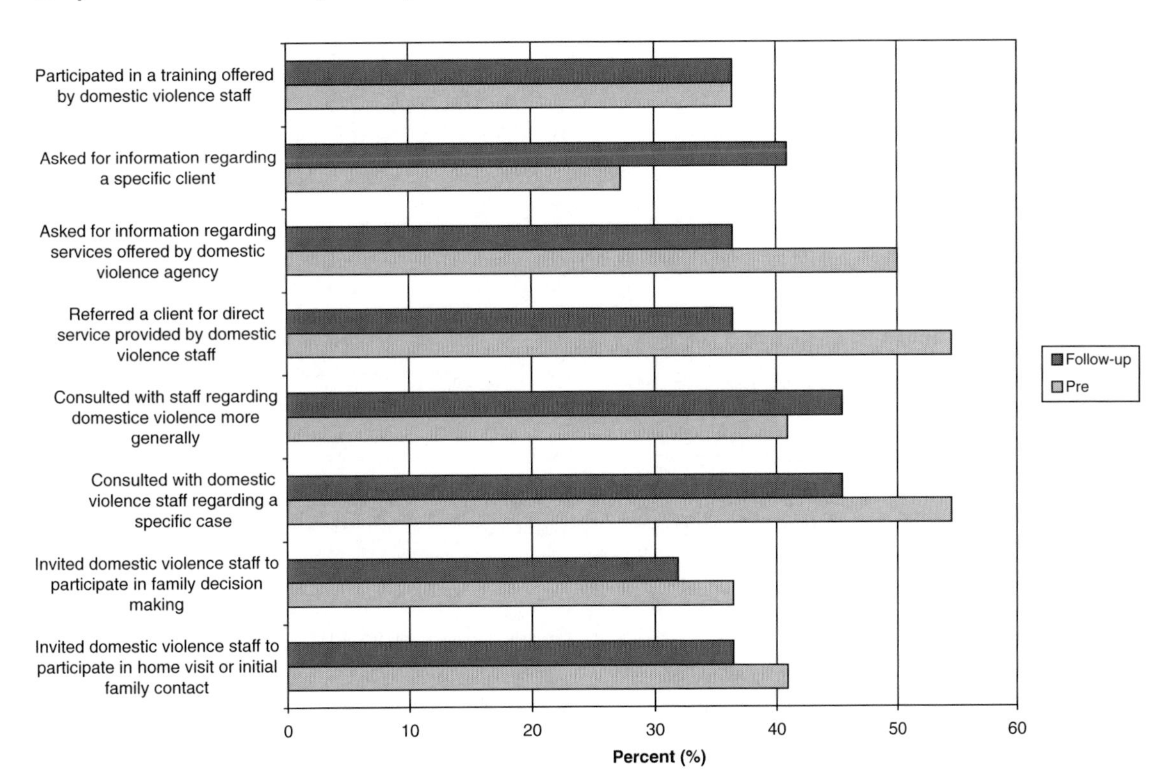


RAND *TR750-C.4*

**Figure C.5**
**Domestic Violence Staff Reported Practice Changes in Working with Child Welfare Staff (n = 15 who completed all three survey waves)**

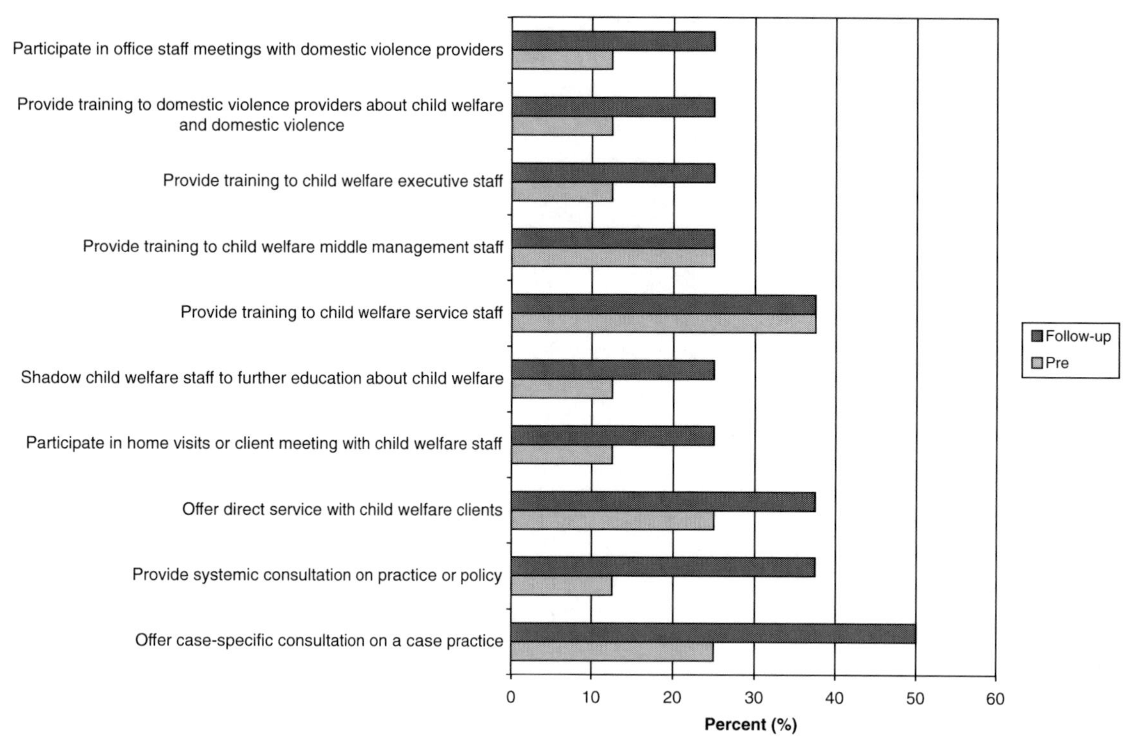


RAND *TR750-C.5*

responses are reported for the baseline and three-month follow-up surveys only. For child welfare workers, the reported collaboration remained consistent or slightly decreased except in two areas: (1) asked for information regarding a client and (2) consulted with domestic violence staff more generally. For domestic violence workers, there was more change particularly in the percentage reporting that they were providing case-specific consultation and providing systemic consultation on a relevant policy or practice.

## Kalamazoo: Head Start School Intervention Project

A core element of the Kalamazoo Safe Start program was a curriculum that teachers implemented in Head Start classrooms. Thus, teachers were trained prior to the school year on issues for children exposed to violence and the content of the curriculum. The curriculum training was provided by Kalamazoo Safe Start staff, developers of the Head Start School Intervention Project (HSSIP). Throughout the course of the year, teachers spent time with the site's project team to review the HSSIP curriculum and experiences in the classroom.

The curriculum focused on five core elements that children exposed to violence need for social, emotional, and academic success. First, the curriculum included concepts and activities around *feeling safe* to build a level of safety and calm that is necessary for learning to occur. The second curriculum component focuses on *making and keeping friends* to help children learn different ways to communicate what they are feeling. The third component is *calming mind and body* and instructs students on how to deal with regulating their emotions, such as hyper-alertness and sensitivity to changes within the environments. The fourth component focuses on *feeling good about learning*. The fifth and final component emphasizes *making meaning of experiences*, which helps children to understand that the environment is not always dangerous and that some adults can be trusted.

These core components are included in the five HSSIP units that cover the school year:

- Learning About School (weeks 1–4)
- Learning About Self (weeks 5–11)
- Learning About Community (weeks 12–16)
- Learning About Friendship (weeks 17–22)
- Saying Goodbye (weeks 23–26).

For the training evaluation, school staff experiences with the curriculum were assessed before, immediately after the training, and at the end of the school year to determine what knowledge was gained and retained as a result of their training and experience with the curriculum.

#### Participant Characteristics

Sixteen staff members participated in the training during the assessment year (2006–2007), and all 16 completed the pre- and post-training surveys. Nine (56%) completed the follow-up survey at the end of the school year.

According to the pre-training survey, half of the participating school staff members were teachers or classroom aides, and the remaining staff members were bus drivers (who participate in working with children) (25%) or education coordinators or speech therapists (25%). Most of the staff had been affiliated with Head Start less than six years, though four participants had been involved with Head Start between 11 and 22 years.

#### Changes in Knowledge

Prior to the training, one of the 16 participants reported a great deal of knowledge about children exposed to violence and, immediately post-training, that number increased to six participants (38%). Among the nine staff members who completed the follow-up survey at the end of the academic year, five reported a great deal of knowledge about this population, with the remaining reporting at least some knowledge.

Table C.8 summarizes changes in knowledge among school staff members. In general, knowledge increased as a result of the training, and this was sustained at the year-end survey.

#### Perspectives on Teacher Meetings

The HSSIP intervention also included weekly teacher meetings with the site's Safe Start program staff after the initial training. The follow-up survey included questions about these meetings. Five of the nine respondents strongly agreed that the meetings helped them to feel better about working with children in their classroom, and seven reported that the meetings helped them deal with students who were having a hard time in the classroom. In addition, the respondents reported that the meetings provided an opportunity to deal with their stress (56%).

#### Perspectives on Training

Four of the Kalamazoo training participants completed telephone interviews six months after the training session. Overall, these participants strongly favored the training and felt that it

**Table C.8**
**Pre-Post and Follow-Up Knowledge from the Michigan HSSIP Training (n = 9) (Answers in Bold)**

| Item | % Correct | | |
|---|---|---|---|
| | Pre | Post | Follow-up |
| Typically a child between the ages of 4 and 6 would be able to do the following except *(begin learning right and wrong, know that rules are important and must be followed, form images of themselves based on interactions with others,* ***develop ethnic and sexual identification****)* | 22 | 22 | 22 |
| Which of the following would be appropriate for building a safe environment for children *(approach gently helping to put words with bad feelings;* ***use firm directive and loud voices to command attention****; maintain structure without being overly rigid, speak with affection and calmness in your voice)* | 33 | 44 | 44 |
| Which behaviors suggest that a three year old is having difficulty regulating his/her mood or behavior *(rocking their body only; throwing things only; yelling only; throwing and yelling;* ***All of the above****)* | 78 | 78 | 100 |
| If a child previously exposed to violence follows directions today, then tomorrow seems to ignore the teacher when told to complete a task, it is probably because: *He/she is trying to manipulate the teacher; He/she doesn't have to listen at home; He/she is unable to self regulate and/or pay attention;* ***All of the above****; None of the above* | 22 | 33 | 33 |
| Children who have been exposed to violence may show anxiety by: *Avoiding interaction with other students and teachers; Daydreaming, fidgeting and/or talking; Looking all around the room; Hitting, kicking or biting;* ***All of the above*** | 78 | 78 | 100 |
| Children who have been exposed to violence are likely to have difficulty communicating/interacting with others. This statement is: **True**/False | 89 | 100 | 100 |
| J'Clare and Steven are fighting over a toy. J'Clare had the toy first, but Steven wanted to take a turn too. J'Clare runs to the teacher crying and says "Steven took my toy away and I want it." Which response is the best example of active listening? *"J'Clare, go tell Steven to give you the toy back";* ***"J'Clare, you sound pretty upset about that";*** *"J'Clare, It's nice to share."; "Steven you should not take that toy from J'Clare now please give it back"; "J'Clare and Steven, you have to learn how to share those toys."* | 33 | 78 | 100 |
| Reading aloud develops: *A child's interest in reading; A child's interest in school and learning; A child's ability to experience calmness and regulate their movements; A child's ability to communicate with others;* ***All of above*** | 89 | 100 | 100 |
| Circle all of the items that would be considered core elements for a classroom intervention for children exposed to violence. *Having rigid rules;* ***Developing relationships with teachers; Making meaning of experiences; Ensuring safety;*** *Learning how to not fidget;* ***Enjoying learning****; Making sure there is full student participation; Having a quiet environment* | 33 | 33 | 33 |
| Working with children who have a history of exposure to traumatic events requires the caretaking adults to: *Affirm the child's coping skills by enforcing more rules; Engage in a power struggle with the child to remind them you are in control; Remind the child that expression of their feelings is not appropriate now;* ***View children's behaviors as survival rather than willful disobedience;*** *Recognize that the child should follow requests based on their age; Build the child's coping skills by demanding that they act their age* | 44 | 100 | 100 |

provided them with some answers regarding why some children were having a difficult time in the classroom. Further, they reinforced the view that the ongoing teacher consultation sessions were helpful in sharing ideas and concerns among staff, and offering time to relax and discuss classroom stressors.

## San Diego: Safe Futures

One of the key training activities for the San Diego Safe Start site was the Safe Futures training, a set of modules for Early Head Start and Head Start staff that focused on supporting children and families affected by domestic violence. Safe Futures was developed by the Administration for Children, Youth, and Families, U.S. Department of Health and Human

Services. The curriculum uses a framework that includes prevention, early intervention, and crisis intervention strategies in working with families affected by domestic violence. Safe Futures focuses on building competencies to perform the following activities (ESI Safe Futures Trainer's Manual, 2005):

- Implement strategies with all families to prevent domestic violence.
- Identify and respond to children and families dealing with domestic violence
- Intervene safely and effectively with children and families in crisis using a team approach.
- Build strong community networks to prevent domestic violence and better support families experiencing violence.
- Develop and implement management systems that support high quality services to children and families experiencing domestic violence.
- Nurture and promote mental wellness of self, as well as other staff, so that they are able to work effectively with families experiencing domestic violence.

San Diego Safe Start engaged in the Safe Futures training with the idea that those trained in the concepts would then train others in their respective organizations or conduct trainings on the Safe Futures concepts with community groups (i.e., train the trainer). Both the initial Safe Future training and subsequent community training sessions were included in the training evaluation.

### Initial Safe Futures Training

#### Participant Characteristics

Twenty program staff members initially received the Safe Futures training (over a three-day training period). Ten percent were nurses, 30 percent were social workers, and the remainder were administrative staff. Twenty-five percent had conducted individual therapy for children, and 20 percent had conducted parent-child dyadic therapy. Most of the staff had some experiencing working with children of all ages (70% elementary; 75% middle school; 85% high school). Seventy-five percent of the participants had attended a training session about working with families experiencing domestic violence prior to the Safe Futures training. Prior to the training, 40 percent had conducted a training session for others on the topic, but only 25 percent felt somewhat or very comfortable doing this. Half of the participants reported working with this population in more than half of their cases.

#### Changes in Knowledge

Prior to the training, 30 percent felt that they knew a great deal about the topic of families and domestic violence, and 40 percent felt they knew a great deal about children who had been exposed to domestic violence. After the training, 83 percent reported a great deal of knowledge about this population. Table C.9 summarizes changes in knowledge at the assessment time points among those who completed all survey waves. Since the session took place over three days during a two-month period, a pre-post survey was administered during each session. The follow-up survey for Session 1, however, did not take place three months later. Because of logistical issues, it took place when the participants came together again for participation in Session 2, approximately two months later. The follow-up questions for Session 2 were administered three months after this session

Overall, knowledge improved with the training, and that knowledge level was maintained at follow-up. The main challenges were with content that focused on statistics, such as

**Table C.9**
**Pre-Post and Follow-Up Knowledge from the Safe Futures Training**

| Item | % Correct | | |
|---|---|---|---|
| | Pre | Post | Follow-up |
| **Session 1** | | (n = 17) | |
| Children under 5 are disproportionately present in households experiencing domestic violence. (True) | 71 | 88 | 94 |
| Domestic violence is a learned behavior. (True) | 94 | 100 | 100 |
| Domestic violence always includes physical violence. (False) | 94 | 95 | 100 |
| Economic abuse can include giving a partner an allowance. (True) | 71 | 94 | 100 |
| Thirty-five percent of women report abuse during pregnancy. (False) | 12 | 24 | 29 |
| Approximately 3 percent of surveyed women report being abused or raped in their lifetime. (False) | 12 | 24 | 59 |
| Resiliency is the ability to not have stressful events affect you. (False) | 59 | 59 | 71 |
| A child's reaction to violence can be a function of the time elapsed since exposure to the event. (True) | 71 | 94 | 94 |
| For a preschooler who has been exposed to violence, symptoms may include trouble concentrating and withdrawal. (True) | 94 | 100 | 94 |
| In 20 percent of homes in which there is domestic violence, there is also child abuse. (False) | 29 | 59 | 53 |
| If a family or woman is contemplating leaving an abusive situation but is not quite ready, basic skills development can be useful to help them consider the benefits of leaving. (True) | 29 | 94 | 94 |
| **Session 2** | | (n = 15) | |
| If the family is in the stage of precontemplation, they see no need to change. (True) | 33 | 100 | 93 |
| If the family is in the stage of planning, it is important that they never relapse. (False) | 67 | 93 | 87 |
| Crisis intervention can be provided by the family worker, home visit(or, mental health consultant, or other type of community partner. (True) | 93 | 100 | 100 |
| It is important to consider the lethality of a domestic violence situation by looking at risk factors such as access to a gun, stalking, or suicide threats. (True) | 93 | 100 | 100 |

the percentage of households with both domestic violence and child abuse. Table C.9 shows these results for both Session 1 and Session 2.

### Community Trainings

During the follow-up survey for the initial Safe Futures training, five participants reported that they had conducted a training session for staff at their organization or for a community agency. These participants distributed short surveys to their training participants to determine how well the "train the trainer" model worked and to assess the dissemination of Safe Futures content to other organizations and individuals working on these issues. The surveys were conducted before and immediately after the training.

### Participant Characteristics

Twenty individuals participated in the community training evaluation. These participants were foster parents (50%), health care providers (40%), and volunteers who work with families experiencing violence (10%). Overall, the trainers focused on the Safe Futures basic content of domestic violence and how to support families, with less emphasis on legal issues, management issues, and specific support to children.

**Figure C.6**
**Community Participants, Perspectives on Working with Families Experiencing Domestic Violence (Before and After Safe Futures Training) (n = 20)**

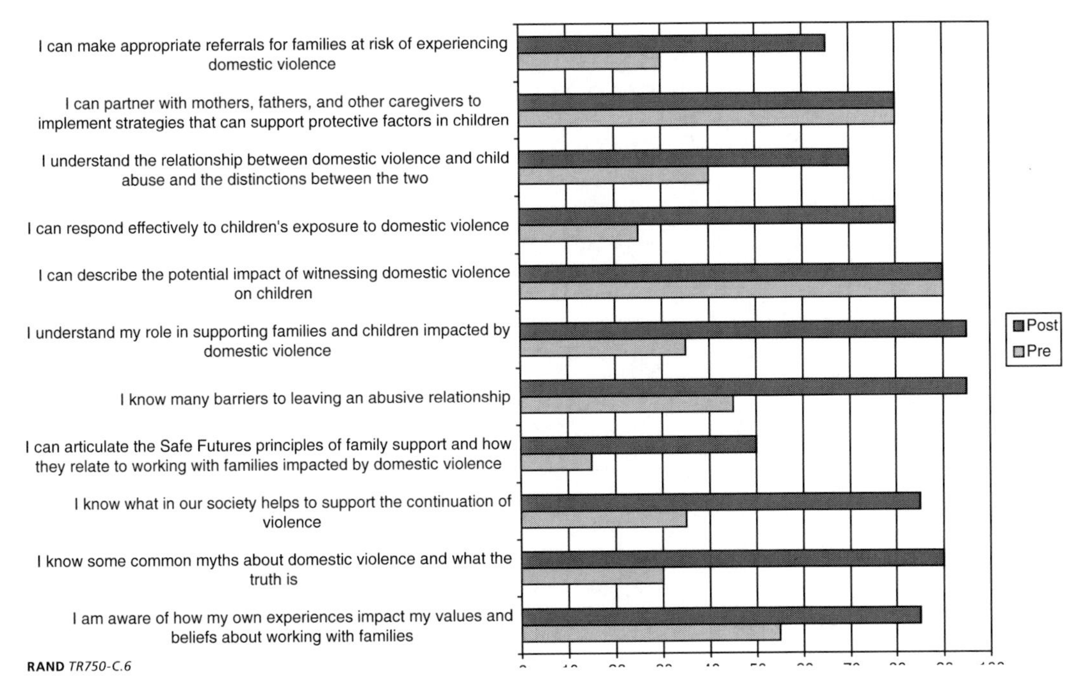


RAND *TR750-C.6*

### Training Experience and Knowledge

Prior to the community training, 15 percent of participants reported a great deal of knowledge about children exposed to violence, and only 10 percent had worked with this population. Half of the participants had at least some experience in working with families confronting domestic violence. After the training, 95 percent of participants anticipated that they would be able to use what they learned in the training to work with families experiencing or at risk for domestic violence.

The participants were also queried about their perceived knowledge about issues related to domestic violence before and immediately after the training. Most of these items were informed by the Safe Futures training module assessments. Figure C.6 summarizes these findings. Overall, perceived knowledge in identifying strategies to work with families at risk for or experiencing domestic violence increased markedly as a result of the training. In particular, participants reported knowing more about the barriers preventing people from leaving abusive situations and understanding their role in supporting families experiencing violence.

## San Diego: Trauma-Focused Cognitive-Behavioral Therapy

Another key component of San Diego Safe Start was training for clinicians in the principles of Trauma-Focused Cognitive-Behavioral Therapy (TF-CBT). TF-CBT was designed for use with children and adolescents who have developed clinical levels of postraumatic stress disorder (PTSD). The therapy can be provided to children ages 3–18 and their parents by trained mental health professionals in individual, family, and group sessions in outpatient settings. It targets symptoms of PTSD, which often co-occurs with depression and behavior problems.

The therapy seeks to teach children skills to cope with the difficulties this disorder creates. TF-CBT involves individualized therapy sessions in which children are given emotional skills training and later, with the help of trained therapists, children begin to confront the traumatic experience that was linked to their PTSD symptoms.

The TF-CBT training also included a focus on assessment tools such as the Trauma Symptom Checklist and the Children's Depression Inventory. San Diego Safe Start used this opportunity to instruct participants about these tools.

### Participant Characteristics

Thirteen individuals participated in the TF-CBT training evaluation. Half of the participants were marriage and family therapists, and the remainder were clinical psychologists or clinical social workers. Prior to the training, all participants had experience providing individual therapy for children and for parents, and most had experience providing joint parent-child therapy (92%). Most participants had worked with middle school age children and older, but less had experience working with infants/toddlers (42%) or preschool age children (75%). Seventy-five percent of participants had attended a training session on working with families experiencing domestic violence prior to the TF-CBT training. Before the TF-CBT training, half of the participants reported a great deal of comfort using standardized assessment tools to guide the development of a client's treatment plan (a core component of TF-CBT); only 42 percent thought that these assessments were very beneficial in guiding treatment planning and decisions, and 33 percent used these assessments in their current practice.

Prior to the training, 67 percent of participants indicated that they focused a great deal on trauma when treating children exposed to violence, and 25 percent reported using dyadic techniques frequently. A third reported using cognitive behavioral techniques in most cases.

### Changes in Knowledge

Participants were queried about whether they knew the clinical cut-off scores for various assessment tools. Table C.10 summarizes these findings. In general, knowledge about these scales improved directly after the training only for the Child Behavior Checklist and Trauma Symptom Checklist for Children. These questions were asked only in the pre- and post-surveys; hence, they are reported separately below.

**Table C.10**
**Changes in Knowledge About Assessment Tools (n = 13)**

| Item | % Correct | |
|---|---|---|
| | Pre | Post |
| Child Behavior Checklist | 0 | 25 |
| Trauma Symptom Inventory | 75 | 75 |
| Trauma Symptom Checklist for Children | 75 | 83 |
| Children's Depression Inventory | 92 | 92 |
| Parenting Stress Index | 83 | 33 |
| Child Sexual Abuse Behavior Inventory | 75 | 75 |
| Family Assessment Measure | 75 | 75 |
| The Child's Dissociative Checklist | 8 | 0 |
| Center for Epidemiologic Studies–Depression Scale | 67 | 91 |

**Table C.11**
**Pre-Post and Follow-Up Knowledge from the TF-CBT Training (n = 6)**

| Item | % Correct | | |
|---|---|---|---|
| | Pre | Post | Follow-up |
| Cognitive coping techniques do not involve direct discussion of emotional reactions to abuse. (True) | 17 | 17 | 17 |
| Cognitive coping uses thought-stopping techniques to distract the child away from them. (False) | 33 | 17 | 0 |
| During progressive muscle relaxation, children are asked to relax muscles through deep breathing. (False) | 33 | 50 | 17 |
| In cognitive processing about the traumatic events, parents should be encouraged to not directly challenges the child's inaccurate thoughts. (False) | 17 | 67 | 50 |
| Children from Asian and Hispanic groups are more likely than other groups to describe stress reactions in terms of physical symptoms. (True) | 67 | 100 | 100 |
| You should remind a child that the abuse isn't their fault even if they never thought the abuse was their fault in the first place. (False) | 17 | 67 | 50 |
| If a child has a hard time discussing their own feelings, it is helpful to encourage them to discuss the feelings of other children or imaginary characters in books. (True) | 100 | 100 | 100 |
| Psychoeducation for traumatized children includes education about traumatic events, mental health issues, and safety planning. (True) | 83 | 100 | 100 |
| Clinicians should not do a trauma narrative if the child gets very upset when talking about the abuse. (False) | 17 | 83 | 33 |
| Helping a child to create and discuss a narrative of the traumatic experiences is a critical process for helping to control intrusive thoughts and disturbing imagery. (True) | 83 | 100 | 100 |

The main focus of the training was on TF-CBT, and we asked participants to respond to a series of knowledge-based questions before and after the training as well as during the three-month follow-up survey (Table C.11). In general, knowledge improved right after the training, but, at follow-up, respondents did not recall information about cognitive coping techniques. However, it should be noted that our response rate was not good: less than 50 percent completed follow-up surveys.

Two participants were included in key informant interviews in order to understand the benefits of the training, what could be improved, and how participants have used the information in their work with children exposed to violence. Based on these two interviews, clinicians reported less favorable attitudes about TF-CBT. They also reported that incorporating TF-CBT with the types of approaches they are accustomed to using from their clinical training was somewhat difficult. Further, they thought that TF-CBT may not be the most appropriate intervention, given their clients' treatment needs.

## Overall Changes in Comfort in Working with Children Exposed to Violence

In addition to the changes in knowledge and reported practices as a result of these site-specific trainings, participants across all site trainings were queried about their general comfort in working with children exposed to violence, parents, and the parent-child dyad. These questions were meant to help understand at an aggregate level how these training opportunities improved the perspectives and ability of program staff to work with this population.

Overall, comfort levels did not improve markedly at post-training or follow-up (among those completing those surveys), but the general comfort level in working with these

**Figure C.7**
**Comfort in Working with Children to Develop Skills Related to Violence Exposure (n = 6)***
**(1 = not comfortable, 4 = very comfortable)**

*N = 6 FOR THE NUMBER OF PARTICIPANTS WHO COMPLETED THE TF-CBT TRAINING

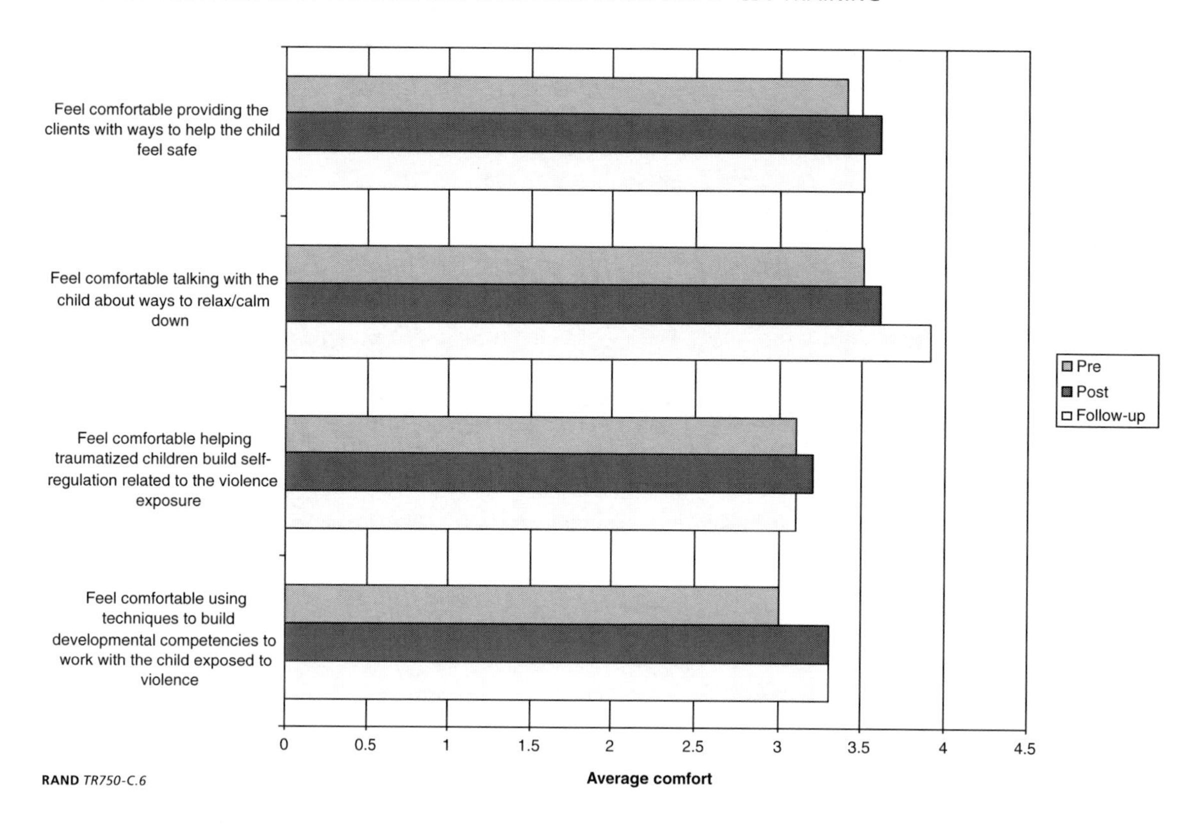


RAND *TR750-C.6*

populations was sustained over the course of the training assessment period. Figures C.7, C.8, and C.9 summarize comfort with employing strategies to address child issues, parent issues, and conflict in the parent-child dyad. Participants reported comfort in helping children to feel safe and to relax, but comparatively less comfort in building skills such as self-regulation or developmental competencies (Figure C.7). Staff also reported more comfort in talking with parents about why a child is behaving in a certain way due to the violence exposure (Figure C.8). Finally, most participants noted greater comfort in helping children and mothers feel closer. The greatest change from baseline to follow-up was in helping staff (and mainly therapists or clinicians) intervene with children and mothers differently when each family member had different needs and agendas (Figure C.9).

## 4. Summary and Conclusions

Overall, the Safe Start sites emphasized training their clinical and administrative staff in recruitment and retention strategies as well as in new treatment approaches. For the training on engaging families in mental health services, improvements in knowledge and reported comfort in using these strategies were maintained at follow-up surveys. However, knowledge retention for the new intervention approaches three months later (e.g., ARC, CPP) was more difficult. In addition, while general comfort levels in working with children exposed to violence started at moderate to high levels pre-trainings, increases in these comfort levels were not pronounced. While it is difficult to compare these findings with other staff training evaluations because items were created newly for each Safe Start training, significant modification of staff perspectives particularly after one or two trainings is typically difficult (Hosany et al., 2007; McCann and Bowers, 2005; Donoghue et al., 2004). Further, our findings should be considered in the context of low survey retention rates at follow-up, which precluded some analyses of change over time.

**Figure C.8**
**Comfort in Working with Parents to Understand Child Exposure to Violence (1 = not comfortable, 4 = very comfortable) (n = 6)***

*N = 6 FOR THE NUMBER OF PARTICIPANTS WHO COMPLETED THE TF-CBT TRAINING

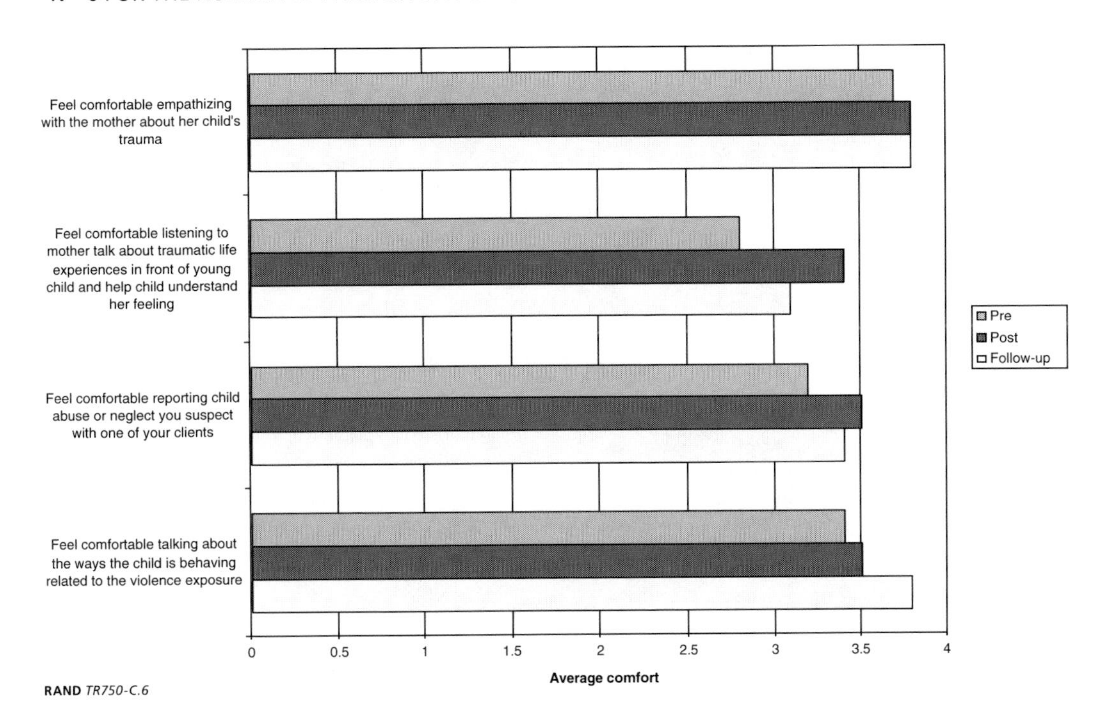


RAND *TR750-C.6*

**Figure C.9**
**Comfort in Working with Parent-Child Dyads in Addressing Violence Exposure Issues (n = 6)***
**(1 = not comfortable, 4 = very comfortable)**

*N = 6 FOR THE NUMBER OF PARTICIPANTS WHO COMPLETED THE TF-CBT TRAINING

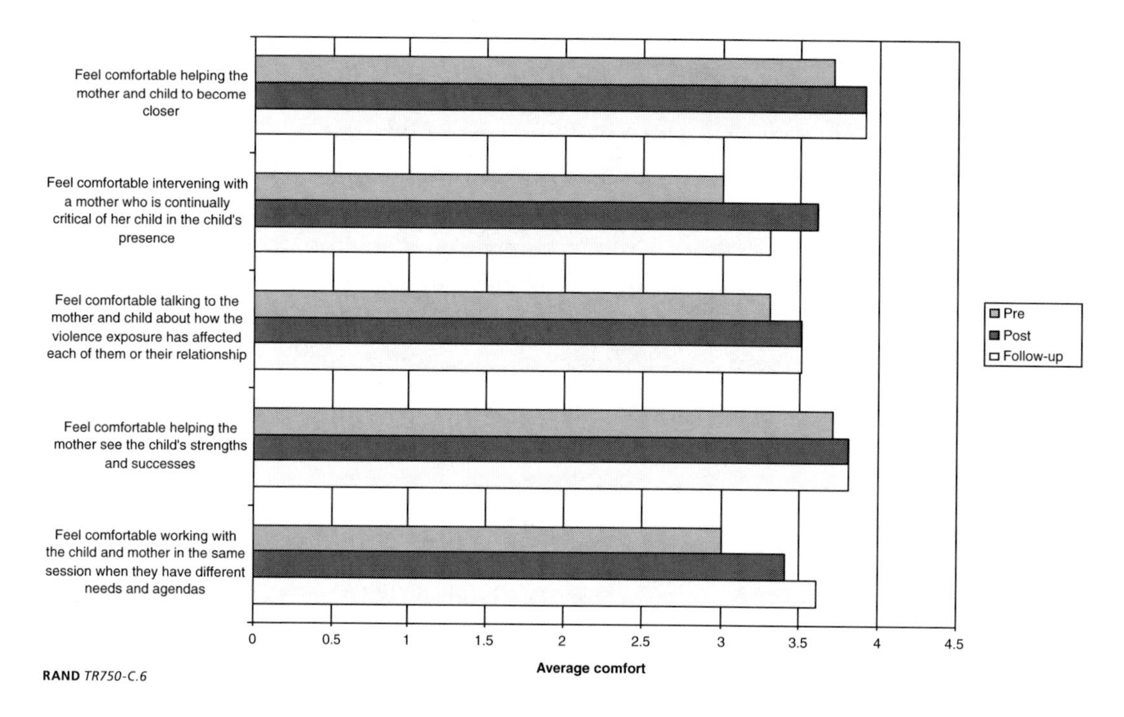


RAND *TR750-C.6*

# References

Achenbach T. (1991). *Manual for the Child Behavior Checklist/4-18 and 1991 Profile.* Burlington, VT: University of Vermont, Department of Psychiatry.

Adams S, Osofsky J, Hammer JH, Graham M. (2003). *Program Evaluation: Florida Infant and Young Child Mental Health Pilot Project.* Florida State University Center for Prevention and Early Intervention.

American Academy of Pediatrics, "National Center for Medical Home Implementation," website, 2010. As of March 22, 2010: http://www.medicalhomeinfo.org/

Annie E. Casey Foundation. (2004). *Residents Engaged in Strengthening Families and Neighborhoods.* Baltimore, MD.

Artemis Center for Domestic Violence Alternatives. (2004). Funding Proposal to the Office of Juvenile Justice and Delinquency Prevention. CFDA [Catalog of Federal Domestic Assistance]: Safe Start: Promising Approaches for Children Exposed to Violence. Artemis Center for Domestic Violence Alternatives, Dayton, OH.

ASDC—*See* Association for the Study and Development of Community.

Association for the Study and Development of Community (ASDC). (2005). *National Evaluation of the Safe Start Demonstration Project: Volume I: Cross-Site Process Evaluation.* Gaithersburg, MD.

Association for the Study and Development of Community (ASDC). (2007). *Safe Start Initiative: Demonstration Project Phase I—Process Evaluation II (2000–2005), Report 2006-3.* Gaithersburg, MD.

Baum K. (2005). *Juvenile Victimization and Offending, 1993–2003.* Bureau of Justice Statistics Special Report NCJ 209468. U.S. Department of Justice, Office of Justice Programs.

Benamati J. (2002). Systemic Training to Assist in the Recovery from Trauma (START) for Residential Staff (Curriculum). (Contact drjoebenamati@yahoo.com for information regarding this training.)

Bingenheimer JB, Brennan RT, Earls FJ. (2005). Firearm Violence Exposure and Serious Violent Behavior. *Science,* 308: 1323–1326.

Bloom SL. (2005). Introduction to Special Section: Creating Sanctuary for Kids: Helping Children to Heal From Violence. *Therapeutic Community: The International Journal for Therapeutic and Supportive Organizations,* 26(1): 57–63.

Bruner C. (2006). Social Service Systems Reform in Poor Neighborhoods: What We Know and What We Need to Find Out. In Fulbright-Anderson K and Auspos P (Eds.), *Community change: Theories, Practice, and Evidence.* Washington, DC: Aspen Institute.

Calvo NP, Serrano L, Katz L, Morgan R. (2008). Heroes Program Manual: Safe Start Promising Approaches Initiative for Children in Crisis: A Group Therapy Manual for Children Exposed to Domestic Violence. Unpublished manual.

Centers for Disease Control and Prevention. (2008). Youth Risk Behavior Surveillance–United States, 2007. *Morbidity and Mortality Weekly Report* Surveillance Summaries, June 6, 57(SS-4): Table 17.

Chadwick Center for Children and Families, Assessment-Based Treatment for Traumatized Children: A Trauma Assessment Pathway (TAP), no date. As of March 25, 2010: http://www.chadwickcenter.org/Assessment-Based%20Treatment.htm

Chaffin M, Silovsky JF, Funderburk B, Valle LA, Brestan EV, Balachova T, Jackson S, Lensgraf J, Bonner BL. (2004). Parent-Child Interaction Therapy with Physically Abusive Parents: Efficacy for Reducing Future Abuse Reports. *Journal of Consulting and Clinical Psychology*, 72(3): 500–510.

Chatterji P, Caffray CM, Crowe M, Freeman L, Jensen P. (2004). Cost Assessment of a School-Based Mental Health Screening and Treatment Program in New York City. *Mental Health Services Research,* 6(3): 155–166.

Chen HT. (1990). *Theory-Driven Evaluations.* Newbury Park, CA: Sage Publications.

Children's Advocacy Center of Erie County. (2004). Funding Proposal to the Office of Juvenile Justice and Delinquency Prevention. CFDA Title: Safe Start: Promising Approaches for Children Exposed to Violence. Erie, PA.

Cohen I, Rodriguez M, Green G. (2005). *Group Curriculum for Children 4–6 Years Old Who Witnessed Domestic Violence.* Cambridge, MA: The Guidance Center.

Cohen J, Mannarino A, Deblinger E. (2003). Child and Parent Trauma-Focused Cognitive Behavioral Therapy Treatment Manual. Unpublished manual.

Consortium for Children in Crisis. (2004). Funding Proposal to the Office of Juvenile Justice and Delinquency Prevention. CFDA Title: Safe Start: Promising Approaches for Children Exposed to Violence. Miami, FL.

County of San Diego. (2004). Funding Proposal to the Office of Juvenile Justice and Delinquency Prevention. CFDA Title: Safe Start: Promising Approaches for Children Exposed to Violence. County of San Diego, San Diego, CA.

Department of Health and Human Services, Administration on Children, Youth and Families. (2009). *Child Maltreatment 2007.* Washington, DC: U.S. Government Printing Office.

Dinkes R, Kemp J, Baum K. (2009). *Indicators of School Crime and Safety: 2008* (NCES 2009–022/ NCJ 226343). National Center for Education Statistics, Institute of Education Sciences, U.S. Department of Education, and Bureau of Justice Statistics, Office of Justice Programs, U.S. Department of Justice. Washington, DC.

Donoghue A, Hodgins G, Judd F, Scopelliti J, Grigg M, Komiti A, Murray G. (2004). Training Case Managers to Deliver Focused Psychological Strategies. *International Journal of Mental Health Nursing,* 13: 33–38.

Dumka LE, Garza CA, Roosa MW, Stoerzinger HD. (1997). Recruitment and Retention of High-Risk Families into a Preventive Parent Training Intervention. *The Journal of Primary Prevention,* 18(1): 25–39.

Durlak JA, DuPre EP. (2008). Implementation Matters: A Review of Research on the Influence of Implementation on Program Outcomes and the Factors Affecting Implementation. *American Journal of Community Psychology,* 41: 327–350.

East Bay Community Foundation Safe Passages Initiative (2004). Funding Proposal to the Office of Juvenile Justice and Delinquency Prevention. CFDA Title: Safe Start: Promising Approaches for Children Exposed to Violence. Oakland, California.

Edgewood Center for Children and Families. (2004). Funding Proposal to the Office of Juvenile Justice and Delinquency Prevention. CFDA Title: Safe Start: Promising Approaches for Children Exposed to Violence. San Mateo County, CA.

Educational Services, Inc (ESI). (2005). *Safe Futures Trainer's Manual: Supporting Children and Families Affected by Domestic Violence.* Washington, DC.

Fantuzzo JW, Fusco RA, Mohr WK, Perry MA. (2007). Domestic Violence and Children's Presence: A Population-Based Study of Law Enforcement Surveillance of Domestic Violence. *Journal of Family Violence,* 22(6): 331-40.

Family Service of Rhode Island. (2004). Funding Proposal to the Office of Juvenile Justice and Delinquency Prevention. CFDA Title: Safe Start: Promising Approaches for Children Exposed to Violence. Providence, RI.

Federal Bureau of Investigation. (2006). Crime in the United States. Uniform Crime Reporting Program. Washington, DC: U.S. Department of Justice, Federal Bureau of Investigation.

Finkelhor D, Ormrod R, Turner H, Hamby SL. (2005). The Victimization of Children and Youth: A Comprehensive, National Survey. *Child Maltreatment,* 10(1): 5–25.

Finkelhor D, Ormrod R, Turner H, Hamby SL. (2009). Violence, Abuse, and Crime Exposure in a National Sample of Children and Youth. *Pediatrics,* 124(5): 1411–1423.

Fixsen DL, Blase KA, Naoom SF, Wallace F. (2009). Core Implementation Components. *Research on Social Work Practices,* 19(5): 531–540.

Ford JD, Russo E. (2006). Trauma-Focused, Present-Centered, Emotional Self-Regulation Approach to Integrated Treatment for Posttraumatic Stress and Addiction: Trauma Adaptive Recovery Group Education and Therapy (TARGET). *American Journal of Psychotherapy,* 60: 335–350.

Fusco RA, Fantuzzo JW. (2009). Domestic Violence Crimes and Children: A Population-Based Investigation of Direct Sensory Exposure and the Nature of Involvement. *Children and Youth Services Review,* 31: 249–256.

Gance-Cleveland B. (2007). Motivational Interviewing: Improving Patient Education. *Journal of Pediatric Health Care,* 21: 81–88.

Gilbert R, Widom CS, Browne K, Fergusson D, Webb E, Staffan J. (2009). Burden and Consequences of Child Maltreatment in High-Income Countries. *Lancet,* 373: 68–81.

Graham-Bermann SA. (2000). Evaluating Interventions for Children Exposed to Family Violence. *Journal of Aggression, Maltreatment & Trauma,* 4(1): 191–216.

Graham-Bermann SA, Seng JS. (2005). Violence Exposure and Traumatic Stress Symptoms as Additional Predictors of Health Problems in High-Risk Children. *The Journal of Pediatrics,* 146(3): 349–354.

Greenberg MT, Domitrovich CE, Graczyk PA, Zins JE. (2005). *The Study of Implementation in School-Based Preventive Interventions: Theory, Research, and Practice.* Rockville, MD: Center for Mental Health Services, Substance Abuse and Mental Health Services Administration.

Grienenberger J, Popek P, Stein S, Solow J, Morrow M, Levine N, Alexander D, Ibarra M, Wilson A, Thompson J, Lehman J. (2005). Reflective Parenting Program Workshop Training Manual. Unpublished manual. Los Angeles, CA: Wright Institute Los Angeles.

Groves BA, Gewirtz A (2006). Interventions and Promising Approaches for Children Exposed to Domestic Violence. In Feerick MM and Silverman GB (Eds.), *Children Exposed to Violence*: 107–133. Baltimore, MD: Paul H. Brookes Publishing Co.

Harachi TW, Catalano RF, Hawkins JD. (1997). Effective Recruitment for Parenting Programs within Ethnic Minority Communities. *Child and Adolescent Social Work Journal,* 14(1): 23–39.

Hembree-Kigin T, McNeil CB. (1995). *Parent-Child Interaction Therapy.* New York: Plenum.

Hood KK, Eyberg SM. (2003). Outcomes of Parent-Child Interaction Therapy: Mother's Reports of Maintenance Three to Six Years after Treatment. *Journal of Clinical Child and Adolescent Psychology,* 32: 419–29.

Hosany Z, Wellman N, Lowe T. (2007). Fostering a Culture of Engagement: A Pilot Study of the Outcomes of Training Mental Health Nurses Working in Two UK Acute Admission Units in Brief Solution-Focused Therapy Techniques. *Journal of Psychiatric and Mental Health Nursing,* 14: 688–95.

Hyde M, Kracke K, Jaycox L, Schultz D. (2007). The Safe Start Initiative: Advancing System and Practice Responses to Children Exposed to Violence. *Protecting Children,* 22(3–4) (Special Issue: Exposure to Violence): 80–95.

Infoplease.com, "QuickFacts from the US Census Bureau: New York," 2009. As of March 22, 2010: http://www.infoplease.com/us/census/data/new-york/bronx/

Institute for Family Centered Services (IFCS), Inc. (2004). Funding Proposal to the Office of Juvenile Justice and Delinquency Prevention. CFDA Title: Safe Start: Promising Approaches for Children Exposed to Violence. Denver, North Carolina.

Jaycox LH, Stein BD, Kataoka SH, Wong M, Fink A, Escudero P, Zaragoza C. (2002). Violence Exposure, Posttraumatic Stress Disorder, and Depressive Symptoms Among Recent Immigrant Schoolchildren. *Journal of the American Academy of Child and Adolescent Psychiatry,* 41(9): 1104–1110.

Jouriles EN, McDonald R, Spiller L, Norwood WD, Swank PR, Stephens N, Ware W. (2001). Reducing Conduct Problems among Children of Battered Women. *Journal of Consulting and Clinical Psychology*, 69: 774–85.

Kalamazoo Assault Intervention Program. (2004). *Domestic Violence Complaints Requested and Authorized Per Month, 1998–2003*. Kalamazoo, MI: Kalamazoo County Prosecutor's Office.

Kernic, MA, Holt, VL, Wolf, ME, McKnight, B, Huebner, CE, and Rivara, FP. (2002). Academic and School Health Issues Among Children Exposed to Maternal Intimate Partner Abuse. *Archives of Pediatrics and Adolescent Medicine*, 156(6): 549–55.

Kinniburgh KJ, Blaustein M, Spinnazola J. (2005). Attachment, Self-Regulation, and Competency. *Psychiatric Annals*, 35(5): 424–430.

Kiracofe L, Mack A, Blashill M, Pond C, Atchison B, Hyter Y, Henry J, Richardson M. (2005). *Head Start School Intervention Curriculum: Interventions with Children Exposed to Violence*. Kalamazoo, MI: Western Michigan University.

Kracke K, Hahn H. (2008). The Nature and Extent of Childhood Exposure to Violence: What We Know, Why We Don't Know More, and Why It Matters. *Journal of Emotional Abuse*, 8(1): 29–49.

Lansford JE, Dodge KA, Pettit GS, Bates JE, Crozier J, Kaplow J. (2002). A 12-Year Prospective Study of the Long-Term Effects of Early Child Physical Maltreatment on Psychological, Behavioral, and Academic Problems in Adolescence. *Archives of Pediatrics & Adolescent Medicine*, 156: 824–30.

Leiter M, Harvie P. (1996). Burnout Among Mental Health Workers: A Review and a Research Agenda. *International Journal of Social Psychiatry*, 42(2): 90–101.

Lieberman AF, Van Horn P. (2005). *Don't Hit My Mommy: A Manual for Child-Parent Psychotherapy with Young Witnesses of Family Violence*. Washington DC: Zero to Three.

Lieberman AF, Van Horn P. (2008). *Psychotherapy with Infants and Young Children: Repairing the Effects of Stress and Trauma on Early Attachment*. New York: The Guilford Press.

Lynch M. (2003). Consequences of Children's Exposure to Community Violence. *Clinical Child and Family Psychology Review*, 6(4): 265–74.

Macy DJ. (2007). Remembering the Collective Body: A Dynamic Understanding of Attunement and Healing. *Journal of Pedagogy, Pluralism and Practice*, 12: 1–23.

Macy RD, Macy DJ, Gross SI, Brighton P. (2003). Healing in Familiar Settings: Support for Children and Youth in the Classroom and Community. In Macy RD, Barry S, Noam GG (Eds.), *New Directions for Youth Development: Theory, Practice, Research*: 51–79. San Francisco: Jossey Bass.

Marans S, Berkman M. (1997). Child Development-Community Policing: Partnership in a Climate of Violence. Juvenile Justice Bulletin.

Massachusetts Department of Public Health, Bureau of Health Statistics, Research, and Evaluation. (2000). *Weapon Injury Data*. Boston, MA.

Massachusetts General Hospital. (2004). Funding Proposal to the Office of Juvenile Justice and Delinquency Prevention. CFDA Title: Safe Start: Promising Approaches for Children Exposed to Violence. Massachusetts General Hospital, Boston, MA.

McCann E, Bowers L. (2005). Training in Cognitive Behavioural Interventions on Acute Psychiatric Inpatient Wards. *Journal of Psychiatric and Mental Health Nursing*, 12: 215–22.

McCart MR, Smith DW, Saunders BE, Kilpatrick DG, Resnick H, Ruggiero K. (2007). Do Urban Adolescents Become Desensitized to Community Violence? Data from a National Survey. *American Journal of Orthopsychiatry*, 77(3): 434–442.

McDonald R, Jouriles EN, Skopp NA. (2006). Reducing Conduct Problems Among Children Brought to Women's Shelters: Intervention Effects 24 Months Following Termination of Services. *Journal of Family Psychology*, 20(1): 127–136.

McKay M, Pennington J, Lynn CJ, McCadam K. (2001). Understanding Urban Child Mental Health Service Use: Two Studies of Child, Family, and Environmental Correlates. *Journal of Behavioral Health Services and Research*, 28(4): 1–10.

McLoyd VC. (1990). Impact of Economic Hardship on Black Families and Children: Psychological Distress, Parenting and Socioemotional Development. *Child Development*, 61(2): 311–346.

Mercy JA, Saul J. (2009). Creating a Healthier Future Through Early Interventions for Children. *Journal of the American Medical Association*, 301(21): 2262–2264.

Morris E. (2009). *Youth Violence: Implications for Posttraumatic Stress Disorder in Urban Youth*. Issue Report from the National Urban League Policy Institute. Washington, DC.

Multnomah County. (2004). Funding Proposal to the Office of Juvenile Justice and Delinquency Prevention. CFDA Title: Safe Start: Promising Approaches for Children Exposed to Violence. Multnomah County, OR.

National Child Traumatic Stress Network. (2008). *CPP: Child Parent Psychotherapy*. Raleigh, NC. As of March 10, 2010: http://www.nctsnet.org/nctsn_assets/pdfs/promising_practices/cpp_general.pdf

NCTSN—*See* National Child Traumatic Stress Network.

New York Presbyterian Hospital. (2004). Funding Proposal to the Office of Juvenile Justice and Delinquency Prevention. CFDA Title: Safe Start: Promising Approaches for Children Exposed to Violence. Bronx, NY.

Northnode, Inc. (2007). *Group Services for Children Affected by Domestic Violence: An Interactive 12-Week Group Curriculum for 8 to 12-Year-Old Children*. Roslindale, MA.

Osofsky JD, Kronenberg M, Hammer JH, Lederman C, Katz L, Adams S, Graham M, Hogan A. (2007). The Development and Evaluation of the Intervention Model for the Florida Infant Mental Health Pilot Program. *Infant Mental Health Journal*, 28(3): 259–80.

Painter WE, Smith MM. (2004). *Wheels of Change—Family Centered Specialists Handbook and Training Manual*. Richmond, VA: Institute for Family Centered Services.

Safe Passages. (2004). Funding Proposal to the Office of Juvenile Justice and Delinquency Prevention. CFDA Title: Safe Start: Promising Approaches for Children Exposed to Violence. Oakland, CA.

Safe Start Center (2008). *Safe Start: Promising Approaches Communities: Working Together to Help Children Exposed to Violence*. Washington, DC.

San Diego Domestic Violence Council. (2009). What is the San Diego Domestic Violence Council? As of March 15, 2009: http://www.sddvc.com/

Simpson JS, Jivanjee P, Koroloff N, Doerfler A, Garcia M. (2001). *Systems of Care: Promising Practices in Children's Mental Health, 2001 Series—Volume III: Promising Practices in Early Childhood Mental Health*. Washington, DC: U.S. Department of Health and Human Services.

Schoenwald SK, Hoagwood K. (2001). Effectiveness, Transportability, and Dissemination of Interventions: What Matters When? *Psychiatric Services*, 52: 1190–1197.

Schwartz D, Gorman AH. (2003). Community Violence Exposure and Children's Academic Functioning. *Journal of Educational Psychology*, 95(1): 163–73.

Slade A. (2006). Reflective Parenting Programs: Theory and Development. *Psychoanalytic Inquiry*, 26(4): 640–657.

Southern Methodist University. (2004). Funding Proposal to the Office of Juvenile Justice and Delinquency Prevention. CFDA Title: Safe Start: Promising Approaches for Children Exposed to Violence. Southern Methodist University, Dallas, TX.

St. Barnabas Hospital. (2004). Funding Proposal to the Office of Juvenile Justice and Delinquency Prevention. CFDA Title: Safe Start: Promising Approaches for Children Exposed to Violence. Bronx, NY.

Stith S, Pruitt I, Dees J, Fronce M, Green N, Som A, Linkh D. (2006). Implementing Community-Based Prevention Programming: A Review of the Literature. *The Journal of Primary Prevention*, 27(6): 599–617.

Straus MA, Gelles RJ. (1990). *Physical Violence in American Families: Risk Factors and Adaptations to Violence in 8,145 Families*. New Brunswick, NJ: Transaction Books.

Stroul BA, Friedman RM. (1996). The System of Care Concept and Philosophy. In Stroul BA (Ed.), *Children's Mental Health: Creating Systems of Care in Changing Society*: 3–21. Baltimore, MD: Paul H. Brookes Publishing Co.

Taylor N, Gilbert A, Mann G, Ryan BE. (2005). *Assessment-Based Treatment for Traumatized Children: A Trauma Assessment Pathway.* San Diego, CA: Chadwick Center for Children and Families.

Texas Council on Family Violence (June 2006). Family Violence in Texas Fact Sheet. Austin, TX.

Toledo Hospital. (2004). Funding Proposal to the Office of Juvenile Justice and Delinquency Prevention. CFDA Title: Safe Start: Promising Approaches for Children Exposed to Violence. Toledo, OH.

U.S. Census Bureau, homepage, no date. As of March 22, 2010: http://www.census.gov

U.S. Department of Justice, Office of Violence Against Women. (February 2007). The President's Family Justice Center Initiative, Best Practices. As of March 15, 2009: http://www.ovw.usdoj.gov/docs/family_justice_center_overview_12_07.pdf

Webster-Stratton C. (1994). Advancing Videotape Parent Training: A Comparison Study. *Journal of Consulting and Clinical Psychology,* 62(3): 583–93.

Webster-Stratton C. (1998). Parent Training with Low Income Families: Promoting Parental Engagement through a Collaborative Approach. In Lutzker JR (Ed.), *Handbook of Child Abuse Research and Treatment: Issues in Clinical Child Psychology*: 183–210. Plenum Press, NY.

Western Michigan University. (2004). Funding Proposal to the Office of Juvenile Justice and Delinquency Prevention. CFDA Title: Safe Start Promising Approaches for Children Exposed to Violence. Kalamazoo, MI.

Widom CS, Hiller-Sturmhofel S. (2001). Alcohol Abuse as a Risk Factor for and Consequence of Child Abuse. *Alcohol Research & Health,* 25: 52–57

Zinzow HM, Ruggiero KJ, Resnick H, Hanson R, Smith D, Saunders B, Kilpatrick D. (2009). Prevalence and Mental Health Correlates of Witnessed Parental and Community Violence in a National Sample of Adolescents. *Journal of Child Psychology and Psychiatry,* 50(4): 441–450.